ROYAL GEOGRAPHICAL SOCIETY

WITH THE INSTITUTE OF BRITISH GEOGRAPHERS

EXPEDITION MEDICINE

EDITED BY

DAVID WARRELL AND SARAH ANDERSON

SECOND EDITION

FULLY REVISED AND UPDATED

P
PROFILE BOOKS

First published in Great Britain in 1998 by
Profile Books Ltd
58A Hatton Garden
London EC1N 8LX
www.profilebooks.co.uk

This completely revised edition published in 2002

Typeset in Minion by MacGuru
info@macguru.org.uk

Printed in Great Britain by Biddles Ltd, www.biddles.co.uk

A CIP catalogue record for this book is available from the British Library.

ISBN 1 86197 434 5

CONTENTS

INTRODUCTION

"... I marvell much how he ever should have escaped so manie thousands of imminent dangers ... to have become captived ... his throte cut by the prauling Arabians, and wilde mores ... the lyons greedie mouth, and the devouring jawes of the crocodile ..."
(John Pory writing in 1600 about Leo Africanus, an early explorer)

Three centuries after Pory's account, Stanley, during his second trans-African expedition, from Zanzibar to the Congo (1874–7), lost 68% of his party of 356 men. Fifty-eight died in battle or were murdered, 45 succumbed to smallpox, 21 to dysentery and 14 to drowning, while 1 was killed by a crocodile, 2 died of fever, 5 were executed and the residue were lost, became insane or were victims of cannibals, opium or starvation. Expeditions were dangerous events in those days. Although some of these conditions remain a hazard to expeditions in the twenty-first century, we are now in a much stronger position than Leo Africanus or Stanley to minimise the risks through careful planning based on knowledge.

An expedition is an organised and usually challenging journey with the defined purpose of exploration, research, education or discovery. Such demanding activity will depend for its success on the health and attitude of mind of its members. To achieve this it is necessary to identify and understand the medical issues that are essential for planning and undertaking an expedition. *Expedition Medicine* aims to provide information on both prevention and treatment of medical problems in challenging environments. Advanced planning is essential in preparing for potential medical problems on any expedition.

This book provides information for doctors, nurses, paramedics and first aiders, as well as for people who are not medically qualified. Its aim is to be useful for people travelling to remote places, for people going on an expedition and particularly for people chosen to be expedition medical officers. It will help readers to be better informed about medical hazards and their prevention. Most chapters start with general statements requiring little background knowledge of the subject discussed; more detailed medical and technical information then follows.

Expedition Medicine is divided into three sections: Pre-expedition Planning; Field Medicine; and Medical Problems of Environmental Extremes. A glossary has been included to make the book more accessible to non-medical readers.

In this, the second edition of *Expedition Medicine*, we have updated some existing chapters, completely rewritten others – vaccinations, legal liability, common infections, emergency dental treatment, hot deserts and heat-related illnesses, tropical, diving and caving expeditions – and added the following new chapters: "Advice for people with pre-existing medical conditions", "Management of the seriously injured casualty", and "Remote medical emergencies".

Section 1, Pre-expedition Planning, aims to prevent, as far as possible, problems arising in the field. There are chapters on vaccinations necessary for travel, first aid training and recommendations for expedition medical kits, medical insurance, risk assessment and people with pre-existing medical conditions. We feel strongly that no one should join an expedition unless they have had first aid training.

Section 2, Field Medicine, provides practical information for use during an expedition or journey to a remote area of the world. Chapter 9 covers the medical officer's role, Chapter 10 emphasises the importance of camp hygiene and includes practical information on latrines, kitchen cleanliness, food storage, rubbish disposal and camp safety. Chapter 11 provides details about how to provide a safe water supply for the expedition. Chapter 12 is mainly for non-medically qualified people to enable a safe assessment to be made of an injured or ill patient and so lead to appropriate management. Chapter 13 covers first aid and the management of minor injuries in the field. It should be useful for dealing with emergencies where medical help is not immediately available. Despite the best efforts at prevention, illness and injuries sometimes do occur. Chapters 14 and 15 provide information on how to treat a seriously injured casualty and how to manage a medical emergency in a remote setting. Chapters 16 and 17 contain details about communication if evacuation is necessary. Chapters 18, 19 and 20 provide medical information on diagnosis and treatment of common infections and the less common but important tropical diseases. Chapter 21 covers psychological problems that may arise during expeditions and Chapter 22 is a brief summary of dental problems and their management.

Section 3, Medical Problems of Environmental Extremes, deals with the specific problems created by hot desert, tropical, polar and high-altitude environments, in addition to mountaineering, diving, caving and canoeing expeditions.

In short, *Expedition Medicine* aims to improve the confidence, enjoyment and achievement of people who participate in expeditions by helping to prevent medical problems or treat them if necessary. This is not meant to be a theoretical treatise, but a practical guide built from the considerable experience of its contributors. We are not complacent about our book and appeal for readers' and users' feedback to keep the advice topical and relevant in a rapidly changing world of exploration and discovery.

DISCLAIMER

The contents of this book are not tailored to any particular factual situation. Emergencies in the wilderness are unpredictable and varied in their circumstances. Medical officers should use their reasonable judgement and skills in the prevailing circumstances. The authors and publishers cannot accept any responsibility for loss occasioned by any person acting or refraining from acting as a result of the material in this publication.

Sarah Anderson
David Warrell
September 2002

SECTION 1

PRE-EXPEDITION PLANNING

1 WHAT IS EXPEDITION MEDICINE?

David Warrell, Sarah Anderson and Chris Johnson

An expedition is an organised journey with a purpose. This purpose can be exploration, achieving a particular aim such as reaching the summit of a mountain, scientific research, surveying for minerals or a test of endurance. In the nineteenth century expeditions consisted of rugged Victorians seeking to map and claim some remote piece of land for their Crown and country. In the twentieth century expeditions increasingly had a scientific purpose, but in the populous world of the twenty-first century personal development and cultural exchange are becoming the predominant reasons for travel. Exploration and adventure travel are now big business. While some groups still raise their own funds for independent travel, large charitable and commercial organisations send thousands of young people overseas each year. With specialist tour companies now offering vacations to remote places, the boundary between an expedition and a leisure trip is becoming blurred. North Americans recognise this and call what we are describing in this book "wilderness medicine".

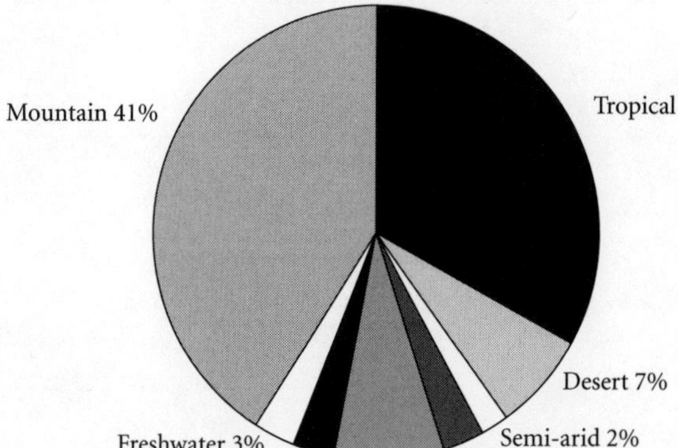

Figure 1.1 *Environments visited by British expeditions (source:* Journal of the Royal Society of Medicine *2000; 93:557–562)*

Expeditions take place throughout the world, but mountains and tropical jungles are the most popular destinations for British expeditions (Figure 1.1). By their very nature, expeditions are more likely to involve exposure to environmental extremes and new and unusual hazards than other types of travel. However, the fact that they are organised implies that those who take part in them can anticipate and prepare for at least the predictable hazards. This book is about the branch of medicine concerned with maintaining health, physical and psychological, under the special stresses and challenges of an expedition. As expeditions usually travel to remote areas where hospitals or even rural health centres are rarely found, the responsibility for dealing with medical problems will fall on the members of the expedition.

Expedition safety

The explorer's worst nightmare may be to catch a dreaded tropical disease or to be attacked by a ferocious wild animal, but for most expedition members the reality is more mundane (Table 1.1). Gastroenteritis, cuts, sprains, bruises and altitude sickness are the common reality. In some countries insect-borne diseases such as malaria and dengue are a real hazard. The risks of serious problems such as road traffic accidents – possibly before or after the expedition proper – mountaineering disasters, drowning and violence can be minimised by advanced planning.

Except in extreme environments death is uncommon. One in six of those attempting to reach the summit of Everest will die, and one in a hundred people travelling to high polar latitudes or climbing above 6,000m in the Himalayas will die. However, few expedition members visit these extreme environments and studies performed at the Royal Geographical Society suggest that travelling with a well-organised expedition is no more dangerous than attending a scout camp or visiting a rock festival in the UK. (Source: *Journal of the Royal Society of Medicine* 2000;93:557–562)

TABLE 1.1 **EXPEDITION MORTALITY**

Perceived	*Real*
Exotic infections:	Gastroenteritis
viral haemorrhagic fevers – Lassa, Ebola, etc.	Falls and other injuries
plague	Altitude, heat stroke
rabies	Infections (malaria, HIV, etc.)
sleeping sickness	Road traffic accidents
Attacks by large animals	Drowning
Venomous bites and stings	Homicide
Cannibals	

However, these figures presuppose proper planning and risk management. Planning the medical provisions for an expedition should start well in advance (Table 1.2). Preventing or minimising risks is based on a careful analysis of the geographical area to which the expedition will travel and a study of its terrain, altitude and climate at the time of year chosen for the expedition. The aims and activities of the expedition may create special risks. In selecting members for an expedition, experience, possession of the necessary skills (for example, diving, caving and mountaineering) and a reputation for psychological stability under stress are among the most important criteria.

TABLE 1.2 **MEDICAL ASPECTS OF PLANNING AN EXPEDITION**
Assessment of risks
Team selection
First aid training
Preventive medicine
Medical kit
Knowledge of special health problems
Medical back-up

On bigger expeditions there needs to be medical input during the selection of the team. It is important to identify expedition applicants who may have special problems (Table 1.3). Such problems need not prevent a person joining an expedition, but the stress of travel in remote areas can cause previously stable medical conditions to become dangerously unstable, and could in certain circumstances cause danger to everyone in the group. There are no absolute answers about who should travel; individuals have a right to decide their own attitude to risk, but should not expect others to risk their lives to save them from foolhardiness if things go wrong.

TABLE 1.3 **EXPEDITION MEMBERS' SPECIAL PROBLEMS**
Pregnancy
Immunosuppression (by drugs or diseases)
Chronic illness (diabetes, epilepsy, asthma, ischaemic heart disease, etc.)
Psychiatric problems
Physical/mental handicap
Alcohol/drug abuse

All expeditions should have a designated medical officer and as many members as possible should attend first aid training, which, ideally, should be aimed at the particular needs of the expedition. The minimum this training should cover is clearing the airway, controlling blood loss, treating shock, relieving pain and ensuring the safe evacuation of the injured. The design of first aid training and preventive medicine is based on the assessment and awareness of the particular risks of the expedition. Knowledge of local medical problems in the chosen geographical area will indicate appropriate vaccinations and prophylactic drugs. All members should have a pre-expedition dental check-up and, if possible, unresolved surgical and medical problems should be dealt with well in advance of the expedition. Medical hazards can often be prevented by behaving sensibly, although excessive caution may be considered out of keeping with the "macho" ethos of expeditions. Food and water hygiene is central to the prevention of time-, energy- and morale-wasting gastrointestinal (gut) infections.

Expedition medical kits need to be much more comprehensive than those carried by ordinary tourists. Lightweight emergency insulation must be taken if there is any risk of exposure in severe weather conditions, and an adequate water supply must be assured or taken if the expedition is to desert areas. A lightweight collapsible stretcher should be included for mountaineering and caving expeditions. A few instruments, such as scissors, and a generous supply of large triangular and crepe bandages and adhesive plasters are also important. Expeditions should take a minimum of three sets of syringes, needles and intravenous drip sets in case members have to have blood tests, or emergency treatment, at hospitals that cannot afford disposable equipment. Such items and drugs may cause problems with customs officers at frontier posts. It may be helpful to have a covering letter on official notepaper signed by a doctor, which explains the purpose of the medical equipment.

Local medical back-up must be arranged in advance through the expedition's local agent. The hospitals or medical stations nearest to the site of the expedition must be identified and, if possible, assessed in advance. An emergency plan should be drawn up for evacuation of severely ill or injured expedition members. In some areas, such as East Africa, organisations such as "Flying Doctor" services (AMREF) may agree to be responsible for evacuation of casualties. Medical insurance cover for the expedition must be generous and allow for medical care and, if need be, repatriation of injured expedition members.

Expedition medicine is not just about the treatment of disease; it should permeate all areas of the expedition. Health criteria must be considered when the location of the base camp is decided and the activities on the trip planned. Food, sanitation and psychology are part of the medical officer's work. The medical officer will fulfil many roles on the expedition and will certainly be expected to be a nurse as well as a doctor. At times this may involve listening to and encouraging those who are finding the expedition stressful. The need to accompany a casualty during evacuation may mean that certain personal goals are not attained, and the medical officer should remain sober enough throughout to deal with any accidents.

Correctly practised, expedition medicine should not constrain the enthusiasms and ambitions of an expedition but, by anticipating preventable medical problems, enhance the achievement and enjoyment of all the participants.

2 VACCINATIONS

Richard Dawood

Vaccines offer reliable protection against a limited range of important disease hazards. Where travellers sometimes go wrong is to assume that, once they've had the injections, there's nothing more to be done. Few things could be further from the truth. An important benefit of being vaccinated is the opportunity to discuss a wider range of health concerns and precautions that will keep you healthy during your trip.

Travel vaccines can be obtained from your general practitioner, university occupational health department or a specialist travel clinic Try to make arrangements at least six weeks before departure, to allow time for vaccines requiring more than one dose, and to avoid having to travel with a sore arm or other side-effects. In the UK, there were severe shortages of yellow fever vaccine during 2000 and 2001, of rabies vaccine in 2000, of the oral polio vaccine in 2001 and of the booster dose of the diphtheria vaccine. An important reason for being vaccinated well in advance of travel is to allow enough time for any supply problems to be overcome.

Certificates and regulations

Yellow fever remains the only disease for which international, WHO-approved vaccination certificates still apply as a condition of entry to some countries. Travellers to Saudi Arabia during the Haj (pilgrimage to Mecca) may be asked to show a vaccination certificate for the currently prevalent strain of meningitis. Long-term travellers to certain countries may very occasionally also be asked to show a so-called "AIDS-free" certificate or HIV test result. These requirements contravene WHO international regulations, but there is not much that most travellers can do about them.

Choosing which vaccines to have

Few of the travel vaccines that are used are required formally as a condition of entry, but are based on recommendations that take account of the likely risks to your own health: where you are going within a particular country; how you will be travelling; how long you will be staying; and whom to ask for advice.

TABLE 2.1 PRE-TRAVEL VACCINATIONS

Vaccination	*Primary course*	*Booster*
Routine		
Diphtheria	3 doses at monthly intervals	Single low dose if > 10 years
Haemophilus influenzae b	2–3 doses 2 monthly	Single dose
Influenza	Single dose	Yearly
Pneumococcal	Single dose	Repeat in those at high risk
Polio (Sabin)	Monthly intervals	3 doses at 10 years
Polio (Salk)	As above	10 years
Tetanus	3 doses at monthly intervals	10 years (max. 5 doses)
Travel		
Hepatitis A (Havrix Monodose)	Single dose	6–12 months, then 10 yearly
Hepatitis B	0, 1 and 6 months	3–5 yearly
Japanese B encephalitis	3 doses on days 0, 7 and 28	1 year and then 4 yearly
Meningococcal	Single dose	3 yearly
Rabies[1, 2]	3 doses on days 0, 7 and 28	2–3 yearly
Tick-borne encephalitis	2 doses 1–3 months apart	1 year
Tuberculosis (BCG)	Single dose	None
Typhoid – killed bacteria	2 doses 1 month apart	3 yearly
Typhoid – live attenuated strain	4 doses on alternate days	5 yearly
Typhoid – capsular	Single dose	3 yearly
Yellow fever	Single dose	10 yearly

From the *Concise Oxford Textbook of Medicine.*
1 Should not be given into buttock; deltoid or anterior thigh preferred.
2 Efficacy reduced if given with chloroquine antimalarial prophylaxis.

In the UK, the Department of Health issues guidelines, and the WHO also issues information. Many GPs, travel clinics and other sources formulate their own policies, based on Department of Health and WHO guidelines.

On an expedition, participants inevitably compare the vaccines and medication they have received; inconsistencies are common, leading to unnecessary anxiety, and can undermine confidence in the advice that has been given.

The best option is for an expedition's medical officer to draw up some general guidelines or a formal policy, seeking specialist advice if this is needed. It is always very bizarre when one half of a group has been protected against a particular disease and the other half has not. The best care comes when one clinic or practice takes responsibility for the entire group. If this is not possible, the medical officer should circulate copies of guidelines to all expedition members to present to the individual clinics or practices that will carry out immunisation.

In the UK, not all travel vaccines can be provided on the NHS, and travel vaccines are becoming increasingly costly – a factor that needs to be considered as part of an expedition's overall budget.

INDIVIDUAL VACCINES FOR TRAVEL

Cholera

The old injected cholera vaccine provided no useful protection and is no longer available. Two new oral cholera vaccines have become available in some countries, though not yet in the UK. These vaccines are currently suitable only for use in disasters or refugee camp situations, when the risk of an outbreak is very high. There is no longer a cholera vaccination certificate.

Hepatitis A (Figure 2.1)

Hepatitis A, a food- and water-borne virus, is also common in hot countries and countries with poor hygiene. Modern hepatitis A vaccines are given in a two-dose regime that provides reliable protection for at least 10 years.

Gamma-globulin injections provided only short-term protection and are no longer given in the UK.

Hepatitis B (Figure 2.2)

Hepatitis B is spread by sexual intercourse and by blood and blood products, including non-sterile medical instruments, and is a hazard in all developing countries.

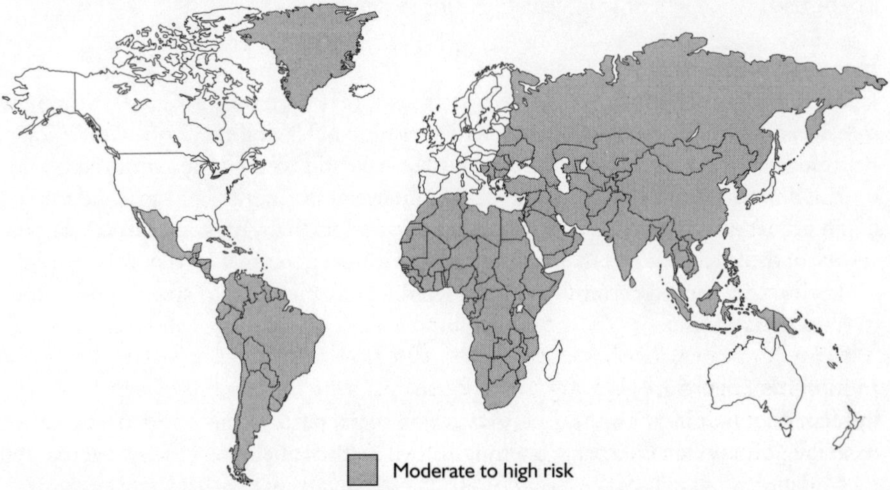

Figure 2.1 *Geographical distribution of hepatitis A virus infection, 2001 (reproduced by permission of the World Health Organization)*

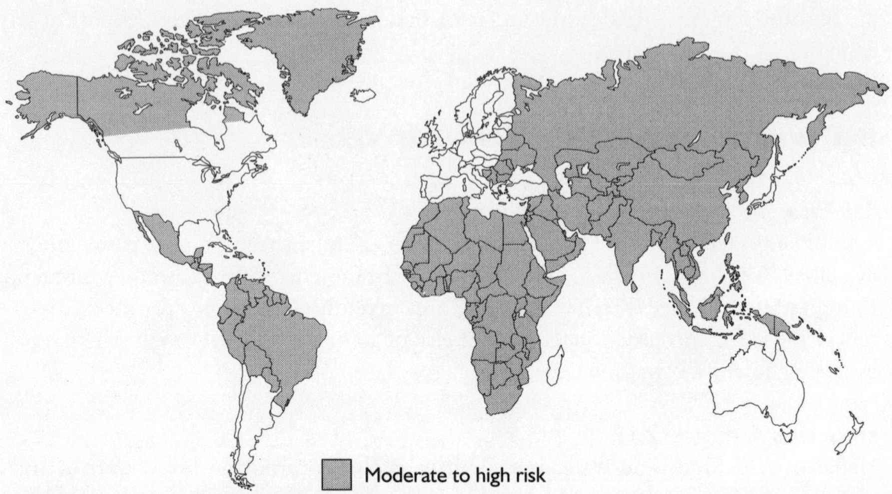

Figure 2.2 *Geographical distribution of hepatitis B prevalence, 2001 (reproduced by permission of the World Health Organization)*

Hepatitis B vaccine is a sensible precaution for anyone planning to spend a prolonged period abroad, particularly if they will be at increased risk of needing medical treatment, especially a blood transfusion.

In addition to the standard methods of giving the vaccine, accelerated schedules can be used when less time is available prior to departure.

Japanese B encephalitis (Figure 2.3)

Japanese B encephalitis is a viral disease transmitted by mosquito bites. Although rare, it carries a high risk of death (around 30%) and of leaving survivors with serious neurological side-effects. It occurs throughout Asia and New Guinea with the greatest risk during the monsoon or rainy season, between the months of April and October. It occurs mostly in rural areas, where farm animals (baby pigs and ducks) are the source of the infection, but in South Vietnam it is now perennial even in urban areas.

The vaccine should certainly be considered by anyone likely to spend much time in rural parts of Asia.

Meningitis (Figure 2.4)

Epidemics of meningitis appear periodically in many parts of the world, particularly in the region known as Africa's "meningitis belt" – the Sahel, from Senegal across to the Sudan.

Most travel clinics are able to provide up-to-date information about areas of risk. Anyone who has had their spleen removed may be more vulnerable to this condition.

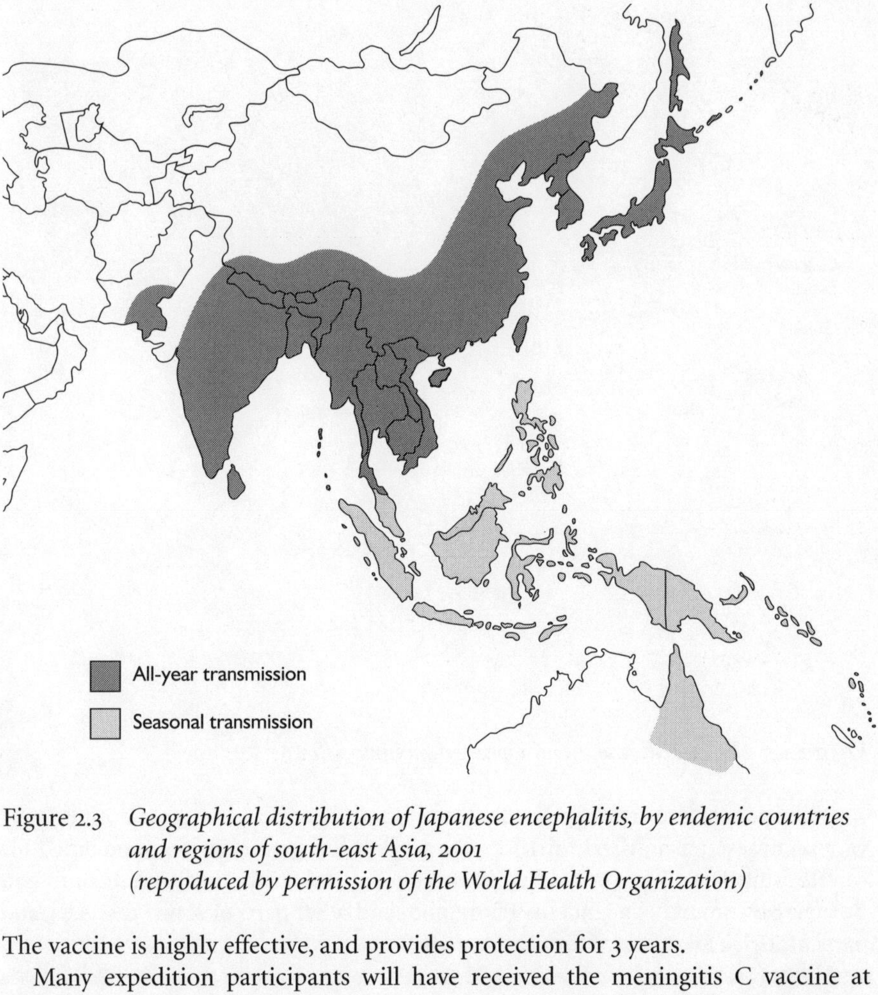

Figure 2.3 *Geographical distribution of Japanese encephalitis, by endemic countries and regions of south-east Asia, 2001 (reproduced by permission of the World Health Organization)*

The vaccine is highly effective, and provides protection for 3 years.

Many expedition participants will have received the meningitis C vaccine at school or college, but this may not cover important travel-related strains: further vaccination is usually needed. Vaccination against the A, C, Y and W strains is currently appropriate for Saudi Arabia, while elsewhere the A + C vaccine will usually suffice.

Rabies (Figure 2.5)

Rabies is spread by bites and by licks and scratches on broken skin by infected animals, and is common in developing countries. Because rabies is such a serious infection, anyone who is exposed needs vaccination and rabies immune globulin (RIG) injections. Good-quality vaccines and RIG are not available in most of the places where rabies is a problem.

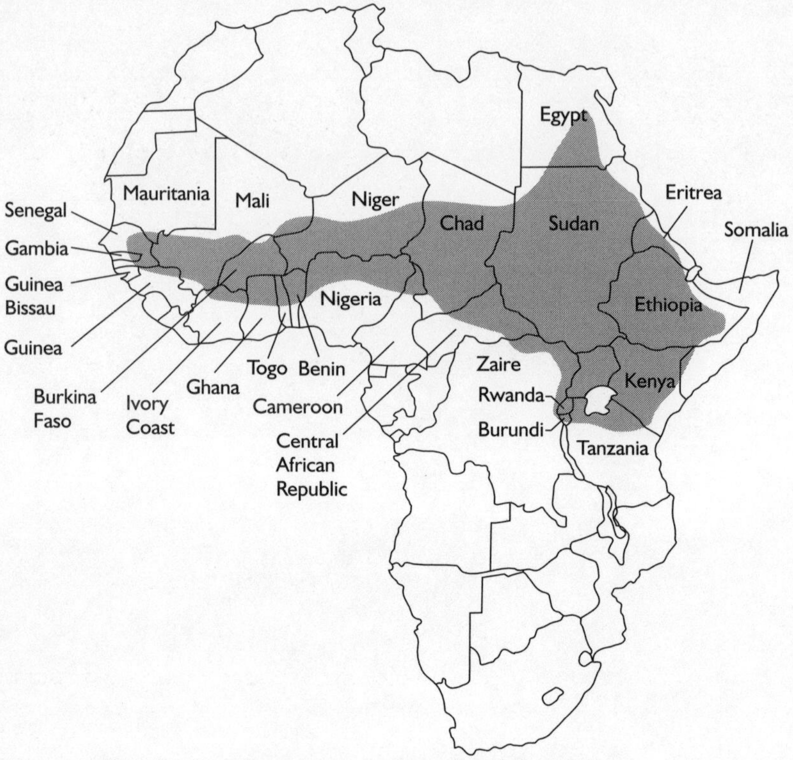

Figure 2.4 *Distribution of meningococcal meningitis in Africa*

Pre-exposure vaccination simplifies the treatment necessary after a bite: fewer vaccine doses and no need for RIG injections. It is increasingly recommended for travellers likely to be exposed, particularly for travel to the Indian subcontinent, Burma (Myanmar), Thailand, the Philippines and other parts of south-east Asia, and parts of Africa and South America.

The new rabies vaccines are safe and cause little or no reaction; ideally, three doses of vaccine are necessary, so some advance planning is required.

Tick-borne encephalitis (Figure 2.6)

This is a viral infection transmitted by ticks throughout coniferous forest areas of central Europe and Scandinavia. It carries a 10% risk of death or disability. The risk is highest on forested hills and mountains between April and November. The risk of infection can be reduced by wearing stout footwear and thick socks, applying an insect repellent and removing ticks promptly.

A vaccine is available from travel clinics for anyone going on hiking trips or proposing to spend much time outdoors.

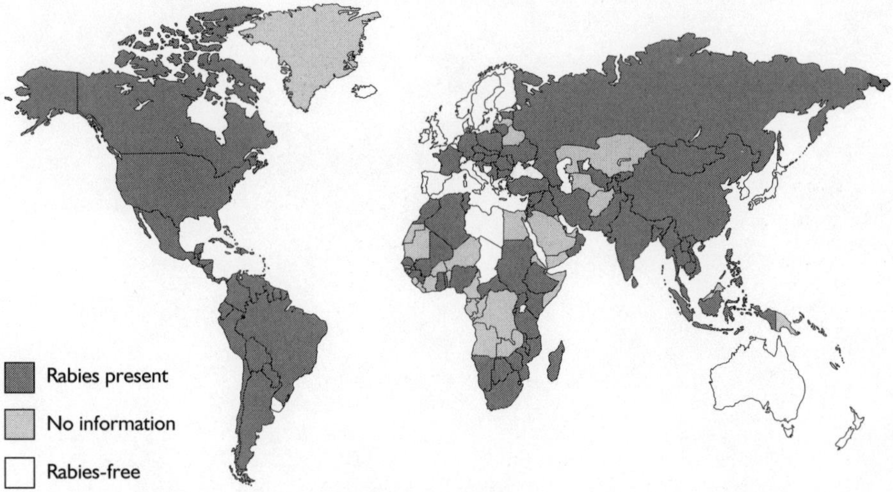

Figure 2.5 *World distribution of rabies, 2001 (reproduced by permission of the World Health Organization)*

Typhoid

Typhoid remains common in all developing countries, and in most hot countries where hygiene is poor. Vaccination is advisable for travel to Africa, Asia and Latin America, and should also be considered for travel to Mexico and the Caribbean. The Mediterranean is becoming increasingly polluted with sewage, and typhoid vaccination is a reasonable precaution for anyone proposing to spend much time in the water there.

Two vaccines are available: an oral vaccine, consisting of three capsules to be swallowed on alternate days, providing full protection for only about 1 year; and an injected vaccine, which provides 3-year protection after a single dose.

Yellow fever (Figure 2.7)

Worldwide, the risk of yellow fever is growing. Recently, a Belgian died of yellow fever acquired in The Gambia. Vaccination against yellow fever is necessary for travel to many parts of Africa and South America, either as a certificate requirement or for personal protection. It is also a certificate requirement in Asia for travellers arriving from affected regions of Africa and South America. The certificate lasts 10 years, but does not become valid until 10 days after vaccination: if you know that you are likely to have to travel at short notice, do have the vaccine in advance.

The vaccine hardly ever produces a reaction, and only a single dose is necessary. Since it is a line attenuated (weakened) virus, it should not be given to pregnant women, young children or people who are immunosuppressed by disease or drugs.

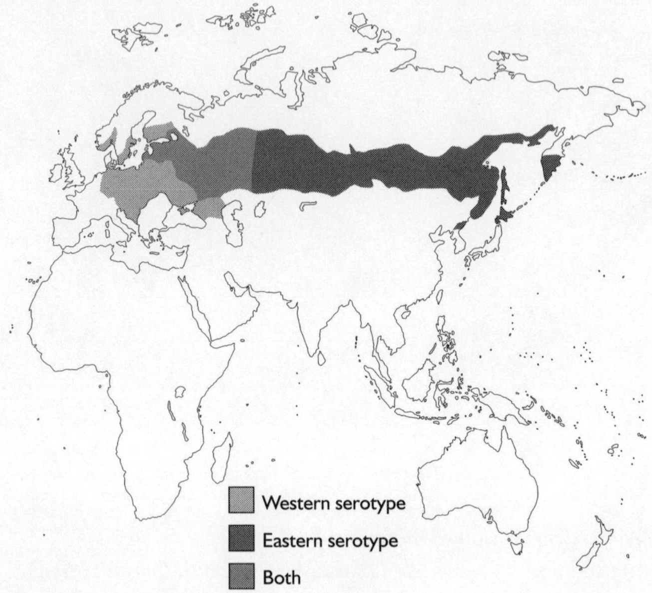

Figure 2.6 *Distribution of tick-borne encephalitis*

Live vaccines should be avoided during pregnancy and in people suffering from reduced immunity – specialist advice may be needed in these as well as in other special situations.

TABLE 2.2 LIVE AND INACTIVATED VACCINES

Live vaccines	*Killed/inactivated vaccines*
Cholera oral (not UK)	Diphtheria
Measles/MMR	Hepatitis A, hepatitis B
Polio oral	Japanese B encephalitis
	Meningitis A + C
Tuberculosis (BCG)	Polio (injected)
Typhoid (Ty 21a)	Rabies
Yellow fever	Tetanus
	Tick-borne encephalitis
	Typhoid (Vi antigen)

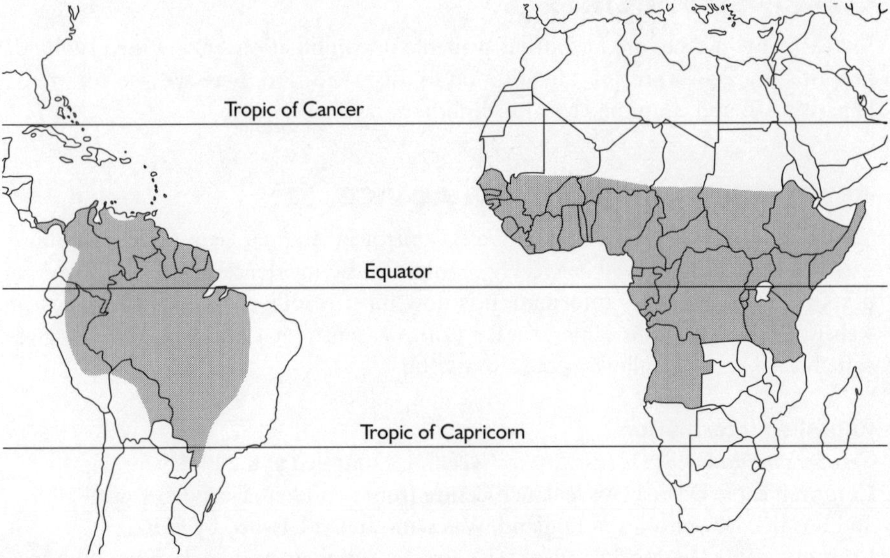

Figure 2.7 *World distribution of yellow fever, 2001 (reproduced by permission of the World Health Organization)*

OTHER ROUTINE VACCINATIONS

Everyone should also be protected against **tetanus** and **polio**, whether they travel or not. Childhood vaccination does not provide lifelong protection, and boosters are necessary every 10 years. North, Central and South America, and the Caribbean, have recently been declared polio-free zones, but a few vaccine-related cases have been reported from the Caribbean and Central America. There are still cases in Africa and Asia, but it is likely that polio will be eradicated worldwide within the next 2 or 3 years.

Diphtheria vaccine is usually given in childhood, but not everyone will have had it. A booster dose can be given in case of doubt, especially for travellers to countries of the former Soviet Union who will be in close contact with local people. Protection from childhood doses is not lifelong and begins to decrease in the mid-30s.

Expedition members travelling to developing countries and who will be in close contact with local people may need specialist advice on the question of **tuberculosis** protection if they did not have BCG vaccination during childhood.

COMBINED VACCINES

Increasingly, vaccines are becoming available in combinations. Combined typhoid/hepatitis A vaccines are a recent addition to this trend, and there are also combined hepatitis A/B and combined tetanus/diphtheria vaccines.

RESOURCES AND FURTHER ADVICE

The WHO and the Centers for Disease Control in Atlanta, Georgia, USA publish useful information as well as weekly reports on the incidence of illness in various parts of the world. This information is now most readily accessible through their websites. The Communicable Disease Control Centre at Colindale, London gives valuable advice. The following are also useful:

Published information

PHLS Communicable Disease Report (weekly). Compiled at the PHLS Communicable Disease Surveillance Centre from confidential reports from PHLS and hospital laboratories in England, Wales and Ireland. Issued by PHLS Communicable Disease Surveillance Centre, 61 Colindale Avenue, London NW9 5EQ. Tel. +44 20 8200 6868

WHO Weekly Epidemiological Record Global Epidemiological Surveillance and Health Situation Assessment, World Health Organization, 1211 Geneva 27, Switzerland
International Travel and Health, published annually by WHO, Geneva, Switzerland
Health Information for Overseas Travel, Lea, G. and Lease, J., HMSO, London, 2002
The Lancet Infectious Diseases, specialist journal, published monthly

Information available by telephone (see also Appendix 5)

Hospital for Tropical Diseases,
Mortimer Market, Capper St, London WC1E 6JA
Tel. +44 20 7388 9600

British Airways Travel Clinics Information Line (run by MASTA)
Tel. +44 1276 685040

Public Health Laboratory Health Centres

London:	Tel. +44 20 7725 2757
Midlands:	Tel. +44 174 326 1336
North:	Tel. +44 191 261 2577
North west:	Tel. +44 151 529 4900

The Fleet Street Travel Clinic
Dr Richard Dawood
29 Fleet Street, London EC4Y 1AA
Tel: +44 20 7353 5678
Fax: +44 20 7353 5500

Information sources on the Internet

World Health Organization (WHO)
www.who.int

Centers for Disease Control (CDC) USA
www.cdc.gov/mmwr

Communicable Diseases Surveillance Centre (CDSC) England and Wales
www.open.gov.uk/cdsc/cdschome.htm

MASTA (Medical Advisory Service for Travellers Abroad)
www.masta.org

Travel Health Online
www.tripprep.com

NHS (Scotland) public access travel health information website
www.fitfortravel.scot.nhs.uk

The Fleet Street Travel Clinic
www.fleetstreetclinic.com
Info@fleetstreetclinic.com

The Travellers' Health website
www.travellers'health.info has news and links to over 200 travel health-related sites.

3 EXPEDITION MEDICAL KITS

Robin Illingworth

There may be some explorers who buy a bottle of aspirin and a tin of Elastoplast while waiting for their plane and bring them back unopened 3 months later. Most expeditions take rather more medical equipment but fortunately need very little of it. However, a few expeditions have major medical problems.

Organising the medical kits for an expedition takes a lot of time and effort if it is done properly. It is particularly difficult to know what to take on a small, light-weight expedition travelling in a remote area and carrying all its equipment. A large expedition can take more medical equipment, but however much is taken one could not possibly deal with every conceivable accident and illness that might occur. Inevitably you have to compromise between taking so little equipment that you cannot deal with even the common medical problems, and taking so much that you are weighed down with an enormous medical kit that is never used. It is pointless to have a medical kit that is so big and heavy that it is left behind because no one can be bothered to carry it, or so comprehensive that items cannot be found when they are needed. However, with careful planning most of the common medical problems can be treated without outside help and first aid treatment for more serious conditions can be given if necessary.

The commonest injuries on expeditions are blisters, minor wounds and small burns. If cleaned and dressed properly these should heal without any problem, but if treated badly they may cause considerable difficulties, especially if the person becomes unable to walk. Some sprains and minor fractures can also be treated quite adequately on an expedition. More serious injuries are fortunately rare; first aid treatment will be required before evacuation to hospital.

The common ailments are aches and pains, sunburn, insect bites and bowel disturbances. These usually get better without treatment but simple drugs provide symptomatic relief. These common conditions are the same wherever you go and so the same basic medical kits can serve for many different expeditions. However, some expeditions will encounter particular medical problems, depending on their area and objectives, and so need extra drugs and medical equipment.

Road travel can be one of the most dangerous parts of an expedition. A road accident might cause serious injuries to several people, completely overwhelming any local medical facilities. Minimising risks while travelling and avoiding injuries and illness during the expedition are far more important than trying to plan medical kits to cover every possible eventuality.

The amount of medical equipment that should be taken on an expedition will depend on a number of factors, including the remoteness from medical aid, the size and duration of the expedition, the mode of travel, the organisation of the expedition (in particular the number of camps and the travelling time between them) and the medical skills of the party.

Remoteness of the expedition from medical aid

The time needed to get help is much more important than the distance to a doctor or hospital, and in a remote area the nearest hospital may be small and poorly equipped. If it is easy to get good medical attention you need take only basic medical equipment. If help is available, but difficult and expensive to reach, you should take more equipment and plan to deal with more of the possible accidents and illnesses without outside help, but also have available a communication system to summon help if needed. However, on some expeditions there is simply no help available and so the party must be completely self-sufficient, and also aware of the likely risks and consequences of any serious injury or illness.

The mode of travel

More equipment can be carried if yaks or lorries are available than if everything has to be carried in rucksacks. Weight is usually the most important factor, but the size and shape of the containers may also be significant. On some expeditions the party walks to base camp while the equipment is taken by lorry or helicopter. If this occurs the party must carry some medical equipment. There is no point in having a medical kit if it is not available when it is needed.

The organisation of the expedition

If camps are a long way apart each one must have a separate medical kit, since drugs and equipment for an emergency are useless if they are not available within a few hours. However, for non-emergency drugs and dressings it may be convenient to have small stocks at outlying camps with a larger reserve stock at base camp to replenish the other medical kits if necessary. Each group of people going away from camp for the day should carry a small first aid kit, so that some basic first aid equipment is always available.

The medical skills of the party and training

There is no point in taking drugs and equipment if you do not know how to use them, since they may be ineffective or even dangerous. A small amount of pre-expedition medical training for the nominated medical officer (MO) in specific procedures, such as suturing, insertion of intravenous lines, local anaesthetic and intramuscular injections, can greatly increase the care offered by non-medical members of the expedition. Everyone should have some first aid training and be able to use basic resuscitation equipment. For every drug in the medical kit there should be specific instructions about when, and when not, to use it, the dose and the possible side-effects. A proper record must be kept when drugs are used. Many expeditions carry drugs that are normally available only on a doctor's prescription; this is reasonable if the drugs are carefully chosen and full instructions are provided, since the potential benefits outweigh the possible dangers. Sometimes medical advice may be obtained by telephone or radio, even from a remote area, and evacuation of the patient to a doctor or hospital may not be needed if the necessary drugs are available.

Cost of medical equipment

If possible the cost of medical equipment should not determine how much is taken in the kit. Some drugs and equipment are expensive, but the cost is small compared with the cost and inconvenience of getting outside help for a condition that could have been treated adequately in camp.

Personal medical kit

Each expedition member should take some personal medical equipment, including Elastoplast or similar dressings, sun cream, lip salve, insect repellent, foot powder, simple painkillers and rehydration sachets (e.g. Dioralyte). For people who need to take a drug regularly it is best if they carry the main supply and someone else looks after a reserve stock. People who are allergic to Elastoplast should take a roll of Micropore tape which does not cause irritation.

Travel to the expedition area

While travelling to the expedition area the main medical kits may be packed and inaccessible, but some medical supplies must be kept available at all times. It is useful to have a small kit containing a few plasters, tablets for headaches, diarrhoea and travel sickness, and water purifying tablets (see also Chapter 11). If travelling outside Europe and North America a small pack of sterile needles, syringes and sutures must be available in case emergency treatment is required.

EXPEDITION MEDICAL KITS

Recommendations for expedition medical kits are based on the kits that have been used on many Brathay expeditions. There are three standard kits: the field kit, the mobile camp kit and the base camp kit. A typical expedition of 20 people to south-east Iceland might have one base camp kit, one or two mobile camp kits and four field kits. Extra drugs can be added and special medical kits made if required for particular expeditions. For example, a Brathay expedition to Sabah (Borneo), involving 18 people as well as local guides and porters, took two base camp kits, one mobile camp kit, four field kits and four extra boxes of drugs, intravenous fluids and other items, a total of 27kg weight of medical kits.

The doses of medication in the following lists are those generally used for an average-sized adult. Specific advice needs to be sought for children since different drugs may be recommended and doses would need to be adjusted for body weight and age. Appropriate substitutions would also be needed if a team member has a known allergy to a drug or dressing.

TABLE 3.1 **DIVISION OF MEDICAL SUPPLIES**

1. Field kit	A basic kit containing limited supplies of first aid equipment to be carried for a small group of people while away from base camp for the day
2. Mobile camp kit	Supplies for each group camping away from base camp a few days at a time.
3. Base camp kit	The main medical kit for the trip. Also used to replenish the other kits and provide a reserve stock of medicines for individual members
4. Accident kit	Part of the base camp kit – a pre-packed emergency kit in case of a serious accident. This needs to be portable and available quickly to team members

Field first aid kit

The field kit contains basic first aid equipment for a small party away from camp for a day. When items are used the kit can be replenished from the base camp kit.

TABLE 3.2 **FIELD FIRST AID KIT**

Item	*Quantity*
Dressing material and equipment	
Large plain wound dressing No. 15 (note 1)	1
Crepe bandage 10cm x 4.5m	1
Triangular bandage	1
Release non-adherent dressing 10cm x 10cm	1
Elastoplast – waterproof and fabric dressings	12
Adhesive tape 1.25cm x 5m	1 roll
Antiseptic swabs (for cleaning small wounds)	6
Steri-strip adhesive sutures (6mm x 100mm) (note 2)	1 sheet
Blood lancets (for blisters or splinters)	2
Safety pins	2
Scissors	1 pair

Disposable gloves (medium)	2
Emergency message form and pencil	1
Medication	
Paracetamol tablets 500mg (note 5)	10
Ibuprofen tablets 400mg (note 5)	10
Chlorpheniramine tablets 4mg (note 6)	4

See notes on pages 29–31.

Mobile camp kit

The mobile camp kit is intended for a group of about six people away from base camp for a few days and carrying all their equipment.

TABLE 3.3 MOBILE CAMP KIT

Item	*Quantity*
Dressing materials and equipment	
Large plain wound dressing, No. 15 (note 1)	1
Medium plain wound dressing, No. 14 (note 1)	1
Release non-adherent dressing 10 x 10cm	2
Triangular bandage	1
Crepe bandage 10cm x 4.5m	1
Elastoplast – waterproof and fabric dressings	12
Steri-strip tapes 6mm x 100mm	10
Elastic adhesive plaster 2.5cm x 5m	1 roll
Savlon or Hibicet antiseptic concentrate (note 3)	20ml
Gauze swabs, 7.5cm x 7.5cm, packets of 5	3 packets
Antiseptic swabs	10
Safety pins	4
Paper clip (note 4)	1
Blood lancets (for blisters or splinters)	2
Scissors	1 pair
Disposable gloves (medium)	2 pairs
Thermometer	1
Cotton-wool-tipped sticks (for removing objects from eyes)	4
Medication	
Painkillers (note 5)	
Paracetamol tablets 500mg	20
Ibuprofen tablets 400mg	10
Co-codamol 30/500 tablets	10
Allergy (note 6)	
Chlorpheniramine tablets 4mg	10
Gastrointestinal (note 7)	
Loperamide capsules 2mg or Lomotil tablets	20

Antibiotics (note 9)	
*Ciprofloxacin tablets 500mg	10
*Erythromycin tablets 250mg	20
Eyes (note 10)	
*Amethocaine eye drops 1%, single dose units	2
*Chloramphenicol antibiotic eye ointment	1 tube
Skin (note 11)	
Silver sulphadiazine cream 20g	1 tube
Optional since need extra skills (note 12)	
*Nalbuphine injection 20mg in 2ml (note 5)	2 ampoules
*Prochlorperazine ampoule 12.5g in 1ml	1 ampoule
Syringe 2ml and needle 38mm x 0.8mm (for injections)	2
Documentation (in a polythene bag)	
Booklet *First Aid on Mountains* by Steve Bollen	
Emergency message form, pencil, notebook	
Instructions on use of drugs and dressings	
Medical history cards for team members (confidentially stored)	

* Available on prescription only.
See notes on pages 29–31.

Base camp kit

The base camp kit is designed as the main medical kit for an expedition of about 20 people for about 4 weeks in an area such as Iceland, where medical help is available within 1 day. Part of the base camp kit is the accident kit, which contains equipment that might be useful at an accident away from camp. This should be kept intact at the top of the box where it may be found quickly in an emergency.

TABLE 3.4 **BASE CAMP KIT**

Item	*Quantity*
Accident kit (in a polythene bag with list of contents)	
Dressing materials and equipment	
Large plain wound dressing, No. 15	2
Medium plain wound dressing, No. 14	2
Small plain wound dressing, No. 13	2
Release non-adherent dressing 10cm x 10cm	4
Triangular bandage	4
Crepe bandage 10cm x 4.5m	2
Elastic adhesive plaster 2.5cm x 4.5m	1 roll
Safety pins	6
Scissors	1 pair

Disposable gloves	4 pairs
Injection swabs	10
Cervical collar adjustable to variable neck lengths	1
Splints if available (note 13)	

Oral and injectable medication (note 12)

*Co-codamol 30/500 tablets (note 5)	10
*Lignocaine (lidocaine) 1% injection (5ml)	2 ampoules
*Nalbuphine injection 20mg in 2ml (with instruction for use) (note 5)	2 ampoules
*Prochlorperazine ampoule 12.5g in 1ml	2 ampoules
Syringe 2ml and needle 38mm x 0.8mm	5

Optional since need extra skills (note 12)

Sutures	3 packets (3/0 and 4/0 nylon)
Suturing instruments (sterile pack with needle holder, fine forceps and scissors)	

Documentation (in a polythene bag)

Medical assessment and accident recording forms (see Appendix 3)
Insurance details, evacuation plan and emergency communication details
Medical history cards for each team member (stored confidentially)
This book *Expedition Medicine*
Instructions on use of drugs and dressings
List of contents of medical kit
Emergency message form, notebook and pencil

Main base camp medical kit

Dressing materials and equipment (in a polythene bag with list of contents)

Antiseptic swabs	20
Savlon or Hibicet antiseptic concentrate	100ml
Cotton-wool balls, sterile, packets of 5	10 packets
Gauze swabs 10cm x 10cm, packets of 5	10 packets
Release non-adherent dressing 10cm x 10cm	10
Release non-adherent dressing 5cm x 5cm	10
Jelonet paraffin gauze dressing 10cm x 10cm	10
Elastoplast – waterproof and fabric dressings (plasters)	60
Elastoplast dressing strip 3.8cm x 1m	1
Steri-strips 6mm x 100mm x 10 tapes	3 packs
Elastic adhesive bandage 7.5cm x 4.5m	1 roll
Adhesive tape 1.25cm x 5m	1 roll
Tubigrip elastic tubular bandage, size C & D	1m each
Crepe bandage (10cm x 4.5m)	3
Eye bath	1
Cotton-wool-tipped sticks (for removing objects from eyes)	10
Eye pad, sterile, No. 16 BPC	2
Disposable gloves	10 pairs
Scissors	1 pair
Splinter forceps	1 pair
Plastic dressing forceps, sterile	2 pairs

Blood lancets	6
Disposable scalpel, No. 15 blade	1
Paper clip	1
Safety pins	6
Polythene freezer bags (note 11)	2
Resuscitation mask (Laerdal mask)	
Medication	
Painkillers (note 5)	
Paracetamol tablets 500mg	100
Ibuprofen tablets 400mg	50
*Co-codamol 30/500 tablets	20
Allergy and asthma medicines (note 6)	
Chlorpheniramine tablets 4mg	50
*Salbutamol inhaler	2
Spacer device (in case of severe asthma attack)	1
*Prednisolone tablets 5mg	50
Gastrointestinal medication (note 7)	
*Hyoscine (buscopan) 10mg	50
*Prochlorperazine (Buccastem) 3mg (note 8)	10
Antacid tablets	50
Loperamide capsules 2mg	60
Senokot tablets	20
Xyloproct ointment	2 tubes
Antibiotics (note 9)	
*Ciprofloxacin tablets 500mg	50
*Co-amoxiclav (e.g. Augmentin) tablets 375mg	60
*Erythromycin tablets 250mg	60
*Flucloxacillin tablets	60
*Metronidazole tablets 400mg	60
Nose, ear and eye	
Otrivine nasal spray 0.1%	1
*Otosporin eardrops	1
*Amethocaine eye drops 1%, single dose units (note 10)	3
*Chloramphenicol eye ointment	1 tube
Skin (note11)	
Calamine cream	2 tubes
Eurax (crotamiton) ointment	2 tubes
Miconazole cream	1 tube
Silver sulphadiazine cream 20g	2 tubes
Other medicines	
Aspirin tablets 300mg (anti-inflammatory or for cardiac pain)	20
Throat lozenges (e.g. Bradosol)	40
*Antimalarial standby treatment (appropriate to area being visited)	2 courses

Optional since need extra skills (note 12)	
Sutures	3 packets (3/0 and 4/0 nylon)
Stitching instruments (sterile pack with needle holder, fine forceps and scissors)	
Injectable medications (note 12)	
*Nalbuphine injection 20mg in 2ml (strong painkiller)	5 ampoules
*Prochlorperazine ampoule 12.5g in 1ml	5 ampoules
*Lignocaine 1% injection 5ml (local anaesthetic and for nerve blocks)	2 ampoules
Syringes 2ml and 5ml plus 38mm x 0.8mm needles	5
Anaphylaxis medications (essential if taking injectable drugs)	
*Adrenaline injection for intramuscular use 1mg in 1ml (1 in 1000)	2 ampoules
(Or EpiPen 0.3mg or child size 0.15mg)	1
*Chlorpheniramine injection 10mg in 2ml (note 6)	2 ampoules
*Hydrocortisone injection 100mg	2 vials
Emergency dental kit (note 14)	1
Diagnostic equipment	
Thermometer (low reading and normal) (note 15)	1 each
Blood pressure instrument (consider if taking fluids)	1 (portable type)
Stethoscope	1
Extra drugs and equipment as required for the particular trip or a specific team member (note 14)	
Paperwork	
Medical history cards for each team member (stored confidentially)	
Insurance details, evacuation plan and emergency communication details	
Instructions on use of drugs and dressings	
List of contents of medical kits	

* Available on prescription only.

Notes to Tables 3.2, 3.3, 3.4

1. **Dressings** – the *plain wound dressings* (sometimes called *sterile compressed wound dressings*) come in three sizes: large (No. 15), medium (No. 14) and small (No. 13). Each consists of a sterile pad (20cm × 15cm in the large dressing) to cover the wound, with a long bandage to hold the pad in place. They are intended as first-aid wound dressings but could also be used to fasten the legs together after a fracture, the soft pad being placed between the knees or ankles. These dressings are compressed to take up the minimum of space. They are available from Data Southern Enterprises Ltd. *Ambulance dressings* are similar to *plain wound dressings* and are more widely available but they are less tightly compressed and so take up more space: the *No. 2 ambulance dressing* is equivalent to the *No. 15 plain wound dressing*, and the *No. 1 ambulance dressing* is the same as a *No. 14 plain wound dressing.*
2. **Steri-strips** – adhesive tapes can be used to close some wounds which would otherwise need

to be sutured. The wound must first be carefully cleaned and the skin dried. Steri-strips should not be placed encircling a finger since they may restrict the circulation.

3. **Savlon and Hibicet Hospital Concentrate antiseptics** contain chlorhexidine and cetrimide and are used for cleaning wounds. The concentrated solution is diluted with clean water and the wound is cleaned using cotton-wool balls or gauze swabs. Some small wounds can be cleaned by irrigation with water alone, but in dirty wounds the diluted antiseptic acts as soap to help loosen dirt. When the wound looks clean it should be irrigated with water to remove any remaining antiseptic.
4. **Paper clip** – this is used to treat subungual haematomas, a blood blister under the finger nail. If the fingertip is crushed blood may be visible through the nail and the finger throbs painfully. This can be treated by melting a hole through the nail using an opened paper clip heated to red heat in a flame. This is surprisingly painless and gives immediate relief.
5. **Painkillers** – a range of painkillers of different strengths is useful.
   Paracetamol ("acetaminophen" in the United States) is an analgesic which relieves minor pain with minimal side-effects and also reduces fever. The maximum dose of 8 tablets per 24 hours should not be exceeded.
   Ibuprofen is a non-steroidal anti-inflammatory analgesic drug which is useful for pain from sprains or bony injuries. Ibuprofen should not be used in patients with peptic ulcers, nor in asthmatic patients who are allergic to aspirin or related drugs. It sometimes causes indigestion. In severe pain ibuprofen can be taken at the same time as paracetamol.
   Co-codamol 30/500 contains codeine phosphate 30mg and paracetamol 500mg in each tablet; for maximum pain relief two can be taken at a time: this combination provides stronger analgesia than either paracetamol or codeine alone but the codeine may cause drowsiness, dizziness and constipation.
   Nalbuphine (trade name Nubain) is an injectable strong analgesic but is not subject to the legal restrictions covering drugs such as morphine and pethidine which make them impracticable for most expeditions.
6. **Chlorphenamine** (also called chlorpheniramine) is an antihistamine used to relieve allergic reactions and itching from insect bites or stings.
7. **Gastrointestinal medication**
   Loperamide is for controlling diarrhoea. Most cases of diarrhoea last only a few days and do not need drug treatment. Replacing fluids is more important. Loperamide may be particularly useful if diarrhoea occurs while travelling (see Chapter 18 for more information about diarrhoea).
   Hysocine (Buscopan) is used to reduce the smooth muscle spasm associated with gastrointestinal disorders.
   Dioralyte sachets contain a commercial salt–sugar oral rehydration solution. A similar solution can be made from household ingredients using a plastic measuring spoon produced by TALC (Teaching-aids At Low Cost), PO Box 45, St Albans, Hertfordshire AL1 4AX, tel. +44 1727 853869 (see also Chapter 18).
   Xyloproct ointment – for haemorrhoids (piles) and soothing painful anal conditions.
8. **Prochlorperazine** is used to treat nausea and vomiting, either from travel sickness or as a side-

effect of nalbuphine. Prochlorperazine may be given by injection or as a tablet (Buccastem) which should be placed between the upper lip and gum and left to dissolve.

9. **Antibiotics** – it is crucial to be aware if any team member is allergic to penicillin.
   Ciprofloxacin is an antibiotic especially useful for diarrhoea, chest and urinary infections. It is relatively expensive.
   Co-amoxiclav (Augmentin) is an antibiotic useful for treating ear, chest, urinary and gynaecological infections, and infections from animal bites. It must not be used in people allergic to penicillin.
   Erythromycin is an antibiotic useful for throat, chest and wound infections and for those allergic to penicillins.
   Flucloxacillin is a penicillin-based antibiotic useful for skin and wound infections.
   Metronidazole is an antibiotic useful for gynaecological and dental infections and also some forms of diarrhoea (for example, amoebic dysentery and giardiasis).
10. **Eyes** – ***amethocaine*** eyedrops are a local anaesthetic used when examining the eye for a foreign body that cannot be flushed out or if there is an injury. After use the eye must be padded up for a few hours till sensation returns.
11. **Skin** – ***silver sulphadiazine*** cream (trade name Flamazine) is useful for extensive burns. Burns of the hand should be covered in Flamazine, placed in a polythene bag and taped around the wrist. The polythene bag keeps the burn wound clean but allows movement of the fingers and some use of the hand. ***Eurax*** ointment is applied to itching insect bites, ***hydrocortisone*** to patches of eczema, and ***miconazole*** or ***clotrimazole*** will treat the extremely common fungal infections of scalp, feet and skin.
12. **Injections, suturing and intravenous drugs** – these can be safely used on expedition by 'non-medical' people with suitable training. Using these can greatly increase the range of problems that can be successfully treated or stabilised in a remote setting. The fluids are heavy, but in the right hands are indispensable in the event of a major accident or illness. The user must know what to do in case of an allergic reaction and is also responsible for safe disposal of any 'sharps'.
13. **Splints** are fortunately rarely needed, and on most expeditions materials for making makeshift splints will be available. The most versatile ready-made splint is a SAM splint, a sheet of foam-covered aluminium 91cm × 11cm which rolls up to 8cm diameter × 11cm and weighs 140g. This could be used to splint a broken arm or ankle, or as an emergency cervical collar. SAM splints and a video demonstrating how to use them are available from SP Services and other suppliers (see Appendix 5). Fibreglass canoe repair kits could be used to make an emergency splint, but great care should be taken because the heat produced when the material sets can burn the skin.
14. **Dental** – an emergency dental kit includes equipment to apply a temporary filling or a dressing for a damaged tooth. One suitable kit is the Lifesystems Dental First Aid Kit which is available from many travel equipment suppliers. Dental kits for expeditions can also be purchased from The Dental Directory +44 800 585 586 or www.dental-directory.co.uk (see Chapter 22).
15. **Thermometers** – diagnosis and monitoring of hypothermia need a special low reading thermometer. For detecting fever and heat stress, the standard glass mercury thermometers,

although fragile, are probably better than either the temperature-sensitive strips or the electronic machines.

Extra drugs and equipment

Many expeditions require extra drugs and equipment in addition to those listed above, and for a major expedition much more equipment will be needed. If there is a doctor or nurse in the party more drugs and equipment should be taken. However, he or she may not be available immediately when needed and so it is best to have basic medical kits which anyone can use if necessary and a separate kit for the doctor or nurse's use only.

Sterile equipment kits

Expeditions to areas outside Europe and North America should carry packs of needles, syringes and sutures and make sure that they are available and used if medical treatment is needed in an emergency. In many developing countries medical equipment is often reused without sterilisation and there is a high risk of transmission of infection, especially hepatitis and HIV (the AIDS virus). Suitable kits for small expeditions are listed below. Large expeditions will need more equipment and should seek advice well in advance.

TABLE 3.5 **SMALL KIT OF STERILE MEDICAL EQUIPMENT**

Item		*Quantity*
Disposable syringes	2ml	2
	5ml	2
	10ml	1
Injection needles	38mm x 0.8mm (green)	5
	25mm x 0.6mm (blue)	2
	20mm x 0.5mm (orange)	1
Sutures with needles	Novafil 3/0	1
	Novafil 4/0	1
	Softgut (catgut) 3/0	1

TABLE 3.6 **LARGER KIT OF STERILE MEDICAL EQUIPMENT**

(As above, in larger quantities, plus the following)

Item		*Quantity*
Intravenous cannulae (e.g. Venflon) 18g		4
Intravenous infusion sets		2
Intravenous fluid	– sodium chloride 0.9% (saline) 500ml	4
	– gelatin (e.g. Gelofusine) 500ml	2

Additional drugs

Extra drugs will be needed if any expedition members have pre-existing conditions such as asthma or are allergic to foods such as nuts or to any drug in the medical kit. Problems may occur suddenly at any time, often while travelling, when the main medical kits may be inaccessible. Careful planning is essential so that any necessary drugs are available immediately. Reserve supplies must be taken in case the main stock is lost.

An exacerbation of asthma will need treatment with inhalers of salbutamol and ipratropium bromide, preferably with a spacer device, and also prednisolone tablets. Ampoules of salbutamol, aminophylline and hydrocortisone should also be taken if a doctor is available.

Anyone who has had a severe allergic reaction (anaphylaxis) to a food such as nuts must carry adrenaline (epinephrine) for injection and know how and when to use it: a pre-filled syringe such as an EpiPen is the most suitable for emergency use. Repeated doses of adrenaline may be needed and also injections of hydrocortisone and chlorpheniramine.

Wound care

On any expedition suturing equipment and local anaesthetic may be needed for closing wounds, and could be used by non-medical people who have had suitable training. A small brush such as a toothbrush is useful to remove embedded dirt from an anaesthetised wound. Tissue glue (such as Dermabond or LiquiBand) may be used for closing some wounds that would otherwise need to be sutured.

Other equipment

Other items of medical equipment that could be useful if there is a doctor, nurse or paramedic in the party are oropharyngeal and nasal airways, auriscope and ophthalmoscope, urethral catheter, nasogastric tube, and a chest drainage catheter and Heimlich valve for treatment of a pneumothorax. Dental forceps and other dental equipment could be taken if someone has the skills to use them. Intravenous fluids are heavy but indispensable in the event of major trauma or severe illness: the most useful fluids are saline (0.9% sodium chloride) and gelatin (Gelofusine or Haemaccel). Some expedition doctors take enough surgical equipment for an emergency appendicectomy, but non-operative treatment of appendicitis with fluids, analgesics and antibiotics is much safer than emergency surgery outside a hospital. Fluids could be given rectally if intravenous fluids are not available. It is unrealistic to plan for major surgery even if there is a surgeon in the party. Local anaesthesia is adequate for repairing most wounds and can also be used for pain relief, especially femoral nerve block for fractures of the femur, using bupivacaine (Marcain). Midazolam could be useful for reduction of a dislocated shoulder. In the very rare circumstances where general anaesthesia is unavoidable during an expedition ketamine is the most suitable anaesthetic drug.

Extra drugs should be taken if particular medical problems are likely. These are discussed in more detail in Chapter 7.

SPECIAL HAZARDS OF PARTICULAR AREAS AND ACTIVITIES

Tropical areas (see Chapters 19 and 24)

In the tropics infectious diseases are common, especially malaria and bowel infections. Even if antimalarial prophylaxis is taken regularly drugs for treating malaria must be readily available. Tinidazole or metronidazole is useful for amoebiasis or giardiasis (see Chapter 18), chloramphenicol for typhoid and piperazine (Pripsen) for roundworms. Gastroenteritis is a major problem in hot countries. The large amounts of fluid lost from the gut may be replaced by oral glucose and electrolyte solution (for example, Dioralyte) or by a solution of sugar and salt measured with a special plastic spoon (obtainable from TALC, Teaching-aids At Low Cost; see also Appendix 5). Wound infections are common on expeditions to hot, wet places such as tropical rain forests. Many people may need treatment with oral antibiotics such as erythromycin or flucloxacillin. The risk of infection can be reduced by cleaning wounds carefully. Fungal skin infections may require miconazole cream. Clotrimazole vaginal tablets are useful for women suffering from thrush. Snake bite is rare if sensible precautions are observed. Few expeditions need to carry antivenom but expert advice about this should be obtained in high-risk areas (see Chapter 20).

Mountaineering (see Chapter 26)

At high altitudes this activity carries risks of mountain sickness and frostbite as well as the usual hazards of illness, injury and sunburn. Substantial quantities of medical supplies may be needed on a large expedition. The paper by A'Court, Stables and Travis (see Appendix 5) lists the medical supplies taken on the 1992 winter Everest expedition. Pollard and Murdoch's *High Altitude Medicine Handbook* provides further information.

Sailing

Members of sailing expeditions are liable to suffer from chapped hands, salt-water boils and excessive sun. Neutrogena hand cream may be needed in large quantities. Cinnarizine tablets often prevent sea sickness, but occasionally injections of an antiemetic such as prochlorperazine (Stemetil) are required. Salt and water depletion is common while sailing in the tropics. Trauma may occur while sailing in bad weather. Falling overboard in bad weather is likely to be fatal, so life jackets and safety harnesses must be used.

Diving (see Chapter 27)
Diving expeditions share the same problems as sailing expeditions with respect to exposure to sun and water. Ear infections (otitis externa) are particularly common, especially if swimming near coral. Olive oil drops and antibiotic ear drops (such as Otosporin) should be taken.

GENERAL POINTS ABOUT MEDICAL SUPPLIES

Treating the local people
Local people may seek medical attention from a visiting expedition. Plans for this situation should be made in advance: some of the issues to consider are discussed in Chapter 9. People with chronic conditions should be referred to local medical services but those with acute illness or injury may need emergency treatment or evacuation for medical care. Paediatric doses of some drugs may be required. Local people employed as expedition guides or porters should receive the same medical treatment as other expedition members, and additional supplies of dressings, analgesics and antibiotics may be needed to allow for this.

Where to get drugs and dressings
Many of the drugs recommended are available in the UK only on a doctor's prescription. A National Health Service prescription may not be used for drugs for use overseas, but a doctor may write a private prescription to enable travellers to purchase drugs. Some suppliers of dressings and medical equipment are listed in Appendix 5.

Packing and labelling drugs
Blister packs of tablets are convenient for expedition use, but they take up more space than the same tablets in a bottle. Any bottles should be plastic with screw tops and clearly labelled with the generic and trade names of the drug. The labels should be covered with waterproof tape. Instructions about the dose and the indications for using the drug may be included on the labels, but full information must also be available, especially about warnings and common side-effects. The most convenient source of information is the *British National Formulary* which is published twice a year and sent to every practising doctor. The trade names of drugs often differ in different countries. Occasionally, the official names are also different; for example paracetamol in the UK is the same drug as acetaminophen in the United States.

Packing and labelling the medical kits
Medical kits must be packed to protect the contents from water, dirt and damage but should allow items to be found easily in bad weather and poor light. Packing and labelling the kits require thought, time and effort. Many items should be wrapped in

resealable polythene bags, with labels visible to identify the contents without opening the bag. Similar items such as dressings may then be grouped together in a larger polythene bag, again labelled with the contents. Plastic boxes are convenient for small medical kits or for drugs and instruments: if the lid is clear plastic the label may be attached inside so that it is visible without opening the box. The outer container of a medical kit must be durable and weather resistant to protect the contents. The expedition members must be able to identify it as a medical kit but labelling it as such could sometimes attract unwelcome attention or the theft of drugs and medical equipment.

Drug export and import arrangements

There are no restrictions on exporting medicinal products from the UK, except for controlled drugs such as morphine, for which a Home Office certificate is needed and for which there are special storage and prescription requirements. Special permission would also be needed to import such drugs into another country. Even with the relevant documents delays and legal difficulties are likely if morphine or similar drugs are carried. There are equally effective alternatives that are not affected by the same legal and practical problems and these are the medicines recommended here. Expeditions taking reasonable quantities of other drugs are unlikely to encounter problems at customs. A doctor's letter on official headed notepaper listing the drugs and stating that they are for the use of expedition members and not for commercial use can be useful at border crossings. It may be helpful to check in advance with the embassy of the country concerned that there will be no restriction on importing the drugs in the medical kits. A detailed list of the drugs with approval from the relevant embassy is a great asset. British drug export certificates are not needed for expeditions unless the host country specifically requests one. A certificate can then be obtained from the Department of Health (Medicines Division), Market Towers, 1 Nine Elms Lane, London SW1 5NQ, tel. +44 20 7720 2188 ext. 3408.

During the expedition

During the expedition the medical officer should make sure that medical kits are actually available where they might be needed, rather than left behind in base camp. It is best if one person looks after the kits, but everyone should know what is available in case an emergency occurs. Notes must be kept if any drugs are used.

After the expedition

Any comments and suggestions for improving the medical kits should be recorded before they are forgotten. The RGS/EAC would be interested to learn of your experiences and ideas. If most of the items are unused they may be kept for future expeditions, or possibly donated to a clinic or hospital in the expedition area. Most drugs have an expiry date printed on the container. Other drugs and dressings should be usable for at least three years if stored in reasonable conditions.

4 EXPEDITION FIRST AID TRAINING

Jon Dallimore

All expedition team members should have at least basic first aid training – if there is only one trained first aider it might be this person who becomes ill or injured. It is also important to ensure that a trained first aider is available at each project site if the expedition will be operating in several different locations.

The aims of conventional first aid, as taught by such organisations as the St John's Ambulance and the British Red Cross, are to preserve life, limit worsening of the condition and to promote recovery.

TABLE 4.1 **AIMS OF FIRST AID**
• To preserve life • To limit worsening of the condition • To promote recovery

EXPEDITION FIRST AID

The management of sudden illness or injury on an expedition is very different from giving conventional first aid in the UK:

1. First aid is often needed in difficult environmental conditions – heat, cold, at high altitude, in rain or snow.
2. Formal medical care can be delayed for hours or even days because of a hazardous location, poor weather conditions or lack of communication and transport.
3. Some illnesses and injuries, such as altitude sickness and snakebite, are more likely on an expedition than in the UK.
4. Advanced first aid techniques, such as straightening broken limbs or treating infections, may be necessary.

5. Expedition medical supplies and equipment will be limited, particularly for small groups.
6. Some victims will recover without requiring formal medical care or evacuation. However, the basic principles of first aid still apply.

TABLE 4.2 PRINCIPLES OF FIRST AID

- Assess the situation
- Make the area safe
- Assess all casualties
  – start with the A B C of resuscitation
  – identify the injury or illness
- Give easy, appropriate and adequate treatment in a sensible order of priority
- Organise removal of casualty to secondary care where appropriate
- Make and pass on a report

CORE FIRST AID SKILLS

The only way to prepare for accidents on an expedition is to go on a first aid course, while recognising that the situation is likely to be very different from a similar emergency in the UK. You may have to move a casualty with a suspected neck injury because there is a great risk of avalanche, for example. This sort of problem should be dealt with on your first aid course. All members of an expedition should receive training in core first aid skills. Remember that simple techniques such as clearing the airway or stopping heavy bleeding make the difference between life and death, but you will not have time to look these up in a book. The more realistic your first aid training the more likely you are to be able to recall what to do in an emergency situation.

TABLE 4.3 CORE FIRST AID SKILLS FOR ALL EXPEDITION MEMBERS

- Scene and casualty assessment
- Resuscitation
- Control of bleeding and the treatment of shock
- Management of fractures and dislocations
- Care of the unconscious casualty
- Safe movement of the injured patient

BASIC MEDICAL SKILLS

Basic medical skills for expedition medical officers (MOs) and for as many of the expedition team as possible should include core first aid skills, general medical skills (traditional first aid skills), diagnosis and management of common medical problems, diagnosis and management of serious medical problems and diagnosis and management of environmental problems (Table 4.4.) This is a bare minimum for expedition MOs. The MO should know how to diagnose and manage each condition listed.

TABLE 4.4 **BASIC MEDICAL SKILLS**

1 **Core first aid skills**
2 **General medical skills**
Management of
– blisters
– bruises
– sprains and strains
– cuts/grazes
– splinters
– cramp
– burns/scalds
– wound care
– bleeding
3 **Diagnosis and management of common medical problems**
Common infections
Headaches
Asthma
Epilepsy
Diabetes
4 **Diagnosis and management of serious medical problems**
Allergic shock
Abdominal emergencies
Heart and lung conditions
Eye/ear problems
Dental conditions
Chest/abdominal injuries
Head/spinal injuries
Establishing death
5 **Diagnosis and management of environmental problems**
Heat-related illnesses
– dehydration

- cramps
- sunburn
- heat exhaustion/stroke

Cold injuries
- frostnip/bite
- hypothermia
- immersion cold injury
- drowning
- non-freezing cold injury

Altitude problems
Bites/stings
Malaria and other important tropical infections
Leeches
Diarrhoea and its avoidance
HIV and other blood-borne problems

Further information on diagnosis and management of these conditions is found in later chapters of this book and in most general medical textbooks. However, having the confidence to make the right decision is essential and will only come from attending courses and gaining field experience; do not rely on books and manuals alone.

The expedition medical officer, and as many of the expedition team as possible, should attend a specialist course. The advantage of these are that they teach you how to deal with problems that are likely to occur in remote places and often stress more advanced first aid and care to be given during evacuation. However, courses of this kind tend to be quite expensive and may last for several days in order to cover the relevant topics. Alternatively a doctor or nurse accompanying the team may teach the rest of the team about important medical problems. This is often a good team-building exercise and might involve practical sessions on moving a casualty or using splints for fractures.

With the above information we suggest you assess your own capabilities, decide what level of medical skills your expedition requires and what skills you already have, and then look carefully at the various courses available and find one that suits your needs.

FIRST AID COURSES

Listed below are details of a number of organisations that offer first aid courses in the UK. These range from basic first aid to those tailored to expeditions and more advanced paramedic training. When deciding on a first aid course in preparation for becoming an expedition MO, it is worth comparing the suggested "basic medical skills" for expedition MOs with the course syllabus. Please note that this list is not exhaustive. If you know of any other suitable courses that are not listed here, or have more up-to-date information, the Royal Geographical Society – Expedition Advisory Centre (RGS–EAC) would be interested to receive details.

Basic first aid

This is best learnt by attending one of the many standard courses run by the St John's Ambulance or the British Red Cross. The cost of such courses varies in different parts of the country, and information on course dates and times can be obtained by contacting the local branch offices. National offices can provide local branch telephone numbers.

British Red Cross: Tel. +44 20 7235 5454
St John's Ambulance: Tel. +44 20 7235 5231

Many ambulance services also provide first aid instruction and details of the ambulance service training units can be found under the first aid section of the *Yellow Pages.*

Advanced first aid training

The need for this depends on how far from medical help an expedition will be operating. The EAC has sent representatives on the following courses and found them to be particularly relevant to expedition members and medical officers.

Wilderness Medical Training (WMT)

WMT offers advanced first aid training for expeditions operating in remote areas of the world, particularly for those expeditions without professional medical support. The use of antibiotics and other prescription drugs is covered on all courses. Residential courses include "Far From Help" over 3 days and "Advanced Medicine for Remote Foreign Travel" over 5 days; the latter also includes the teaching of invasive techniques (drips, suturing, injections, etc.). The majority of the teaching on WMT courses is delivered by doctors with extensive overseas expedition experience. WMT also runs an annual 5-day conference for expedition doctors in Chamonix, France.

Contact: Barry Roberts
Commercial Director, WMT
The Coach House
Thorny Bank
Skelsmergh
Kendal
Cumbria LA8 9AW
Tel. fax +44 1539 823183

Email: office@wildernessmedicaltraining.co.uk
Website: www.wildernessmedicaltraining.co.uk

Rescue Emergency Care

The REC scheme (Health and Safety Executive [HSE] registered) offers six 2-day modules ranging from basic to expedition first aid. The emphasis across the full range of the modules is effective first aid provision, with the minimum of equipment, in remote environments. In order to achieve this these concept-based courses rely heavily on practical scenarios to introduce an element of realism that expedition doctors, medics and first aiders should be prepared for. Courses are tailored for specific groups such as exploration teams, film crews and mountain rescue teams. The scheme has trainers instructing throughout the UK and the courses are recognised and approved by the British Mountaineering Council, Mountain Leader Training Board, Royal Yachting Association and British Canoe Union.

Contact: Peter Harvey
Wilderness Expertise Ltd
The Octagon
Wellington College
Crowthorne
Berkshire RG45 7PU
Tel. +44 1344 774430, fax +44 1344 774480
Email: REC@wild-expertise.demon.co.uk
Website: www.wild-expertise.demon.co.uk

British Red Cross

The British Red Cross, in addition to basic first aid courses, provides specialist courses for "Outdoor Activity" and "Expedition First Aid". These are modular courses with specialist elements, including casualty handling and specific modules on key environments such as the tropics and cold climates, and key activities such as caving, mountaineering, water sports and pony trekking.

Contact: Lynne Covey
British Red Cross Society
9 Grosvenor Crescent
London SW1X 7EJ
Tel. +44 20 7235 5454

Life Support Training Services (LSTS)

LSTS provides modular courses aimed at those going to remote areas. There is a basic course (2 days) and a choice of advanced courses (3 and 5 days). If there is sufficient demand, i.e. an entire expedition, the courses can be arranged at a venue of your choice with cost by arrangement, depending on numbers and venue. The courses concentrate on practical skills in as realistic a setting as possible.

Contact: Daryl Wight
Life Support Training Services
2 Underhill Cottages
The Hill
Millom
Cumbria LA18 5HA
Tel. fax +44 1229 772708

Orion First Aid

Orion are registered with the HSE to deliver first aid courses to industry and commerce. In addition they also provide first aid courses to the general public that specialise in outdoor pursuits and exploration group organisations. Their instructors have wide-ranging experience, having seen and dealt with frontline trauma injuries, coming from Mountain Rescue, Cave Rescue and NHS paramedics. Courses include: Emergency First Aid, Mountain First Aid, Advanced Mountain First Aid and Expedition Medicine. They also specialise in maritime courses.

Contact: Stan Farrington
Orion First Aid
Brownrigg Guide Road
Hesketh Bank
Nr Preston
Lancashire PR4 6XS
Tel. fax +44 1772 812 277
Website: www.oriontraining.co.uk

Andy Sherriff – Specialist First Aid Training

Training is available to suit all requirements, from basic to highly advanced, whether the expedition be to the high mountains or the tropics. Courses are run as a progression of 2-day units. Expedition members can enter the scheme at "foundation" level or higher, depending on experience and existing first aid training. Current courses include: "First Aid for Mountaineers and Instructors", "Advanced Immediate Care" and "Expedition Medical Care". All courses exceed the requirements for National Governing Body Awards (MLTB, BMC, BCU, etc.). The emphasis of training is towards the delegates gaining the necessary skills to provide appropriate medical care in remote locations, using formal and improvised equipment. Andy Sherriff is a HSE-registered training provider.

Contact: Andy Sherriff Specialist First Aid Training
Nyth yr Hebog
Llandyrnog
Denbigh
North Wales LL16 4HB
Tel. fax +44 1824 790195
Website: www.mtn.co.uk/sherriff

Courses tailored to special requirements
The Ieuan Jones First Aid Course for Mountaineers
Contact: Gerry Lynch
Tel. +44 1248 600589
Mountaineering expeditions might like to attend courses specially run for members of mountain rescue teams (some of the best first aiders in the UK belong to mountain rescue teams).

British Association of Ski Patrollers (BASP)
Contact: Fiona Gunn
Tel. +44 1855 811443

First aid and medical courses are also run by various outdoor adventure and training centres and these should be contacted individually to find out when and what sort of courses they offer. Centres that run first aid courses include:

Glenmore Lodge, Aviemore	Tel. +44 1479 861256
Brathay Hall, Ambleside	Tel. +44 1539 433041
Plas-y-Brenin, Capel Curig	Tel. +44 1690 720366
Outward Bound Schools	Tel. +44 990 134227 (Head Office)
Aberdovey	Tel. +44 1654 767464
Loch Eil	Tel. +44 1397 772866
Ullswater	Tel. +44 1768 486347

Other expedition medicine courses

ExpeMed Expedition Medicine Course, Glasgow
Frontline Medical Services organise 4-day courses for medical professionals who wish to undertake the role of medical officer on expeditions to remote areas. Courses are suitable for doctors, nurses, dentists and paramedics. The aim is to provide training on all aspects of expedition medicine with emphasis on pre-trip planning, casualty management and casualty evacuation. Instructors have backgrounds in medicine, pre-hospital care, rescue and expedition management. Specialist vehicle extrication is provided by Strathclyde Fire Brigade and a full day of outdoor casualty

scenarios and rescue training is provided by the Arrochar Mountain Rescue Team. ExpeMed courses are organised and run by Frontline Medical Services Ltd.

Contact: Stephen Hearns FRCSEd, Dip IMC, Course Director
Tel. fax: +44 1389 877811
Email: expemed@frontlinemedics.com
Website: www.frontlinemedics.com

5 LEGAL LIABILITY

Alistair Duff

Expeditions offer an exciting challenge to their expedition medical officers. While their role is key to the success of an expedition, medical officers may find themselves liable for the care that they give if it is deemed to be inadequate or incorrect.

Fortunately, I am not aware of any case in which a doctor is being sued for treatment given on an expedition and the Medical Defence Union has confirmed that, as of January 2002, there are no such actions involving their members. However, society is becoming more litigious (*Woodroffe Hedley v Cuthbertson, English High Court* 1997) so doctors, and others acting as expedition medical officers, should not be complacent in their role as medical officer. Medical professionals must inform their defence organisation in advance if they intend to act as an expedition medical officer. In most instances they will receive cover against litigation arising from care given on an expedition (possibly for a small additional fee). Since October 1999, the Medical Defence Union provides "Good Samaritan Cover" for every country in the world, including the United States and Canada. Insurance will not take away the danger of being sued, but certainly it should give piece of mind. The most important thing is to check what insurance cover you have before you act as an expedition medical officer.

MEDICAL NEGLIGENCE

To understand the potential risks of taking on the role of expedition medical officer it is necessary to understand the legal terminology involved.

Duty of care

In any potential court action, a "duty of care" must be established between the person giving the treatment and the patient. Clearly, if any doctor treats a patient, whether as an expedition doctor or in a rescue situation, a "duty of care" will be established. It is important to remember that a "duty of care" is not owed to the world at large, but to those who may become injured if the duty is not observed.

Standard of care

Any person acting as an expedition doctor has to exercise the "standard of care" expected of an expedition doctor. A doctor cannot plead, in essence, inexperience. In England "standard of care" is governed by the court's decision in *Bolam v Friern Hospital Management Committee* 1957 (1 WLR 582) in which it says: "The test is the standard of the ordinary skilled man exercising and professing to have that special skill. A man need not possess the highest expert skill at the risk of being found negligent. It is well established that it is sufficient, if he exercises the ordinary skill of an ordinary competent man exercising that particular art."

Inexperience

A doctor who holds himself out as a specialist (for the purposes of this chapter, an expedition doctor) will be held to the standards of a reasonably competent expedition doctor even if he is a novice and even where he is performing the procedure for the first time (see *Jones v Manchester Corporation* 1952, 2 All ER 125 and *Wilsher v Essex Health Authority* 1986, 3 All ER 801).

Different opinions

Where different opinions exist as to the acceptability of a course of action, if a doctor can show that the course he or she followed was one that has the backing of a body of respectable opinion within the profession, then liability will not be imposed merely because the treatment may be disproved by a section of medical opinion. Therefore, if one is able to obtain support from various doctors involved with Medical Expeditions Limited (MEDEX), who run courses and whose members publish books that have itemised lists or follow protocols laid out in the British Antarctic Survey Medical Handbook, this could do much to protect any doctor, paramedic or trek leader. (See *Bolitho v Hackney Health Authority* 1997, 4 All ER 771.)

Emergency situations

Expeditions work in remote areas, often with limited resources. The circumstances in which medical care is provided may influence a court's decision as to what constitutes a reasonable "standard of care". An expedition doctor is highly likely to face what could be described as an emergency situation, and in determining what is reasonable care the court will take account of the particular situation as it presented itself to the defendant as part and parcel of all the circumstances of the case. Clearly the court would take into account the fact that expeditions work in remote areas, that resources are limited and that the setting is not an accident and emergency (A&E) department. This is highlighted by the case of *Wilsher v Essex Health Authority* 1986 (3 All ER 801), where the judge considered that "An emergency may overburden the available resources and if an individual is forced by circumstances to do too many things, the fact that he does one of them incorrectly should not lightly be taken as negligence".

Expectations of expedition members

Expedition members should not expect to receive the same "standard of care" as they would in a hospital A&E department, but should expect to receive a similar standard to that of any competent doctor in a similar situation. Prior to the expedition it is useful for an expedition medical officer to discuss with expedition members what "standard of care" they can expect to receive, given the limitations of the expedition environment. They should also have members fill out a relevant health questionaire.

Expedition leader/paramedic

The "standard of care" expected of a paramedic is not that of a doctor but that of an ordinary skilled paramedic professing to have the special skill of a paramedic. The expedition leader would likewise have to exercise the standard of skill expected of an expedition leader.

Expedition doctor and Good Samaritan acts

Generally speaking, if one were travelling as an expedition doctor, even if there were no payment for your services, there would be no "Good Samaritan Cover". Quite often a doctor will not get paid *per se* but will receive a discount or some other benefit. Generally, Good Samaritan Cover is available only if you are there as an ordinary person (i.e. as a layman) and not as a doctor and decide to treat someone in your party, or you treat someone unconnected with the expedition. Obviously if one is acting under the auspices of a Good Samaritan, the "standard of care" is only that expected from a normal GP if you happen to be a GP.

Appointment as a doctor to a commercial expedition or trek

There is a duty on the part of a commercial expedition or trekking company to appoint a competent doctor if it is appointing one. As a trek company, it should check the doctor's experience. If a doctor is directly employed by an expedition organiser or trekking company, the organisers will be liable for the actions of this doctor. Even if the doctor is held to be an independent contractor, he or she is usually still under the control of the company and it will be responsible for his actions.

Can a doctor avoid liability by disclaimers?

Arguably, if the doctor is not getting paid and has asked every expedition member to sign a disclaimer of liability prior to giving treatment, he or she might avoid liability. Generally speaking, such disclaimers are caught by the Unfair Contract Terms Act 1977 (as amended). Equally, trekking companies sometimes try to persuade clients to sign disclaimers, but these are caught by the Act as the Act applies to anything arising in the course of business and this is generally given a fairly broad interpretation.

This should be compared to the position in the United States and Canada where companies can certainly ask clients to sign disclaimers which, subject to being written clearly and properly, will be effective in absolving the companies of all liability for negligent acts. (See the American case *Patricia Vodopest v Rosemary Macgregor*, Supreme Court of Washington, 8 March 1996 and the Canadian case known as *Bay Street Court Decision*, Supreme Court of British Columbia, 20 September 1996.)

Provision of drugs for expeditions

A doctor (whether or not present on the expedition) who prescribes or advises on the use of drugs on an expedition retains the "duty of care" towards the individual for whom they are prescribed and remains responsible for the effects of these drugs. GPs, giving advice on prescribing to expedition leaders or medical officers, or if they are going to prescribe drugs for use by unknown third parties, should clearly label the drugs, give indications for the use, contraindications and possible side-effects, and state how to use them. Clearly the person then using the drug should be knowledgeable.

The Crown Report (1999) recommends that prescription-only medications (POMs), when given by a person not registered as a medical practitioner, should be governed by written and signed protocols. It is therefore advisable for any expedition medical officer who is not a doctor to have written and signed protocols for all expedition drugs.

SUMMARY

Perhaps the most important thing for anyone contemplating going on an expedition as the medical officer is to ensure that he or she has the appropriate insurance (indemnity) cover. This must be checked with the relevant professional body prior to departure. In addition the medical officer must ensure that the correct procedures are in place for the prescription of drugs by non-medical personnel.

Lastly, those considering acting in a capacity other than a Good Samaritan should satisfy themselves that they are able to deal competently with any medical problems that arise. They should also try to obtain a written letter of engagement, ideally from the expedition organisers, setting out what their duties are, what is expected of them and who is in overall command (especially when relating to medical matters). They should also make enquiries about the company/organisation appointing them as to their reputation and track record, so that they can make an informed judgement whether or not to accept the appointment.

This chapter is a very brief synopsis of some of the legal issues relevant to expeditions but is by no means definitive or exhaustive on what is a complex subject. Clearly, matters should be discussed with the relevant professional indemnity organisations and with their legal advisers before setting out.

6 MEDICAL INSURANCE

Mark Whittingham

Expeditions, almost by definition, seem rarely to have sufficient funds for their true objectives, let alone the "luxury" of insurance. This can easily result in failure to insure adequately. Do not under-insure. Always bear in mind that, if you cannot afford the premium, you are even less likely to be able to afford the potential loss.

Without doubt, the most important thing to remember when arranging insurance is that the law requires the person insuring to disclose all material facts to the insurers whether or not the information is sought by them. Failure to comply with this fundamental tenet of insurance (no matter how unfair it may appear) can have the effect of completely invalidating the insurance contract. For instance, if part of your expedition involves white-water rafting or mountaineering it is important to declare this.

What facets of insurance do expeditions need to consider when arranging expedition medical insurance?

Expeditions should consider the following broad categories of insurance cover.

Medical and additional expenses

This is a most important insurance cover. It usually covers medical and travel expenses for each member of the expedition following accidental bodily injury or illness. These expenses may vary from a doctor's visit through to major surgery and after-care. The UK has reciprocal National Health arrangements with some countries (see below). This category of insurance should include the following:

a) Emergency assistance and repatriation including air ambulance or air transport costs.
b) Emergency dental treatment.
c) Travel and accommodation expenses for people who have to travel to or remain with or escort an incapacitated insured person.

d) Local funeral expenses or transportation of the body to the UK.

- Medical conditions known to exist before the start of the expedition may not be covered. This exclusion may not apply, provided the insured person has been without medical treatment or consultation during the previous 12 months. Expedition members who are in doubt about this exclusion should consult their insurance adviser before departure and/or obtain a medical certificate from their doctor stating that they are not travelling against medical advice. This may satisfy the insurance company's requirements.
- It is important if your travel policy has a 24-hour emergency telephone number for hospitalisation or repatriation that this number is used when an accident or illness occurs. Professional advice may be available about hospitalisation, repatriation or alterations in any travel plan.
- Do not totally rely on the insurer's emergency assistance rescue company; expeditions visit isolated and remote areas and there are no guarantees there will be sufficient local resources. Be sure to have a contingency evacuation plan agreed and arranged beforehand. Insurance companies are no substitute for a sound crisis management plan.
- If foreign nationals are on the expedition they may need to be repatriated back to their own country instead of the UK. Insurer agreement needs to be obtained to this before the expedition commences.
- Cover normally excludes claims associated with HIV-related illness. It is possible to obtain separate "Dread Disease" insurance for nurses, doctors and health workers where a benefit is payable should a person test HIV positive.
- All travel insurance policies have geographical limits. Premiums are lower if cover is restricted to Europe instead of worldwide; however, careful consideration needs to be given to the insurer's definition of Europe.
- No limit less than £2,000,000 per person should be accepted for journeys to the United States. Travellers are recommended to carry proof of medical expenses insurance cover at all times in the United States in case the authorities do not provide treatment.
- Any action taken by the expedition in the field without consultation with the emergency rescue company/insurers may have to be justified to the company afterwards. A diary of events should therefore be kept.

Personal accident

This covers death and disablement following accidental bodily injury. An amount is paid in the event of loss of use of an eye or limb, permanent total disablement or death. Cover should include disappearance, and death or disablement by exposure. The amount paid will be additional to any other personal accident or life assurance that individual members of the expedition have arranged for themselves.

- Benefits should be payable for disability from usual occupation as opposed to any occupation.
- Note that cover should be accidental bodily injury; avoid insurance policies that restrict cover to violent visible or external means.
- Make sure cover is on a 24-hour basis, includes commuting to and from the expedition departure point, and is not restricted to certain activities.
- As expedition members can change, make sure cover is on an unnamed basis for all members, as opposed to named individuals.
- The lower age limit should be carefully checked, because the death benefit will be restricted to a nominal amount for minors below 16 years of age. Some insurers will try to apply the nominal amount to members aged 16 and 17.
- If your insurance policy is a group policy for all expedition members, the insurer may try to apply a limit of liability in respect of more than one individual being injured on an aircraft or other conveyance. Larger expeditions should check the policy wording to make sure any aggregate conveyance limit is adequate.

Public/personal liability insurance

All members must have adequate insurance against any legal liability in the event of an incident occurring, and that includes liability to other members of the expedition.

The legal necessity for public or third-party liability varies greatly from country to country (care should be taken to comply with local laws). This type of cover should include liability for bodily injury or illness caused to anyone. Cover should also include damage to other people's property other than property in the care, custody or control of the expedition. Warning: do not admit liability in the event of an incident, as you may prejudice your rights.

Leaders have greater responsibilities than other members. Leaders of school expeditions should ensure that the school's liability policy extends to include the teachers'/leaders' liability in full and in the region to be visited. If the school's insurance cannot be extended to provide this cover then some other form of liability insurance should be arranged. Check with your insurer that cover also extends to expedition organisers.

- If the logisitics of the expedition are being arranged by a commercial company, special tour operators' liability may be necessary.
- Cover will exclude mechanically propelled vehicles – this includes water-borne craft and aircraft. Separate liability policies will be necessary for all water-borne craft and motor vehicles.
- If hiring a car in the United States or Canada, the indemnity limits will be low; separate top-up cover is normally necessary.

Replacement and rearrangement

You can insure additional travel and accommodation expenses for a replacement expedition member following the death or disablement of an insured person. In addition, this type of insurance would cover the cost of returning the originally insured person to complete the expedition following recovery.

Further points to consider when arranging insurance

1. If you hold insurance in your own name (for example, life, personal accident, all risks) you should notify the destination and details of your expedition activities to your insurers. If you do not, your policy could be invalidated.
2. When relying on an "umbrella" policy (for example, a school or association policy) check that the cover is adequate. Insurance provided by a school's policies will not usually cover boys or girls who left school at the end of the term before the expedition.
3. If you hire local labour, make enquiries about your responsibilities before the expedition starts. In many countries something equivalent to the UK employers' liability insurance, normally known as workers' compensation, may be needed. In most cases this can be arranged locally, before engaging local labour, and exact requirements can usually be confirmed from the host country's embassy. In addition, many expeditions work with local scientists and helpers who should be included in the expedition's liability insurance.
4. Read the insurance policy details carefully, and explain them to all members of the expedition.
5. Take some claim forms with the expedition to complete while the incident is still fresh in your mind. *It is absolutely essential that any claim is reported to the insurer immediately, as an insurance policy may time bar a claim if notified late.*
6. Be careful to declare separately to the insurer any holiday taken after the expedition has finished. Separate cover may need to be arranged as a separate risk from the rest of the expedition.
7. Check your policy will not expire if your expedition is delayed beyond the planned return date, due to circumstances beyond your control. It may be impossible to contact your insurer from the field.
8. Some insurers will try to exclude any cover arising from "war risks". This should be strongly resisted as expeditions often work in politically sensitive areas. A more acceptable wording is an exclusion of war risks by major powers only. If you are in any doubt about the stability of the area you are working in, check with the British Foreign Office or equivalent body overseas and declare the facts to the insurer for written agreement.
9. Insurance Premium Tax (IPT)/VAT. When obtaining a quotation make sure the price you are quoted is inclusive of Insurance Premium Tax. The present IPT rates are as follows: Personal Travel Insurance, 17.5%; Travel Insurances as part of Employment, 5%.

Medical treatment abroad

There are over 40 countries outside the EU with which the UK has reciprocal healthcare agreements that entitle British visitors to emergency medical treatment. A Department of Health leaflet *Health Advice for Travellers* provides vital information on obtaining emergency medical treatment abroad and contains details of how to use Form E111, the passport to free or reduced-cost emergency medical treatment in most European countries. This is an important and complex process and the leaflet is essential reading. To order a copy, phone the Health Literature Line on +44 800 555777 any time, free of charge. Orders for more than ten copies should be placed with the Department of Health, PO Box 410, Wetherby LS23 7LN.

Where to get insurance

Aon Limited organise the official RGS–IBG Expedition travel insurance scheme which is designed to meet the specialised needs of scientific and educational expeditions. Details can be obtained from the Expedition Advisory Centre at the RGS (see Appendix 5), or contact Aon Risk Services Ltd, Richmond House, College Street, Southampton SO14 3PS, tel. +44 238 060 7500, fax + 44 238 063 1055; email: expeditions@ars.aon.co.uk.

Few insurance consultants are qualified to arrange expedition insurance, but among those who have shown an interest in insuring expeditions are:

Campbell Irvine Ltd, 48 Earls Court Road, London W8 6EJ, tel. +44 20 7937 6981, fax +44 20 7938 2250. In the first instance, please submit brief details of the expedition in writing.

Harrison-Beaumont Insurance Services, Witney Bay, Witney, Oxon OX8 6BE, tel. +44 1993 700200, fax +44 1993 700502, email: info@hbinsurance.co.uk, website: www.hbinsurance.co.uk

If obtaining quotations from any other insurance intermediaries, make sure the insurance broker is a Member of the General Insurance Standards Council.

Many clubs and associations have special insurance schemes arranged for their members. These range from mountaineering and hang-gliding to canoeing and caving, and are designed to provide insurance cover for specialist high-risk activities. Beware, some of these schemes have restricted cover.

For mountaineering expeditions

British Mountaineering Council, 177–179 Burton Road, Manchester M20 2BB, tel. +44 161 445 4747, fax +44 161 445 4500, website: www.thebmc.co.uk

For winter sports

Snowcard, Freepost 4135, Lower Boddington, Daventry, Northants NN11 6BR, tel. +44 1327 262805, website: www.snowcard.co.uk

The "Snowcard" is popular with skiers. It provides a "card" in your pocket for proof of insurance, with access to the Assistance International 24-hour telephone service for everyone insured under Snowcard's Flexi-Option Insurance, in case of a serious medical problem. This policy has since been adapted for trekkers and river rafters.

For general insurance

Endsleigh Insurance Services, 3 Kings Street, Watford WD1 8BT, tel. +44 1923 218438, fax +44 1923 218458, website: www.endsleigh.co.uk

Endsleigh's ISIS insurance includes a range of policies from the "Backpacker" to the Premier World-wide policy designed for the specific needs of the independent traveller.

Professional indemnity insurance

Doctors and other medical professionals must not assume that their professional indemnity insurance will provide all the necessary insurance cover for their care of expedition participants or host-country nationals. It is therefore important that expedition doctors discuss which countries they will be visiting with their insurers. In some cases this may require an additional premium.

It is also prudent to ensure that your employers are aware of your plans and have no objections. This is particularly important for doctors employed by the NHS on full-time contracts, as working overseas may not be covered by their insurance.

Specialist insurance cover can usually be obtained for student medical electives, on short- and long-term medical practice overseas.

Medical Defence Union, 230 Blackfriars Road, London SE1 8PJ, tel. +44 20 7202 1500, email: mdu@the-mdu.com, website: http://www.the-mdu.com

Medical Protection Society, 33 Cavendish Square, London W1G 0PS, tel. +44 20 7399 1300, fax: +44 20 7399 1301, email info@mps.org.uk, website: www.mps.org.uk

Finally, if you are dissatisfied with an insurer's service you can ask the Insurance Ombudsman to review your case. His offices are at: City Gate One, 125 Park Street, London SE1 9EA, tel. +44 20 7928 4488. If you contact the above body in respect of complaints, this will not affect any legal right of action you may have later.

7 PRE-EXISTING MEDICAL CONDITIONS

Mukul Agarwal

The lure of wild places is attracting people from an ever-widening range of backgrounds. Some have pre-existing medical conditions or a disability. It is neither necessary nor desirable for people to be excluded purely on the basis of these. With careful risk assessment, preparation and appropriate back-up it is possible for most people to enjoy a wilderness experience and take part in an expedition successfully, enjoyably and safely. This chapter is largely intended to help medical professionals give appropriate advice.

Expeditions visit remote and challenging environments where logistics are difficult and access to medical facilities, personnel and equipment ranges from limited to non-existent. It is the element of remoteness that makes expedition medical advice and preparation different from that for general travel. The medical concerns that surround a person with a pre-existing condition on an expedition are:

- They may not be able to participate fully in the physical and emotional challenges that make up expedition life by virtue of their condition or disability.
- The rigours and living conditions of an expedition may worsen their condition and diminish their own enjoyment and achievement while compromising that of others.
- If they become unwell, facilities may not be available to provide appropriate care.
- They may be at increased risk of an illness that could endanger or compromise them or the expedition.

These concerns are real and valid but their magnitude depends on the exact nature of the individual's condition or disability and on the proposed trip. The chapter that follows starts by presenting a general approach that could be taken, regardless of the condition or disability, before a more detailed consideration of common medical conditions and of disability. The number of possible conditions or disabilities for which advice could be sought is vast. Even for the commonest of these, there is little evidence-based literature on which to base recommendations. A pragmatic approach is presented and the following framework is suggested:

1. Risk assessment
2. Pre-expedition advice
3. Advice during the expedition
4. Post-expedition assessment.

RISK ASSESSMENT

A risk assessment will give some idea of the magnitude of potential medical and logistical problems. It will allow recommendations to be made regarding the degree of pre-expedition assessment and preparation needed as well as the appropriate level of medical support and back-up once in the field. A doctor should review a person with a pre-existing medical condition or disability before they join an expedition and particularly before significantly increasing their level of exercise for pre-expedition training. A summary of this assessment should be sent to the expedition medical officer (MO).

For the potential expedition member with a pre-existing medical condition the emphasis should be on symptoms related to exercise and cardiac risk factors. This may involve investigations like cardiac stress tests, post-exercise spirometry or blood tests, depending on the situation.

For the potential expedition member with a disability the assessment should include consideration of the impact that the terrain and living conditions may have on their usual level of independence and on any mechanical aids they use. For instance, on a sailing expedition, how a person normally independent using a wheelchair would manage in the narrow confines of the boat. On a trekking expedition, what would be the effects for a person with a lower limb amputation and using a prosthesis of walking over uneven ground?

The condition must be stable and not vary day to day. It would be unwise for anyone to consider going on an expedition soon after a serious medical event such as a heart attack, a first seizure or major surgery. As a general guide, waiting until six months after the episode and for the person's return to full fitness seems sensible.

To help assess the risk posed by a pre-existing condition it may be useful firstly to grade its severity and secondly to grade the remoteness of the expedition. Together these help determine the potential risk for serious problems. These risks need to be understood and accepted by the individual and the expedition before they go.

TABLE 7.1 A SIMPLE GRADING SYSTEM FOR PRE-EXISTING CONDITIONS

Mildly affected	A well-controlled and uncomplicated condition amenable to easy self-management, e.g. mild asthma well controlled with inhalers or high blood pressure (hypertension) with no complications
Moderately affected	A condition needing some medical assessment and treatment from time to time, e.g. periodic courses of steroids to control exacerbations of asthma or hypertension with known organ damage
Seriously affected	Previous occurrence or future risk of a life-threatening problem, e.g. recent hospitalisation for asthma or hypertension with a renal transplant on immunosuppressants

TABLE 7.2 A SIMPLE GRADING SYSTEM FOR THE REMOTENESS OF AN EXPEDITION (USING EXPEDITION LENGTH AND THE TIME TAKEN TO ACCESS MEDICAL HELP)

Isolated	Day trip or up to 3 days in the field or medical assistance a few hours away
Remote	Up to a week in the field or medical assistance more than a day away
Wilderness	Greater than a week in the field with medical assistance several days' travel away or unreliable

Terrain and climatic conditions, not just the distance involved, will clearly influence the time taken to get help. A storm, being at altitude or in a forest at night, for example, may mean a helicopter cannot fly in or the expedition team cannot carry out a casualty. These factors and the means by which help will be summoned, e.g. radio, EPIRB (emergency position indicating radio beacon) or satellite phone, need to be considered in a risk assessment. It is best to plan for the worst-case scenarios since medical problems will tend to occur when physical or environmental pressures are greatest.

Using these simple grading systems allows some practical recommendations to be made regarding medical support on the trip. As the potential seriousness increases, it would be appropriate to recommend that the MO accompanying the expedition have a professional medical background or be a doctor with relevant skills. Additional medical supplies may need to accompany the team and suitable evacuation plans to be made. A thorough risk assessment helps plan for these scenarios and any additional costs involved.

There may be times when the potential risks of participating in an expedition seem to outweigh the benefits perceived by the MO. It falls to the individual with the pre-existing condition or disability and to those accompanying him or her to decide whether to accept these risks and how to act on the advice received.

GENERIC PRE-EXPEDITION ADVICE

- Arrange for a pre-travel assessment (as detailed above) by an appropriately knowledgeable person at least 6 months before departure.
- Allow time to optimise the condition with particular attention to any medications that affect the exercise capacity of the individual.
- Prepare a medical self-management plan and an emergency management plan for the individual.
- Encourage people with a pre-existing medical problem to build up their exercise level gradually to that anticipated for the expedition, initially in surroundings where help is easily available. This will give experience of managing medications and exercise in conditions like asthma and diabetes.
- Encourage individuals with a pre-existing medical problem gradually to build up their time spent in the wilderness, initially with short, low-intensity trips to develop experience of managing in these surroundings.
- Seek help and modify strategies should any problems arise during the initial training.
- Plan the expedition itinerary taking into account the possibility of ill-health. It is wise to have rest days interspersed through the trip that could be used in case of ill-health or if the itinerary needs to be changed. Most expeditions have tight time constraints.
- Decide on the appropriate level of medical support needed to accompany the expedition (this does not necessarily mean a doctor is needed).
- Prepare an evacuation plan, together with a communication list for contacting help.
- Arrange comprehensive and appropriate *medical insurance* and *repatriation cover*. Medical insurance with emergency assistance and repatriation is essential. Those with pre-existing medical conditions must declare them; unless the insurance company has explicitly agreed to provide cover for someone with such a condition they are likely to decline the bill should problems arise. Bespoke cover may need to be arranged at extra expense (see Chapter 6).

- Organise for a letter on headed notepaper from the person's family doctor summarising details of their condition and treatment together with equipment needed, e.g. syringes, which can be shown to officials if questioned or to in-country doctors should the need arise.
- Train all expedition members in relevant first aid for potential emergencies, for example the management of a fit or how to give adrenaline in case of anaphylaxis (as the MO you may want more advanced skills in resuscitation and drug administration).
- Encourage people with a pre-existing medical condition to carry more than enough medication for the entire trip, in divided lots, in case their luggage gets misplaced or damaged, and to carry some medication on them at all times (see Chapter 3).

GENERIC ADVICE TO REDUCE POTENTIAL PROBLEMS DURING AN EXPEDITION

- Encourage people with a pre-existing medical condition to carry with them at all times written details of their condition, treatment and contact details and to consider a means of easy identification such as a MedicAlert bracelet.
- Keep a simple diary, to record doses taken (as doses can easily be missed).
- Expeditions often begin with a long plane journey and the rapid change in time zones means the timing of medication needs to be changed, particularly those taken with meals. Flying west results in a long day and flying east a short one. It is recommended that people who take medication should stay on home-time for the duration of the journey and take doses at the usual time, with a snack if necessary, and adjust timings on arrival at the destination. The few days 'in town' before the expedition heads 'up-country' is often the best time to adjust doses. When travelling eastward it may be easier to shorten the time slightly between doses during travel.
- Monitor the condition carefully and enjoy a trouble-free trip but seek help early should there be any problems.
- Organise a buddy system whereby an expedition member with a pre-existing medical problem has a nominated partner who keeps an eye on them. This can be a good security net as long as it is not too intrusive or inflexible. Being overprotective will not be popular.

GENERIC POST EXPEDITION ADVICE

- Encourage the person to have a medical reassessment on returning home.

- Forward copies of any MO medical records to the person's family doctor.
- Forward copies of your report to the RGS so that your experiences can help fellow travellers in the future.

SPECIFIC ADVICE FOR COMMON PRE-EXISTING CONDITIONS

Asthma

This is probably the commonest pre-existing medical condition that will be encountered, especially on youth trips. The concern on an expedition is that a person with asthma may be restricted physically by their symptoms or have an asthma attack that is difficult to control.

Risk assessment

The extent of asthmatic problems will vary enormously between sufferers. The mildest will have some symptoms on vigorous exercise that are easily controlled, the more severe will need periodic courses of oral steroids to control an exacerbation, and the most severe will have suffered a life-threatening episode in the past or will have symptoms refractory to treatment. Any triggers should be carefully noted. It is difficult to predict what will happen to the asthma during the trip. The best guide to likely response is past history.

Respiratory infections picked up during the outbound journey and exposure to unaccustomed levels of pollution, exhaust fumes, dust and cigarette smoke may make asthma worse soon after arrival. Scuba diving poses special risks for people with asthma because inhaling seawater may induce bronchospasm. Despite the cold and dry air of mountains, symptoms may improve, perhaps because the allergen load is lower. Remember in the tropics that there is an increased risk of chest infections.

Pre-expedition

- Optimise asthma control: spirometry or peak expiratory flow rate (PEFR) monitoring before, during and after exercise, to the intensity needed for the trip, is useful to help adjust medication. Remember, exercise-induced symptoms are often worst 10 minutes after exercise.
- Consider a written management plan for the person, based on past peak flow measurements, with clear guidelines on when to step up treatment and when to ask for help.
- Review medications: first-line treatment for exercise-induced symptoms are salbutamol and cromoglycate taken 5–10 minutes before exercise with the addition of regular inhaled steroids if needed. Encourage people with asthma to carry their own supply of medication for the full expedition.

- Aspirin-like drugs can cause a sudden worsening of some people's asthma. Ensure these are avoided on the trip as painkillers for people with asthma. Such drugs should be well labelled so they are not used unwittingly.
- Train all expedition members in the first aid management of an acute asthma attack (sit the person up, give multiple doses of inhaled bronchodilator via a large volume spacer device and consider a short course of oral corticosteroid to curtail an exacerbation).
- All people with asthma should receive all relevant vaccinations and take antimalarials. Consider suggesting that they receive influenza and pneumococcal vaccines to reduce the chance of chest infections. (The flu season in the southern hemisphere is May to September and the relevant vaccine will need to be specially arranged.)

TABLE 7.3 **ADDITIONS TO THE EXPEDITION MEDICAL KIT FOR PEOPLE WITH ASTHMA**

- Lightweight peak expiratory flow (PEF) meter, e.g. Mini-Wright meter
- PEF charts
- Spacer device for the delivery of inhaled medications during an exacerbation
- Spare inhalers – salbutamol and beclomethasone
- Prednisolone 5mg tablets x 50 and instructions for use

Consider oxygen, an Ambu-bag and injectable medications for a person with severe asthma, and a doctor on the trip

During the expedition

- Ensure that individuals carry inhalers in their hand baggage (this is allowed in the cabin).
- Continue regular medication with PEF monitoring and adjust according to the self-management plan. It is best to step up treatment early rather than wait.
- During an exacerbation avoid swimming, ascending to higher altitude or anything that causes breathlessness.
- Triggers should be avoided if possible. Facemasks can be helpful for cold-induced symptoms. Smoking of any substance should be avoided as it increases the risk of an exacerbation and of chest infections.
- For management of an asthma attack see Chapter 15.

Epilepsy

Travellers with well-controlled epilepsy are not necessarily at increased risk during an expedition. Specific concerns are that the person may have a fit and need medical attention, that the fit may occur in a dangerous location or may not be self-limiting, and that the medications may cause adverse effects (some antimalarials e.g. chloroquine and mefloquine, and some antibiotics, e.g. ciprofloxacin, may provoke fits). In addition, diarrhoea may result in reduced absorption of anticonvulsants.

Risk assessment

Any previous history of a fit is important in the assessment of someone planning to join an expedition. Epileptic fits can recur, particularly if the initial episode was without a clear precipitant like a head injury or illness. A thorough medical assessment after a first fit, together with a 6-month observation period to see if the fit recurs, seems a sensible precaution before travelling to a remote location. For those who have had more than one fit it is important to evaluate the degree of control and predictability of the fits with or without medication. In most cases the cause of the epilepsy will not be known but in a small percentage it will be linked to a structural or genetic abnormality, and it is important to assess whether any other elements of this condition have a bearing on the expedition plans.

There is no reason why a person with well-controlled epilepsy should not participate in an expedition. It is important, however, that rules regarding driving, operating machinery and participating in dangerous activities (e.g. in mountaineering or scuba diving) are observed as they would be at home, for the safety of all concerned. A very careful assessment is needed if the person has unpredictable fits or temporal lobe epilepsy, or has had status epilepticus at any time. There may be very real risks if a person has a fit on an expedition while riding on the back of an open vehicle, swimming or rafting, or during climbing.

Pre-expedition

- Review medications: remember that optimisation of seizure control and achievement of therapeutic blood levels of anticonvulsants will take time and may need specialist input. Exercise does not affect blood levels of anticonvulsants.
- Train all expedition members in seizure first aid with the possible administration of rectal diazepam if the fit lasts longer than 5 minutes.
- If travelling to a malarious area, review antimalarial medication: chloroquine and mefloquine can precipitate fits; doxycycline, Maloprim (pyrimethamine and dapsone) or proguanil can be used, depending on the local drug-resistance patterns. Remember that phenytoin, carbamazepine and barbiturates can reduce the blood levels of doxycycline through hepatic

enzyme induction and that several common drugs can affect anticonvulsant levels, e.g. erythromycin and omeprazole. Such drugs need to be well labelled so they are not used unwittingly in people with epilepsy.

- Vaccinate as normal.

TABLE 7.4 **ADDITIONS TO THE MEDICAL KIT**
• Appropriately sized Guedel airway x 1 • Rectal diazepam tubes x 4–10mg each (2 carried in the person's medical kit at all times and 2 in the base camp kit • Possibly intravenous diazepam (with oxygen and an Ambu-bag) if a doctor is part of the expedition team

During the expedition

- Adjust timing of doses on passing through time zones as discussed earlier in this chapter.
- Encourage avoidance of known triggers if possible. Potential triggers are TV screens, flashing lights, excess alcohol and being overtired.
- Fits often occur at the time of falling asleep and waking and when medication has been taken erratically. The changes in time to a person's normal medication routine during the long journey out or back may predispose them to a fit.
- If a fit occurs, move the person only if they are in a dangerous situation, e.g. on a road. Loosen their clothing but do not put anything in their mouth or restrain them from moving. Try to protect the face from rubbing on the ground and monitor how long the fit lasts. If it is longer than 5 minutes, give rectal diazepam. After a fit the person is often exhausted, confused, sleepy or temporarily weak and will need to rest for several hours (see Chapter 15).

Post expedition

- Encourage the individual to see his or her family doctor and have anticonvulsant dosages re-evaluated.
- If a fit has occurred during the expedition a written summary of circumstances, duration and action taken should be sent to the person's own doctor.

Diabetes

Travelling rarely causes problems for people with diabetes as long as they and their expedition team are confident in monitoring and adjusting the diabetic control and accept the slightly increased risks involved. The main concerns for a person with diabetes on an expedition are:

- The storage and availability of medication and monitoring equipment.
- The increased risk of hypoglycaemic ("hypo") episodes with changes to time zones, diet and exercise, compared to their normal lifestyle, particularly in insulin-dependent diabetics.
- The increased risk of infections and of complications should they become unwell.
- The increased risk of a life-threatening event for people with long-standing diabetes, such as a heart attack or stroke, which would be difficult to manage in a remote place.

Risk assessment

Every person with diabetes should have a medical review and examination with a doctor well before the expedition. The emphasis during the consultation should be on symptoms with exercise, cardiovascular risks and the presence of organ damage, including the sensation and blood supply to the feet and eyesight. Any findings here will need further assessment.

A young, insulin-dependent person is less likely to have complications than someone who has had the disease for over 10 years. Adjustment of insulin will be the main issue. In the older, non-insulin dependent person organ damage is often present at diagnosis. Those with any evidence of organ damage need to be carefully assessed; an ECG is recommended in those with diabetes for greater than 15 years and those over 35 years old. A formal exercise test looking for silent cardiac ischaemia may be helpful.

The expedition should strongly consider taking a doctor or other medical professional as MO, who is able to give injectable medications should the need arise.

Pre-expedition

- Review medications and optimise diabetic control. For insulin-dependent diabetics it may be preferable to be on a four-times-a-day regime of pre-meal insulin as this gives greater flexibility with meals and the effects of exercise.
- Reinforce the message that people with diabetes must never stop their insulin completely or they will rapidly decompensate.
- Ensure they are aware that if they are vomiting and unable to keep down food they must seek help immediately, as intravenous fluids and injectable antiemetics for treatment of the vomiting may be needed.

- As fitness improves during exercise, insulin sensitivity increases and people with diabetes will notice better control and reduced need for medications and insulin. It is important that the blood is adequately monitored and doses are lowered appropriately, otherwise hypoglycaemia is a risk.
- Obtain a letter from the patient's family doctor detailing the condition and need for syringes (this letter should be carried at all times by the patient).
- Train all expedition members in diabetic first aid, the recognition of a "hypo" and the administration of oral sugar or injected glucagon as needed.
- Vaccinate and recommend antimalarials as normal.
- Inform the food purchaser and cook of the need for a diabetic diet. This may need to be planned for and will not always be possible, especially if the expedition does not have its own kitchen facilities.

TABLE 7.5 **ADDITIONS TO THE MEDICAL KIT FOR EXPEDITIONERS WITH DIABETES**

- Oral glucose tablets and glucose gel (e.g. Hypostop) carried by the person at all times and also available in the base camp medical kit
- Injectable glucagon kits and instructions for use in an unconscious patient with a low blood sugar can also be useful if immediately available (can easily be given intramuscularly)
- Appropriate antisickness medication in tablet and injectable or suppository form
- Intravenous glucose and fluids
- A plentiful supply of extra insulin and glucose
- Other supplies: blood and urine testing strips, syringes, a "sharps" bin, finger-pricking device and blood sugar meter (with spare batteries)

During the expedition

- Adjust timing of doses – stick with the home-time regime until arrival at the final destination and then adjust by a few hours per dose. The insulin dose could be reduced if doses are moved closer together and a small supplement taken with a snack to lengthen the interval.
- If the expedition has its own kitchen staff they may be able to produce a diabetic diet. Otherwise the person with diabetes will need to choose food appropriately from what is on offer.
- Encourage people with diabetes always to carry a snack in case meals are unexpectedly delayed or sugar levels are low.
- Maintain reasonable control by regularly monitoring blood sugar and

adjusting doses if on insulin. (A change in timing of food intake, different ingredients and different activity patterns can impair control.)
- It will probably be very difficult for the person with diabetes to maintain the "tight" control possible at home. "Looser" control for a few weeks is not harmful in the long term as long as control is reasonable and hypos are not occurring. It may be better to aim to run blood sugars a little "high" since the main danger in the field is from hypoglycaemia.
- Exercise will affect blood sugar levels. Ensure careful monitoring of sugar levels in the pre-expedition period, before, during and after similar intensity exercise. This should give some idea of how to adjust carbohydrate intake and insulin. On average, before moderate exercise of an hour or two, a reduction of insulin dose of up to 30% will be needed, together with a snack of about 50g of complex carbohydrate. For longer exercise a reduction in insulin dose, together with 20–50g of carbohydrate per hour is needed.
- If unwell encourage a person with diabetes to see the expedition medical officer early.
- People with diabetes are more susceptible to infections (skin, urinary and gut) so encourage vigilance with diet and in monitoring skin for early signs of infection.
- Encourage people with diabetes to inspect and clean their feet daily. Toenails

TABLE 7.6 **CARRYING AND STORING INSULIN**

- There are many different types of insulin and they are not interchangeable
- Ideally insulin is stored in a refrigerator at around 4°C (but not frozen) and will remain effective for up to 2 years. If stored in less than ideal conditions (as is likely on an expedition) insulin decays faster and becomes less effective but will continue to be usable. At a storage temperature of 30°C it is effective for about 2 months. If there are "clumps" in the insulin or it is discoloured it should not be used. The only way to get around the varying efficacy of the insulin is to carry out 4- to 6-hourly blood or urinary glucose monitoring and adjust the amount taken accordingly
- Always keep insulin in hand baggage on the flight, as it is likely to freeze in the hold and may get delayed or lost. Cabin staff will often agree to put it in the plane's fridge. (Since 11 September 2001, some airlines, such as BA, require a letter of authorisation for needles to be carried in the cabin)
- For long journeys a polystyrene container or vacuum flask designed to carry food can be used. If cool packs are used ensure the insulin doesn't freeze
- X-rays do not affect the insulin

need to be short. Ensure that any wound infection is treated promptly with antibiotics and dressings.
- People with long-standing disease or with certain types of insulin do not get typical "hypo" warning symptoms when their sugar level is low. It is crucial to know if this is the case for an individual and to measure the blood sugar if anything "doesn't seem right".

Note: The main hazard for people with diabetes on an expedition is hypoglycaemia. Always ensure that they are carrying food as well as emergency sugar and that someone is with them who knows how to diagnose and treat hypoglycaemia.

Hypertension

In itself hypertension (high blood pressure) is not a problem for people joining an expedition, but its complications, such as a heart attack or stroke and the side-effects of medication, may be a cause for concern.

Risk assessment

Hypertension with no signs of end-organ damage does not increase risk but patients with evidence of such damage and particularly those with organ failure (e.g. heart failure, kidney failure and ischaemic heart disease) do have a risk of major problems. The stresses, physical and emotional, of an expedition may be sufficient to uncover latent disease. Prior to travel hypertensives should be capable of exercising symptom free to the intensity that will be required on the expedition.

Pre-expedition

- Organise a full assessment of cardiac risk factors and symptoms. A stable blood pressure pre-trip is essential. An ECG is desirable for all people with hypertension, with formal cardiac exercise testing if there are symptoms on exercise or multiple risk factors.
- Review medication and blood electrolytes. Several antihypertensive drugs can affect exercise capacity. Beta-blockers can cause muscle fatigue and lethargy as well as limiting the maximum heart rate response during exercise. They decrease blood flow to the extremities, which will be of concern in those going to cold environments. Calcium channel blockers affect heart rate on exercise, can give dependent oedema and cause flushing that may be particularly uncomfortable in hot climates. Diuretic drugs have the obvious inconvenience of increasing urinary flow but may lead to hypotension if the person is already dehydrated by exercise, diarrhoea or inadequate fluid intake.
- Effects of exercise and training: exercise and weight loss are treatment strategies for the control of hypertension. As fitness increases pre-expedition

weight often decreases and together these may mean the blood pressure is lower. The amount of medication may need to be reduced. Post-exercise hypotension may also occur with angiotensin-converting enzyme (ACE) inhibitors and calcium channel blockers, particularly if the person is dehydrated.
- Hypertensive patients should receive vaccinations as normal, but care should be taken when prescribing antimalarials. There are concerns about the interaction of beta-blockers and the antimalarial, mefloquine.
- Train all expedition members in basic cardiopulmonary resuscitation (CPR).

TABLE 7.7 **ADDITIONS TO MEDICAL KIT FOR THOSE WITH HYPERTENSION OR ISCHAEMIC HEART DISEASE**

- Aspirin 300mg tablets for cardiac events
- Glyceryl trinitrate (nitrolingual GTN) spray for angina
- Equipment for resuscitation and blood pressure monitoring

During the expedition

- Monitor closely any new symptoms, particularly on exercise
- Do not ascend further, dive or travel to more remote locations if there are new or worsening symptoms

Post-expedition

- Encourage the individual to have a medical review, to optimise control and to check electrolytes.

Ischaemic heart disease

Ischaemic heart disease (IHD) becomes increasingly common as the age of the expedition member rises. On many expeditions it will be the doctor and expedition leader who have the greater risk of IHD. The risks and effects of medication are similar to those discussed for hypertension above. The danger that latent symptoms will be uncovered due to the stresses, physical and otherwise, of expedition life is also similar. Careful assessment pre-expedition and cautious increase in exercise is important, with immediate attention should new symptoms be uncovered.

Even after heart attacks, by-pass operations, coronary angioplasty or stenting it is possible to undertake expedition travel as long as there are no residual ischaemic symptoms and the person can tolerate the required level of activity symptom free.

There will remain a certain increased risk that cannot be eliminated. The remaining advice is as detailed above for hypertension.

Chronic lung disease

Those with significant chronic lung disease are not commonly involved in expeditions. The effects will depend mostly on respiratory exercise tolerance. Aircraft are pressurised to about 2,500m of altitude, which should not give any problems to all but the most severely compromised.

Additional concerns for this group of people are the management of an acute exacerbation with or without infection, a pneumothorax or cardiac disease. These risks should be thoroughly assessed pre-expedition and antibiotics, steroids and inhalers similar to those advised for asthma should be available. Someone with significant respiratory disease will walk and perform other physical activities more slowly than someone with normal lungs, especially at altitude, and this should be taken into account when planning the expedition itinerary.

SPECIFIC ADVICE FOR EXPEDITIONERS WITH DISABILITIES

Over the last few years there has been a growing interest in wilderness travel from people with disabilities. The medical establishment may have been guilty of "benevolent" overprotection of people with disabilities in the past; now they have an important role in increasing access for those people who wish to participate in expeditions and in demystifying medical issues and disabilities. By assessing the abilities different people possess, MOs and expedition leaders can help individuals with disabilities participate successfully in an expedition and help the expedition identify appropriate and challenging projects.

The major challenge is to design an expedition that tests abilities and resources while maintaining a person's independence and dignity by accommodating any adaptations he or she requires. One aspect in which expeditions are unlike competitive sport is that the "playing field"need not be exactly the same for each participant. The relative strengths and skills of the individual expedition members combine to make the expedition team and disability need not be relevant.

There are only a few medical issues that differ for people with disabilities. As for able-bodied expeditioners, trauma, blisters, bites and infections remain the most common reasons for consultation and the majority of preventative care is the same. The striking difference may be the way in which a person with a disability achieves the tasks of daily living. "Normality" for this person may be mobility with a prosthesis or in a wheelchair, communication with adaptive techniques and eating with modified implements. Table 7.8 suggests areas of ability that the MO should explore with an individual. The specific expertise of healthcare professionals, such as occupational therapists, physiotherapists, nurses, rehabilitation physicians, prosthetists,

TABLE 7.8 **AREAS OF ABILITY TO EXPLORE WITH AN INDIVIDUAL**

Transfers	How do they move from one surface to another in a safe manner? For example, floor to chair or on and off the toilet
Mobility	How do they move from one place to another and are any aids required to do this safely, e.g. wheelchairs, prosthetic limbs, calipers or walking aids? It is important to note that techniques used over short distances may be different to those used over longer ones: a person may be able to take a few steps inside but need a wheelchair outside. Levels of endurance and fatigue should also be considered
Self-care	How are toileting, bathing, grooming, dressing and eating achieved? Are assistance or adaptive aids required?
Continence	How is bowel and bladder continence achieved? For instance, is intermittent self-catherisation or a bowel regime needed?
Skin care	Is extra care needed for insensate areas, wounds or vulnerable skin, e.g. pressure areas, the skin below the level of a spinal cord lesion or the skin on an amputation stump?
Communication	How is effective two-way communication achieved – are sign language, large print or other aids needed? Are there any sensory impairments, such as vision and/or hearing?
Cognitive and behavioural issues	Does the individual have any impairments of thinking, behaviour or psychological health, e.g. intellectual disability in a person with cerebral palsy?
Medical issues and effects of medications	Does the individual have any associated medical conditions or medications, e.g. a person with cerebral palsy who also has epilepsy, or an amputee with diabetes? Each of these pre-existing conditions would need to be assessed as discussed earlier in this chapter

recreation officers and neuropsychologists, may be needed to help make these assessments.

The different terrain and environments faced on an expedition may alter the disability and therefore a person's experience, for better or worse. A person with a hearing impairment may have difficulty lip-reading in a foreign language but on a diving expedition has no disability underwater, as everyone uses dive sign language. On the other hand, a wheelchair user's usual level of mobility may be very limited by the uneven ground on a mountain trekking expedition yet they may not have the same degree of difficulty on a sailing or horse-riding trip.

TABLE 7.9 **POTENTIAL CHALLENGES FACED BY EXPEDITIONERS WITH A DISABILITY IN A VARIETY OF ENVIRONMENTS**

Environment	*Potential challenges*
Airports and plane trips	Long distances to traverse inside the airport; dehydration, excessive pressure to vulnerable skin areas and bladder/bowel management problems during long delays; difficulty boarding small craft; difficulty of transferring or of being assisted in the narrow aisles, toilets and seats of planes
Car, train or bus journeys	Difficulties getting in and out of vehicles, limited availability of space; long journeys with limited breaks on scheduled services, security problems for vital equipment
Hotels	Lack of disability access; steep stairwells with no lifts; squat toilets; marble or polished floors; less-than-ideal hygiene conditions; unfamiliar locations/languages for the visual or hearing impaired
Campsites	Transfers, especially floor to chair in sleeping and mess tents; difficulties of self-care with pit latrines and improvised bathing facilities, unmarked hazards like cliff edges or water nearby; finding the way around camp; disposal of soiled dressings or continence items
Mountain or polar regions	Exposure of insensate skin to sun, cold or wind; effects of the uneven terrain on mobility, rescue and safety concerns
Sailing, diving or river trips	Safe transfers on and off boats; transfers and movement in the cramped conditions onboard; the effects of water motion on balance; rescue and safety concerns, corrosive effects of salt water on mechanical aids
Tropical or desert regions	Dehydration and heat illness; increased risk of skin damage and infection of moist vulnerable skin; mobility problems on uneven or overgrown terrain; hygiene problems with limited water supplies

The effect of a new environment on the expeditioner's abilities needs to be considered. The trip often starts with negotiating an airport and a plane flight, followed by a stay in a hotel, then a road/train journey before heading into the field. The help of various professionals may again be useful during this assessment process. Table 7.9 covers briefly some of the environmental issues an expeditioner with a disability may face during an expedition.

By working through Table 7.9, the feasibility of an individual participating in a proposed expedition, the problems they will need to overcome and the amount of support that will be needed should become evident. Solutions will need to be found to each of these problems for the trip to be safe, enjoyable and dignified for the person involved and the team as a whole. The steps mentioned earlier in the chapter with regard to trying out these strategies on smaller trips close to home apply equally well here.

SUMMARY

This chapter has provided a framework for assessment of the needs of expeditioners with pre-existing medical conditions and of those with disabilities. Some indication has been given of the kinds of difficulties that may be faced and some practical solutions have been suggested. It is hoped this will allow people from a broader range of backgrounds to experience the joy of a wilderness experience, to participate in the shared purpose and camaraderie of an expedition, and to return safely. Often much more is possible than thought at first glance. Remarkable journeys have been undertaken in the past by people who just happen to have a pre-existing medical condition or a disability. Long may this continue.

8 RISK ASSESSMENT AND CRISIS MANAGEMENT

Clive Barrow

"Climb if you will, but remember that courage and strength are nought without prudence, and that a momentary negligence may destroy the happiness of a lifetime. Do nothing in haste; look well to each step; and from the beginning think what may be the end."
From Scrambles Amongst the Alps *by Edward Whymper, 1860*

Risk assessment is increasingly becoming a prerequisite for organisers of expeditions and outdoor activities in the UK and overseas. It is now a legal requirement for commercially organised outdoor activities for under 18s in the UK. There is currently no law in this country governing the organisation of expeditions overseas. Many see this as a good thing. Fortunately, the number of serious incidents among participants in overseas expeditions is very small; at 0.3 per 1,000 person-days (source: *Journal of the Royal Society of Medicine* 2000;93:557–562). Recently published data on medical problems seen on expeditions are shown in Table 8.1.

However, the climate of opinion in the UK is changing in several ways:

- The public is more circumspect about safety and risk as a result of increased media coverage of expedition or outdoor activity accidents.
- As a nation, the UK is adopting a more litigious culture in line with the United States.
- Expectations of safety amongst the parents and guardians of young people are becoming higher as a result of the introduction of stringent safety procedures and Health and Safety regulations in educational establishments.

Given this risk-adverse climate, planners and leaders of all overseas expeditions should be conducting a systematic, careful and responsible safety management assessment. Risk assessment is the first and perhaps most important part of this. This chapter is intended to provide a brief practical guide to risk assessment coupled with

TABLE 8.1 **INCIDENCE OF EXPEDITION MEDICAL PROBLEMS**

Category	*Sub-category*	*Number of incidents*	*Incident total per category*	*Incidence per 1,000 person-days*
Gastrointestinal	Gastrointestinal	275	275 (33%)	2.12
Medical	General medical	98	179 (21%)	1.38
	Malaria	23		
	Dengue fever	7		
	Skin	31		
	Pharmaceutical	16		
	Psychiatric	4		
Orthopaedic	Orthopaedic	22	142 (17%)	1.10
	Back	16		
	Trauma	104		
Environmental	Environment	1	117 (14%)	0.90
	Sun / Heat	40		
	Cold	13		
	Water	5		
	Altitude	58		
Fauna	Animal	19	63 (8%)	0.49
	Insect	44		
Feet	Feet	30	30 (4%)	0.23
Surgical	General surgical	6	29 (3%)	0.22
	Dental	10		
	Eye	13		
TOTAL		**835**		**6.44**

Taken from *Journal of the Royal Society of Medicine* 2000; 93:559.

the key considerations involved in crisis management planning for medical officers. Expedition leaders will use similar ideas to those outlined below but on a larger and more general scale.

RISK ASSESSMENT

Hazard and risk on overseas expeditions

Hazard and risk are inherent in everything we do and the degree of hazard and risk is dependent on the activity and environment in which that activity takes place. In the UK the degree of risk is considerably less than overseas, particularly in developing countries where our knowledge of and our ability to control the environment are less strong. Risk assessment of overseas projects must therefore consider a wider array of hazards, and must always allow for the unexpected (see Table 8.2). The expedition organiser must always be prepared to adopt alternatives and/or completely abandon an activity if the risk assessment suggests that control measures cannot reduce the risk to an acceptable level.

In attempting to qualify and quantify risk, it is important not to worry unnecessarily about trivia. A risk assessment that is too cluttered with minor concerns will be discarded in the field as a bureaucrat's folly, and will be of less value than not doing one at all. Any severe and persistent risk must appear in the risk assessment document, together with appropriate control measures.

Acceptable risk

On an overseas expedition, risk can never be completely eliminated. Indeed, it is through the management of both perceived and real risks that expeditions of all types can be of such beneficial effect to the participants. Most expedition organisers speak of reducing risk to an *acceptable* level. This is extremely difficult to define since opinions about acceptability may differ greatly among individuals. The experience, age, ability and technical competence of the participants on an expedition or overseas project must be considered, since this will affect the level of risk considered acceptable. When considering the concept of acceptable risk, think first of to whom the risk should be acceptable? To whom are you accountable? Examples might include your peers, participants, parents, school governors, local education authorities, teachers, sponsors, research bodies etc. In order to qualify acceptable risk in the context of your own project or expedition, it is important to ask key individuals and groups what they feel is acceptable to them. Don't ever assume! The greater the challenge and promise of achievement (e.g. first conquest of a new mountain peak), the greater the acceptable risk.

Control measures

Control measures are the backbone of the risk assessment process. They are what the expedition leader or medical officer (MO) initiates to reduce or eliminate a particular risk. Some examples would be as follows:

- Providing first aid training before the expedition starts.
- Getting immunised before exposure to disease.
- Preventing bites by disease-transmitting insects.

TABLE 8.2 HAZARD AND RISK ON OVERSEAS EXPEDITIONS

Hazard	*Risk*
1. The team	
Health and fitness (including previous/existing medical conditions)	Increased risk of health problems on expedition leading to serious illness/death
Attitude and behaviour	Increased risk of ignoring control measures resulting in illness/injury
Experience and training	Lack increases risk in all activities
Personal equipment	Serious injury/illness due to inadequate equipment/equipment failure
2. The environment	
Mountains/sea/desert/jungle	Altitude sickness/drowning/heat problems
Climate and weather conditions	Heat and cold-related injury/death
Wildlife (including insects)	Attack/poisoning through bites/stings/disease
3. Health	
Endemic disease (dengue fever/ Japanese encephalitis)	Serious illness or death
Malaria	Serious illness or death
AIDS/HIV	Serious illness or death
Polluted water	Serious illness
Contaminated food	Serious illness or death
4. Local population	
Political climate	Political instability/coup/kidnapping/ imprisonment (e.g. UK plane spotters in Greece!)
Attitudes to foreigners/cultural differences	Attack/rape/theft/access to drugs
Hygiene/living conditions	Disease
5. Expedition activity	
Trekking/climbing/mountaineering	Altitude sickness/falls from height
River crossing	Serious injury/drowning
Water-based activities (diving/kayaking/sailing)	Drowning/leptospirosis
Underground activities (caving/cave-diving)	Drowning/suffocation/starvation
Equipment failure/inappropriate use	Serious injury/death
Games/sports activities	Injury/incapacitation
6. Travel and camp life	
Transport (public/private)	High risk of serious injury/death
Road/water conditions	Increased risk of accidents
Other road users	Increased risk of accidents
Camp hazards (stoves/fires/flooding/ avalanche/wildlife)	Burns/drowning/suffocation/injury/death
Accommodation/hotels	Fire/electrocution/serious injury/disease/ mugging/attack

In most cases, many control measures can be implemented before the expedition as part of the planning process. However, once the expedition or project actually starts there may be many more control measures to consider.

The five steps to risk assessment

The UK Health and Safety Executive refers to the process as one of five steps. These are as follows:

1. Identify the hazards and associated risks.
2. Identify who is potentially at risk and how.
3. Identify the precautions or control measures to minimise the risk, including any further action required to reduce the risk to an acceptable level.
4. Record your findings.
5. Review the risk assessment periodically.

This process is clear and straightforward and can be applied to any expedition overseas.

A convenient format for risk assessment is a table with each of the five steps as a column heading (Table 8.3).

TABLE 8.3 **RISK ASSESSMENT**

Hazard	*Risk level*	*Control measure*	*Additional action*	*Review mechanism*
Data collection activities Trekking/river crossing	High	• Careful route selection • Use of guides • Competent, experienced group leaders • Use of ropes/training in river crossing techniques • No activity after dark • Safety and medical kit carried at all times • Group risk assessment before each day's activity	Leader/staff approve activity or, if necessary, halt progress if new risk arises, rendering it unsafe to proceed	Post-expedition report with information about incidents and changes to risk assessment

Involving others in the risk assessment process

Never presume that members of an expedition team will observe or abide by the contents of a risk assessment in which they have had no involvement. The key to effective risk assessment stems from clarity and commitment on the part of all of those who may potentially be at risk. It is strongly recommended, therefore, that team members play a part in compiling the assessment at some stage of the planning process. This risk assessment is an essential part of turning a piece of paper into a living process for managing day-to-day risk on an expedition.

Reviewing a risk assessment

Because of frequent changes in environment, the risk assessment must be reviewed regularly to remain effective. Changes to the assessment on paper are useless if they are not properly communicated to staff and participants, or if staff and participants cannot see a reason for the changes.

Golden rules of risk assessment

Always consider the CRISIS acronym when conducting your risk assessment(s).

C Clarify the hazards and risks
R Reassess and revise it where necessary
I Involve all participants in the process
S State it simply in writing
I If it's too risky – don't do it!
S Share the knowledge and experience

CRISIS MANAGEMENT

An expedition crisis generally involves an accident, illness or injury to expedition members. Crisis management comprises those processes and systems developed to foresee, avoid and, in the worst case, manage a crisis on an overseas expedition.

The principle adopted in crisis management planning is always to concentrate on the worst-case scenario. It is the expedition leader's role in planning an expedition to foresee and avoid a crisis in the making and to facilitate the handling of a crisis if it occurs.

The role of the MO in crisis management is to:

- organise adequate medical training for all expedition members, including him- or herself;
- provide an appropriate medical kit;
- investigate the availability of local medical support (doctors/hospitals);
- investigate access to casualty evacuation locally, nationally and internationally;
- consider the use of an international assistance agency or emergency centre.

To be able to achieve the above, attention must be paid to the skills of the expedition members and accompanying staff. There must be sufficient first aid skills among the team to deal with the immediate care of a casualty. Several courses are now available, from organisations such as Wilderness Medical Training (see Appendix 5), which concentrate on more advanced medicine for remote foreign travel for competent first aiders.

The investigation and enlistment of locally and nationally available medical support form another essential part of the MO's role. Embassies in the host country often have lists of recommended doctors and dentists in the capital city, but rarely have information about the more remote areas likely to be frequented by expedition teams. For this reason, detailed research is necessary to produce a support network of medical contacts in the areas in which the expedition will be operating, perhaps through an appointed local agent. Support may come from local aid projects with medical back-up, clinics and dispensaries, local hospitals, or, on a national basis, the GPs and hospitals commonly used by the expatriate population of the country. It is important to identify a recommended dentist.

Communication is an important part of crisis management and the more options that are researched and made available the greater is the chance of establishing and maintaining links with the outside world. Essentially, the expedition team relies either on its own communications brought in from overseas (radios, distress beacons, satellite telephones) or on local systems (telephone, runner, telex, local radio communications and, increasingly, email). In practice, some or both will be involved, depending on the nature of the expedition and the size/budget of the organiser.

Whatever the size of the expedition, it must have a 24-hour contact in the UK capable of responding and assisting in a crisis. For smaller or one-off trips abroad, this may be a family member or colleague who is fully conversant with the expedition medical and contacts network, as well as its itinerary and emergency procedures. This individual must have contact details for all next of kin/closest relatives of all expedition members (including staff). For larger organisations, this back-up may take the form of a duty officer and/or assistance agency or emergency centre. The function of the UK back-up is to liaise with all the relevant parties in the UK. This may include relatives, sponsoring organisations, insurers, assistance agencies and the press. The potential scope and extent of this role in a crisis require the UK back-up to be highly capable and responsible, and fully briefed by the expedition's organiser. Further information on communication and practical crisis management can be found in Chapter 16.

An example of a crisis management plan can be found in Appendix 2. It gives one way of implementing a process to ensure that the most important areas of the crisis management plan have been considered and action taken. This crisis management plan is of the type used by expedition leaders, so some areas may not be relevant to MOs/staff.

TABLE 8.4 EMERGENCY COMMUNICATION NETWORK

Casualty
↓
Expedition leader
↓
Local representative/doctor (contacted by runner, radio, local transport)
↓
Assistance agency/national contact point (contacted by telephone/radio/telex/fax)
↓
UK back-up link/emergency centre (contacted by satellite distress beacon/telephone/telex/fax/email)
↓
Media/public/relatives (contacted by telephone)

SUMMARY

It is important to reiterate the small number of serious accidents recorded on overseas expeditions to date. Well-planned expeditions conducted by suitable and properly trained teams with the right back-up stand a very small chance of sustaining a tragedy. The potential benefits for participants and host country alike of expeditions still far outweigh the risks of disaster. Through practical risk assessment and sensible crisis management planning, the balance can be continually weighted in the right direction.

SECTION 2

FIELD MEDICINE

9 THE ROLE OF THE EXPEDITION MEDICAL OFFICER

Sarah Anderson

The expedition medical officer (MO) is the guardian of an expedition's health. The MO's primary role is to prevent expedition members becoming ill and secondly to treat those who have had an accident or become unwell. This does not necessarily mean that the MOs must treat everything that is presented to them, but rather that they must use their knowledge and authority to advise on the best course of action.

As MO you are unlikely to be very busy with medical problems but if someone is ill or injured you may be the only person who can deal with the situation. These can be stressful times, with no senior cover to turn to for advice and no one to relieve you for a break. Good communication among you, your patient and other expedition members is essential, as is strong decision-making, based on the knowledge and facilities available to you.

To help prepare yourself for the role of expedition MO you will need carefully to research the area to which you are travelling and the likely medical problems that you will encounter, prepare yourself physically and consider attending relevant courses. These might include courses in first aid, advanced life support, basic dental skills or a Diploma in Tropical Medicine and Hygiene (DTM&H).

The roles and responsibilities of the expedition medical officer are best divided into three areas: pre-expedition, during the expedition and post-expedition.

PRE-EXPEDITION

These thirteen pre-expedition responsibilities of the expedition MO should help prevent ill health in the field. Medical screening of all expedition members is essential so that you can provide pre-travel advice to individuals as dictated by their past medical history and expand the expedition first aid kit as necessary. Medical screening can be undertaken by asking each member of the expedition to complete a personal medical questionnaire (see Appendix 1). Three copies of the personal medical questionnaire should be made, one to be left in the UK with a nominated contact and two to be

TABLE 9.1 ROLE OF THE EXPEDITION MEDICAL OFFICER PRE-EXPEDITION

- Advise and brief the team on medical issues
- Undertake medical screening of all expedition members
- Encourage all participants to have a pre-expedition dental check-up
- Provide advice on immunisation requirements (see Chapter 2)
- Provide advice on the need for malaria prophylaxis (see Chapter 19)
- Organise first aid training (see Chapter 4)
- Provide education on health and hygiene issues (see Chapter 10)
- Prepare the expedition medical kits (see Chapter 3)
- Undertake a risk assessment and prepare associated documentation (see Chapter 8)
- Anticipate and plan how a severely ill or injured expedition member might be evacuated
- Prepare a communication network in case of evacuation (see Chapter 16)
- Organise medical insurance with full emergency evacuation cover (see Chapter 6)
- Improve your own knowledge of local medical problems and find out about local medical facilities

taken on the expedition, one of which can be used in an emergency, if evacuation is required. In addition, you should ask each expedition member to document his or her blood group. This can be obtained free by donating blood at a local blood donor centre.

DURING THE EXPEDITION

Once the expedition arrives in the field the need to protect the health of expedition members continues. If the expedition is to be happy and successful this must be done without causing antagonism.

Camp health and hygiene

As the MO you are responsible for base camp health and hygiene. This includes regular checks of latrine and kitchen hygiene, food storage and rubbish disposal. If anything is substandard it should be brought to the attention of all expedition members and steps taken to rectify it. Strict adherence to the rules of camp and personal hygiene is essential to minimise the risks of gastroenteritis, the most common complaint of all expeditions.

TABLE 9.2 **ROLE OF THE EXPEDITION MEDICAL OFFICER DURING THE EXPEDITION**

- Reiterate the rules of camp and personal hygiene (see Chapter 10)
- Continue to reinforce these at regular intervals during the expedition
- Ensure a safe water supply
- Consider conducting a brief medical review of each expedition member on arrival
- Revise basic first aid and management of minor injuries with all members of the expedition
- Practise a mock evacuation
- Place expedition medical kits and communication network papers in a designated place
- Ensure the safety of expedition members
- Organise a routine for patient consultations
- Reassess the risks posed by the natural environment and alter emergency plans as appropriate
- Write up accident reports as necessary
- Review evacuation plans

Consultations

During the expedition, one of the main roles of the MO is to provide a consultation service for non-urgent problems. How you do this will depend on the size and structure of your expedition. In general, it is sensible to allocate a regular time of day when you are exclusively available for confidential consultation. Before or after meals often works well. It is important to ensure complete privacy; this is not always easy on an expedition but should be your aim. All consultations should be briefly recorded, as should the treatment that you give. Consider conducting a brief medical review of each expedition member on arrival. This will enable you to update participants' records with new problems or drugs and clarify anything in the pre-expedition medical questionnaire.

Treatment

Most expedition MOs are simply equipped due to the size and mobility of their expedition. This can mean that few diagnostic aids are available. MOs should ensure that they have medical supplies sufficient for treating minor illnesses and are able to provide emergency care for more serious conditions until a patient can be evacuated.

Most problems are straightforward and trivial and can be dealt with on the spot. The role of the MO is therefore uncomplicated: to make a diagnosis and treat. Most doctors develop a sense of when something apparently trivial is actually a manifestation of something more serious. In the usual urban surroundings help is available to confirm intuitive feelings or doubts; however, in the field it is not, and as expedition MO you therefore have to assume the worst possible scenario. This may mean causing a lot of inconvenience and concern, for example, by sending someone with stomach ache to hospital with possible appendicitis, or making someone with a headache descend 1,000m. You will arouse grumbling and hostility if the person recovers without intervention, but you really have no choice other than to take the safest course of action. If you are not reasonably sure that there is no serious disease you cannot gamble and afterwards, even if the patient does get better without intervention, they may still have had the early stages of disease.

MOs are also there to offer reassurance. People come with genuine symptoms, although in most cases it is merely natural concern about symptoms, the minor significance of which may not be apparent to the sufferer. You will not know what the situation is until you have made a serious attempt at a diagnosis, so never fail to take this step. If you think nothing is wrong, friendly reassurance is important. You should endeavour to treat even natural grumblers properly, because indifference or contempt will eventually leave them suffering in silence, and prevent them consulting when they really need to. Remember that psychological or psychiatric problems, fears and tensions may manifest themselves as physical symptoms.

There is always the problem that illness in an expedition member may adversely affect the expedition as a whole. Expedition members, not least the patient, may try to persuade you to allow activities to go on when this would not be in the patient's best interest. It is important not to yield to this persuasion because it may harm the patient and it may also, in some circumstances, jeopardise the whole expedition. The authority of the expedition rests mainly on the reputation, credibility and good personal relationships the MO is able to build up with the other expedition members.

Expeditioners tend to be self-sufficient people, and the circumstances of an expedition often reinforce this. There is a tendency for MOs to overdo the self-sufficiency; this can lead to them attempting to solve all problems single-handedly. Always ask yourself whether extra help and advice are available and if they would be useful.

All patients rightly expect that when they give the MO information, or a diagnosis is made or suspected, it will be confidential. People also have a right to refuse treatment, even if, in the MO's view, this will not be in their best interest. However, the General Medical Council has made it clear that doctors also have a duty to the public at large. On expeditions circumstances could arise where confidentiality might need to be broken and the expedition leader informed that an individual is concealing an illness or refusing treatment, so that the health and safety of other expedition members is not jeopardised.

Consent

Without consent treatment is assault. Consent to emergency life-saving treatment is usually presumed by the law if the patient is unconscious or too ill to consent. The law presumes that a reasonable man would wish his life to be saved. In the case of a doctor or healthcare professional acting within his or her sphere of clinical competence, consent is usually implied, i.e. the patient does not resist the treatment and therefore is presumed to consent. In other situations where treatment carries considerable risk, or is controversial, informed expressed consent should be obtained. For consent to be informed the individual must understand the proposed treatment and the risks involved in accepting or refusing that treatment. This means that the patient should be made aware of material risks and common or serious side-effects, as well as the likely consequences should treatment be withheld. Verbal consent, especially in an expedition setting, is usually adequate. For an individual over 16 years of age, only that individual is able to give consent. Remember, patients have the right to refuse treatment. Children under 16 can consent to medical treatment themselves if, in the opinion of the doctor, they are capable of understanding the nature and consequences of that treatment. However, when taking under-16s on an expedition it is wise to gain written permission from the parent or guardian that medical care can be given, if it is thought to be in the child's best interest. If written parental permission is not available, and a minor needs medical attention, treatment can be given if he or she is judged to be capable of consenting. If the child is not judged capable of consenting then actions taken will be judged against what a prudent and careful parent would consent to in the same situation. The child should, however, be given information that is relevant to his or her age and understanding.

Accident reports

There is the potential for an accident on any expedition; one of the roles of the expedition MO is to write up an accident report if this becomes necessary. Information should be collected on: the site and time of the accident; the people involved; who else was present; what happened; what action was taken; and what the outcome was.

Evidence from the RGS expedition database published in the *Journal of the Royal Society of Medicine* (2000;93:557–562) states that 59% of medical incidents seen on expeditions are preventable; one third (33%) are due to gastrointestinal disorders; 20% are due to "medical" problems including chest, ear and skin infections plus a few tropical infections (malaria and dengue in particular); and 17% are "orthopaedic" problems, including knee and wrist injuries.

Remember that the most likely problems you will have to deal with as an expedition MO are *common* medical problems (skin infections, gastroenteritis, minor lacerations) seen daily in a general practitioner's surgery.

Assessing risk

The assessment of risk is made just as well by people who commonly encounter the hazard, such as climbers, cavers and divers, as by MOs. In these activities participants are usually well informed and are trained to advise beginners. Risks can be minimised by the use of sensible precautions such as safety belts in vehicles and hard hats while climbing. Remember while coping with a possible fracture to use improvised splints.

Once in the field, it is important to reassess the risks posed by the natural environment, particularly local flora and fauna, and the climate – both heat and humidity.

One of the many roles of the MO is to be aware of the risks posed by the physical environment. There are, of course, many of these. Situations may arise in the field where the MO will either have to give an opinion about a proposed activity, or give unsolicited warnings when activities have already started. Once in the field assessment of risk by the MO is essential and a crisis management strategy should be prepared (see Chapter 8). Inexperienced people are likely to underestimate risk, particularly where the hazard is not obvious, for example, the risk of sunburn is well known, although many northern Europeans are not aware of how much more intense sunlight is at tropical latitudes and how heat exhaustion can kill.

Evacuation

One of the essential roles of the MO is the ability to make a decision on evacuation. This may be an unusual position to be in, and consideration should be given to:

- the need to choose the safest option when diagnosis cannot be confirmed by colleagues or tests;
- the often conflicting needs of the other expedition members;
- the lack of privacy and confidentiality, which is part of expedition life.

Treating people not on the expedition

In many parts of the world expeditions are perceived by local people to be rich and endowed with clinical skills and drugs. The apparently universal human desire to take medication may be stimulated by the arrival of the expedition, and the slightest hint that you will treat people in the local community may produce a flood of "ill" people. It is tempting to try to "help" and to establish goodwill by offering medicines to all but, before you do, consider the potential harm:

1. You may not understand local people's health problems and therefore misdiagnose.
2. You may endanger your own expedition members by using drugs intended for them.

3. You may be blamed unreasonably for adverse outcomes.
4. You may offend local healers.
5. Treatment may be incomplete and thus ineffective or harmful.
6. You might be exploited for your novelty value.
7. You may induce expectations among local people that the local medical services cannot meet.

Nevertheless, you cannot avoid doing what you can for other people. People, particularly children, who are clearly and severely ill, should be treated, but not necessarily by you. Evacuate the patient if possible. Your authority may help to achieve this. As the expedition MO you should not treat serious chronic disease (especially in adults). You will not have the resources or the time, and it would be better for everyone if the patient were treated by the local health service. The stream of people in whom you can see little wrong, and who mainly request medicine rather than presenting a problem, should be referred elsewhere.

POST-EXPEDITION

Once the expedition has returned home, the role of the expedition MO continues (Table 9.3). Expedition members may require support for new or ongoing medical problems. Do not forget that tropical diseases such as malaria and schistosomiasis may present weeks, months or even years after the expedition has ended. A single case in your expedition should alert you to suggesting the screening of all other members since they are likely to have shared the same risk of exposure. In general the role of the MO will be to direct individuals to the best local health provider to treat the problem. An important role of the MO post-expedition is to complete the Royal Geographical Society's Health and Safety Questionnaire (available on the RGS-EAC website: www.rgs.org/eac). This is essential to help the RGS Expedition Advisory Centre collect statistics on expedition health and safety problems, so that they can bring these to the attention of other expeditions and help them to develop ways to improve the safety of those participating in an expedition.

TABLE 9.3 **ROLE OF THE EXPEDITION MEDICAL OFFICER POST-EXPEDITION**

- Repeat advice on malaria prophylaxis if appropriate
- Provide health and medical advice and support as necessary
- Complete the RGS Health & Safety Questionnaire and return to the EAC

10 BASE CAMP HYGIENE AND HEALTH

Hokey Bennett-Jones

Unstinting efforts to maintain a high standard of hygiene will contribute to a lower incidence of gastrointestinal problems and prevent the loss of working person-hours during an expedition. "Be obsessional about camp hygiene." Routine in camp life pays great dividends and responsibility for hygiene, cleaning and safety chores may have to be organised by a strict rota to ensure that standards are maintained throughout the project.

If you cannot help in the choice of a site for base camp, you should at least be aware of its characteristics and therefore any risks and hazards it presents. In planning the layout of the camp, particular attention should be given to the following:

- Water supply
- Latrines
- Areas for washing up, washing clothes, ablutions
- Drains
- Kitchen (smoke, smell and fire risk)
- Food storage
- Rubbish disposal
- Fuel dump and fire precautions
- Areas for eating, working, sleeping and relaxing
- Medical area tent/hut (on the edge of the camp for privacy).

Water supply

Be unremitting in your efforts to maintain a high standard of safe water (see Chapter 11). Find the best source of water. It may, for example, be possible to use rainwater. Before departure, discuss with the leader what safe water regime (rules) needs to be established. On a large expedition someone should be responsible for the water every day. This might be the responsibility of the medical officer (MO) throughout the project, or be organised in rotation, but everyone must be aware of how the system operates. Every member of the expedition must know the difference between safe and unpurified water containers: consider using a simple system of markers. They must also know which source to use for which purpose: for example, not to clean teeth, or wash with untreated water to avoid schistosomiasis contamination.

People use a lot of water. Water will be needed for drinking, washing (people, clothes, cutlery and crockery), cooking, vehicles and sometimes animals. Wherever the expedition – in desert, tropical forest, tundra or at altitude – everyone should drink enough daily fluid for him or her to pass 1 litre of clear urine. This means that their intake will change from day to day depending on workload and speed of acclimatisation.

- Do not underestimate the time it takes to purify water every day.
- Carrying water is hard work. Make sure that your containers are small enough to be carried without too much effort.
- Do not embarrass the local people by making unreasonable demands on limited supplies of water, or be seen to waste it.
- Do not allow expedition members to pollute water supplies, your own or other people's, by being thoughtless.
- Have a back-up system for treating water. All too often the best-made plans go wrong or break down in the field.

Latrines are the subject of much interest, concern and a fair amount of embarrassed mirth. People's bowel habits change on expeditions, one way or the other, and often dramatically. Once again it is necessary to plan which latrine system is appropriate for your expedition. Mobile and short-stay sub-camps can use an earth pit or trench. Sub-camps should dig a trench at least 1.25m deep and about 30cm wide. It may be necessary to construct a grab rail and foot-rest that can be repositioned. Each time the latrine is used, the user should shovel over a coverage of earth from the pile on the edge of the trench. Ash from fires may also be used to help prevent smells.

Long-drop latrines for static base camps should be at least 4m deep and have a seat and fly-proof cover placed over the top. In environments where the soil is unstable, such as sandy desert, consider using old oil drums (lid and base removed and perforated holes halfway up) to shore up the sides, adding a packing of sticks between the edges to stop loose sand filling the drums. Chemical toilets (Elsan type) are not often possible for the expedition camp, but if you are lucky enough to have them there must be adequate provision for the disposal of the contents in a sewage system or deep pit that can be covered. All latrines must be constructed more than 50m away from wells or other water supplies and kitchens.

It is difficult to calculate how many latrines you will need for a big group in a static camp, especially if there are both men and women on the expedition. The efficient working of any camp toilet is of course influenced by the environmental conditions

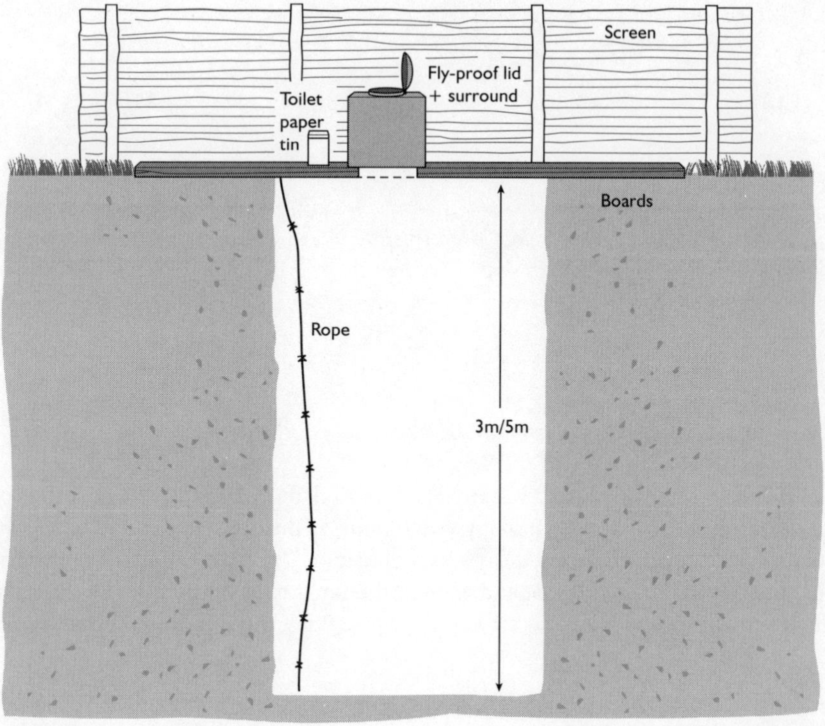

Figure 10.1 *Long-drop latrine for static camp*

of the camp – drainage, porosity of the soil and humidity – and by the number of people using it, so there can be no set formula to help calculate how many to construct. As a rough guide, one long drop for ten people should last two months. A large static camp of some duration may require new long drops to be constructed during the project. If flies become a problem a covering of earth can be shovelled into the long drop after each use, as for an earth trench. Storing toilet paper in a tin stops it blowing away, keeps it dry and keeps the ants out. Arrange hand-washing facilities near to the toilets (the bowl should be a different colour from the ones for kitchen use) and fix the soap on a string. You may need to establish procedures for the disposal of paper, tampons and so on away from the latrine area. Expert advice must be sought by women travelling in areas such as North America where bears are attracted by menstrual flow. Be aware of any expedition members' religious requirements that need catering for when setting up latrines. If local people are to use your facility make sure that they understand how to do so. Problems arise if people try to use Western-style toilets in the local way.

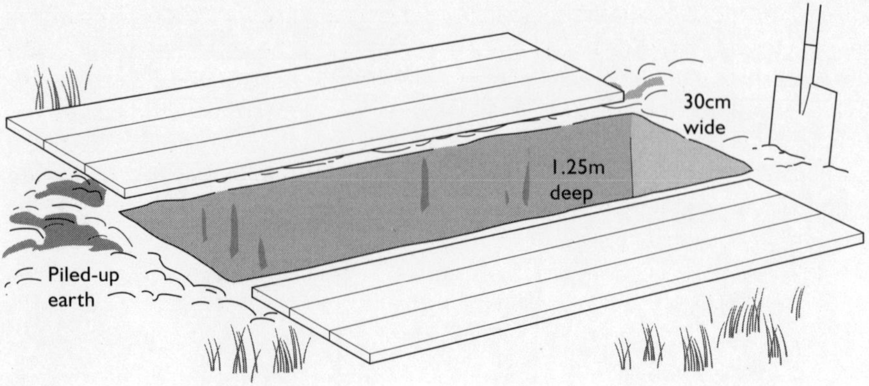

Figure 10.2 *Earth pit or trench latrine for small, mobile camps*

The latrine area needs to be cleaned and dried daily. A long-handled brush is useful for scrubbing the seat with soapy water. Pouring disinfectant down the long drop does not reduce infection and delays decomposition. Try to keep the latrines as dry as possible to discourage flies. Spend time at the beginning of the expedition making sure that seats and lids fit and close properly, making them as fly-proof as possible.

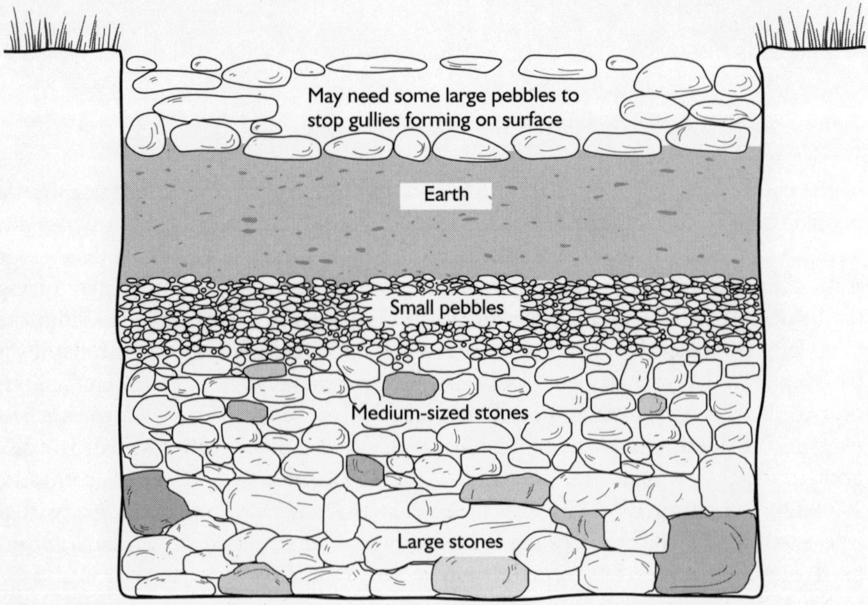

Figure 10.3 *A soak-away pit*

Whatever type of latrine you use you must understand its workings so that any malfunctions can be rectified. It is not a pleasant task to mend or reconstruct toilets when they are in operation. Check at regular intervals that the system is working and is safe. Boards can become slippery, rotten and damaged, and long drop sides cave in. It may be prudent to have a fixed rope down inside the long drop as a safety line. Mesh-covered duckboards around the toilet can be helpful, especially in muddy camps, as inevitably the area becomes squelchy. Ensure the latrine site is clearly marked for night-time visits. Encourage everyone to use a torch to check, particularly under the seats, as snakes and other creatures are frequent visitors to latrines.

If your expedition has built the latrines for your camps you must have a plan for dealing with the area after the expedition is over, leaving it safe and hygienic. This will require some thought and time if the camp has been of any size or duration. In areas of permanent frost, where natural biological breakdown of sewage is impossible, all camp excreta will have to be stored and then taken away.

TABLE 10.1 **CARDINAL RULES FOR LATRINE HYGIENE**
1. Clean seat daily; check operation and safety
2. Keep dry; do not pour down disinfectant
3. Ensure seats and covers are fly-proof
4. Beware of snakes; use a torch at night
5. Ensure adequate hand-washing facilities are available close by

Drains

Even small mobile camps will need to dispose of dirty water somewhere. Without adequate drains your static camp will soon become smelly, and stagnant water is a breeding ground for mosquitoes and infectious diseases. Constructing drains is a time-consuming process. By their very nature they have a tendency to be regularly washed away or become clogged up. For camps that will be used for any length of time, building good kitchen drains and grease traps will pay great dividends in the long term, provided they are used and maintained properly.

Grease traps and soak-aways can get clogged up quickly by a surface layer of food particles, causing the whole system to break down. A good filter, which is small enough to hold back rice and other particles and can easily be cleaned, is a great asset. Making a removable filter of plastic netting or mosquito screen over chicken wire is one possibility. Washing suds and toothpaste can cause problems as they form a slimy surface over soak-aways which then requires regular maintenance to clear.

If you are constructing an improvised shower you will need a mesh-covered duckboard to stand on and a drain and soak-away underneath.

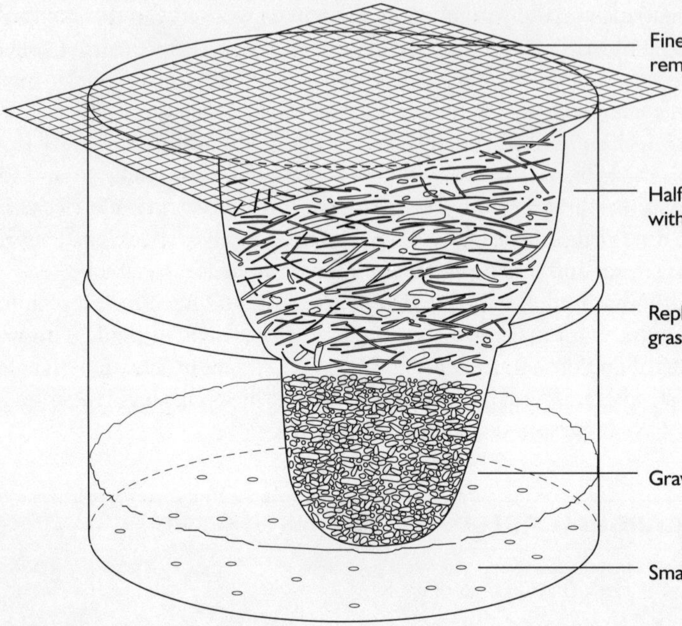

Figure 10.4 *A grease trap*

Rubbish

Rubbish disposal should be tackled as a daily chore to prevent smell, flies and infectious diseases. Rubbish also attracts scavengers if not disposed of properly. It is advisable to burn everything (including the top layer of grass or leaves from the grease trap) before burying it in a deep pit or taking it away for disposal. This includes tins and glass as even hungry expedition members leave unpleasant scraps in the corners of sardine tins. Designate a site away from the main camp to be used as a burning area. A shallow pit may be used to contain the fire. Ensure that plastic and glass containers have had their lids removed prior to burning to prevent small explosions. Flatten things like tins with a mallet. It can be useful to dig a rubbish pit on a slight gradient to promote drainage of rainwater. Beware of using petrol to ignite fires.

Kitchen

Expedition diarrhoea is usually caused by bad hygiene. Again, unremitting efforts to keep a high standard of hygiene in the kitchen will help cut down the person-hours wasted suffering from gut infections. It is imperative that hands are washed prior to all work in the kitchen. One person must be in charge of organising the catering, so that there is no doubt whose responsibility it is to cook each day, and who is to keep the kitchen area clean and tidy. Decide who will do the washing up, where it will be done, and how the cutlery and crockery are stored. On larger expeditions, members may be responsible for washing their own crockery and cutlery. Ensure that all dishes are washed immediately following meals to prevent the attraction of flies and other wildlife. Try, if possible, to wash up in hot water. Organise a clear washing routine, for example a hot soapy wash followed by a cold rinse and dry.

Many expeditions may not have a designated cook and different members of the team may be responsible for kitchen duties each day. Ensure that everyone is aware of the kitchen rules. A written list of the chores that must be completed each day should be available. For example, tabletops and food preparation areas need to be scrubbed daily, aprons washed, and cloths boiled and hung out in the sun to dry.

There must be firm rules about the cleaning and preparation of food, including the preparation of fresh fruit and salads; you may wish to ban lettuce, other broad-leaf vegetables and shellfish completely. Raw food must be prepared, washed or peeled away from already cooked food, taking special care with raw meat. This should be prepared with a separate chopping board and knife kept for this purpose. Food must be properly cooked, served hot on clean plates and eaten promptly; it must not be left lying around or reheated. Make sure the other expedition members know the risks from milk, ice cream, ice and so on, and which foods are unsafe if eaten away from camp.

You will need to consider how to store food. Rodents quickly appear in camp and can severely damage stores as well as transmit disease to humans; for example, the multimammate rat, *Mastomys natalensis*, urinates on food supplies and transmits Lassa fever in West Africa. Large and dangerous animals such as bears may be attracted to camps and vehicles by subtle food odours, with devastating consequences. Food storage in strong metal drums may be the only solution. Hanging insect-proof larder cupboards are useful as they can be packed flat. Refrigerators in the field (whether gas, paraffin or electrically operated) are seldom 100% reliable. They are usually unable to maintain the cold setting of a modern kitchen refrigerator, allowing disease organisms to multiply much faster. Scientific specimens may compete for space in the refrigerator with the food, beer and even the MO's drugs. This must be resisted at all costs. Scientific specimens must be kept in a separate refrigerator if they need to be kept at a low temperature. The camp kitchen refrigerator must be kept clean, with raw meat at the bottom and cooked food above. It must not be overfilled and the door must not be opened and closed too often.

If the expedition has the good fortune to have a cook, be vigilant about standards of hygiene. It is not safe to assume that your cook, whether local or expatriate, has any understanding of the principles of kitchen hygiene. Staphylococcal food poisoning usually results from contamination of, for example, chopping boards, by people harbouring bacteria in their noses. Always bear in mind the possibility that the cook may be a carrier of disease. Consider treating for worms and do not let someone who is ill do the cooking.

TABLE 10.2 CARDINAL RULES FOR KITCHEN HYGIENE
1. Wash hands and scrub nails with soap before starting any work in the kitchen
2. Keep fingernails short and cover wounds with a plaster
3. Wear clean clothes or an apron (available for kitchen use only)
4. Do not use the same chopping board or utensils for raw and cooked ingredients
5. Food should be eaten immediately after it is cooked or, if not, refrigerated or reheated to sterilising temperatures before being eaten

The cooks work long hard hours, getting up before the rest of the team and working late into the night. They are the heart of the expedition and perform a thankless task. On every expedition food will become the all-absorbing topic and higher on the agenda as time passes. However well you have planned to please everyone, there will always be complaints. The cooks can often become the whipping boys – they are moaned at if not actually abused – but an expedition cannot function without food. Cooks need support, and a show of thanks from other members of the team will be much appreciated.

Camp safety

Spend time in camp removing hazards – marking guy ropes and washing lines, fixing handrails or holds and tying back branches where people regularly work or pass. Before pitching tents, check the ground for scorpions (at night they can be made visible with ultraviolet light which makes them fluoresce green) and other biohazards. In some tropical countries, sleeping on the ground entails a definite risk of nocturnal snakebites, by kraits (in Asia) and spitting cobras (in Africa). The risk is reduced by tucking the mosquito net well in under the sleeping bag and by fitted groundsheets, and is eliminated by sleeping in a hammock or raised camp bed. Make sure everyone hangs and uses mosquito nets correctly.

Be aware of anyone using or storing dangerous chemicals. Anaesthetic agents for small mammals and formaldehyde are commonly used on expeditions. If firearms are to be used, training and safe storage must be rigorous. Be especially aware of any scientist working with dangerous specimens (alive or dead). No one should handle venomous animals without previous training. If, for example, a venomous snake is to be handled, advise that it be done early in the day; if anything untoward happens communications and, if necessary, evacuation, are far easier in daylight. Handling dangerous animals, chemicals or machinery must not be allowed after drinking alcohol.

Everyone should know where the camp first aid kit is kept, but make sure all medical equipment and drugs are stored securely. Everything should be packed and labelled clearly with its name, strength and batch numbers. There must be some system for the resupply of individuals' first aid kits. This will enable the MO to keep account of what minor problems members are suffering from and, if necessary, to check wounds and to stop the medical stocks constantly being pilfered or bits of the evacuation kit (e.g., spare torch batteries) being "borrowed". Consider having a book for recording every piece of equipment or dose of drug issued. Make sure that those who are on regular medication know where their spare supply is kept.

Think about the fire risks and what fire-fighting methods are available to you, especially in the kitchen. A fire blanket is needed to deal with frying pan fat fires. Store fuel safely away from the main camping area. Fuel (i.e. lamp fuel) should not be kept in people's tents or in plastic containers. Money spent on clearly labelled metal cans is never wasted. In large camps the siting of the generator is important to reduce the effect of the noise and fumes. Make sure any electric cables and plugs are safe. Check these at regular intervals throughout the project.

TABLE 10.3 **CARDINAL RULES FOR FIRE PREVENTION**
1. Identify risks
2. Publicise extinguisher sites or sand buckets
3. Store fuel, clearly labelled, away from tents
4. Do not keep fuel in plastic containers
5. Regularly check plugs and cables

Remember that the risk assessment done during the planning stages of the expedition and the routine safety rules may need to be modified in the field. Keep a book at the base camp for people to record daily where they are going, with whom and their expected time of return. Try to make sure people have adequate clothing, food and kit for the environment and daily conditions.

Everyone should know the policy and procedure for a late or lost person (see Chapter 8).

Be aware of the first aid skills within the rest of the team. The acclimatisation period and time in base camp offer the opportunity to go over some basic first aid with expedition members, with special reference to local problems such as recognising and managing heat stroke or hypothermia. In the event of the MO having time away from camp for any reason, appoint a second-in-command.

Lastly, you should be aware of any local security risk, for example, driving after dark or whether it is safe to leave anyone alone in camp.

Camp life

A happy, relaxed atmosphere in camp can help support those who are feeling the loss of their usual social props or missing their homes and families. Base camp should be a place for rest and healing, but birthdays in the field are a good excuse for a party to boost morale. The MO can also help morale by taking an interest in, and spending time with, members working on their projects. This will be much easier to achieve if the MO is seen to be mucking in with general camp duties where possible. But the MO must remain available at all times for consultation and be seen to have an unquestionable standard of confidentiality.

Communication with the outside world by letter, radio or phone is very important. Do not underestimate the disappointment if this breaks down.

Meal times are important focal points for everyone and give the MO a chance to check that all are happy and well. The setting of the meal times can be critical and it is always difficult to please everyone and fit in with their work. It is frustrating to have meals consistently late, forcing people to wait around. Young people need food regularly and in large amounts. There will be accidents if they get hungry and tired. Try not to let people skip meals, and if possible make packed lunches for them if their work means they cannot get back for meals.

TABLE 10.4 **MEAL TIMES**

1. Meal times are an important focal point
2. The setting of meal times is important
3. Young people need food regularly
4. Make packed meals if away from base

It is often necessary, on a long expedition, to identify one day of the week (say a Sunday) that is slightly different from the rest in some way, perhaps with breakfast half an hour later. This Sabbath is also useful for those taking weekly antimalarial prophylaxis: "Sunday is antimalarial day." The MO can be responsible for putting out the appropriate pills and seeing that everyone remembers to take them.

Do not forget that large numbers of local people waiting around camp to see the MO can create a risk to the camp hygiene.

Records

Keep details of expedition members and records of all medical consultations. You should already have with you or have taken a detailed medical history of each expedition member, and be aware of what he or she wishes to happen in case of an accident, fatal or otherwise. Hold contact details of members' next of kin and the circumstances in which they should be contacted. Have a secure system for storing notes.

If there is an accident write down what happened in great detail as soon as you can. If you have planned how to cope when things go wrong and you stick to the rules you will not make matters worse. Clear and truthful information is vital. Make sure that the insurance companies are informed promptly. Never destroy any records.

Creating a happy camp life will help maintain the group through and during the aftermath of an accident, and keep it working together as a team for as long as is needed.

The end of the expedition

Lastly, remember to honour any commitment to sponsors and to thank all who have helped you in the host country and elsewhere. Make sure that all members know what to do if they fall ill after returning home, and the length of time for which this applies. Repeat antimalarial advice and check that everyone has enough first aid kit for the last few days in camp and journey home before everything is packed up. Make sure the campsite and the surrounding area are left clean and safe. The final days of the expedition can be dangerous times – people will be tired and with that end-of-term feeling rules are often broken. Be on your guard.

11 WATER PURIFICATION

Paul Goodyer and Larry Goodyer

A safe water supply is an essential part of camp hygiene. Water intake for adults in temperate conditions is around 3 litres per day, but this can rise to as much as 10 litres per day in hot climates because of loss due to sweating. In addition, around 4 litres of water per person per day will be needed for cooking and washing up. Therefore considerable supplies may be required both at base camp and by field parties. In many cases, water obtained from rivers, lakes and ponds, as well as from taps and wells, carries a considerable risk of contamination. Spring water collected away from human habitation may be safer but it would be wise to treat even this water source.

Before treating the water to kill any organisms, organic matter and silt need to be removed. This can pose considerable problems if you are trying to obtain supplies for a large expedition, where sedimentation tanks and large ceramic filters would need to be employed.

Various methods for water purification will be described in this chapter. Some are more suitable for the base camp and others for field workers. Before deciding on the system to use it is also important to consider the likely infective organisms and the risk posed by them to the expedition.

Transmission of disease by water

Numerous organisms and chemical pollutants that may be found in water can lead to human disease. The organisms include bacteria, viruses, protozoa and other parasites, such as schistosomes, guinea worm larvae (in tiny shrimps) and leeches, which vary in the ease with which they can be killed. Water may be boiled or chemicals added for sterilisation, but if sediment is not first removed the sterilisation process may be ineffective. If the expedition is close to mines or factories, chemical pollution must be foreseen and appropriate filtration used.

Removal of sediment and organic matter from water

If the water is cloudy or contains any suspended matter, this must be removed before further treatment. One method is to pass the water through a Millbank bag (Figure 11.1). This is a sock-shaped bag woven so that solids are retained but water flows by gravity through the weave. The bag can be left hanging over a receptacle with occasional top-ups to provide continuous production of filtered water ready for sterilisation. The bag is rugged and easy to clean. Millbank bags are available in two sizes: 2 litres for personal use and 9 litres for large quantities of water. Cloudy water can also be left to stand for some hours for solids to settle, either in a jerry can or in sedimentation tanks, depending on the volume to be treated. Very fine particles, such as "rock flour" in glacial outflow and mica flakes, are gastrointestinal irritants and must be removed by a ceramic filter (Table 11.1). Remember that simply clearing water does not sterilise it and that further treatment will be needed before it may be drunk.

METHODS OF WATER PURIFICATION

Boiling

This is undoubtedly the best method, but it is often inconvenient and wasteful of fuel supplies or natural resources. Water should be kept continuously boiling for 5 minutes, which is sufficient at any altitude. The water must be covered when cooling to prevent recontamination, and it will also taste better.

Iodine

This is the most effective chemical method. Its main disadvantage is that it is unsuitable for some people: those with a thyroid condition or iodine allergy, pregnant women and young children. There are also concerns, largely unfounded, about the long-term use of iodine-treated water. A further drawback is that the cheapest method involves the use of iodine tincture, which must be carried in glass containers – this could be messy and hazardous if they should break. Iodine can be stored in plastic bottles if the bottle has been fluorinated to stop the iodine reacting with the plastic.

There is some discrepancy about the exact amount of iodine to use. Five drops of iodine tincture (2%) to 1 litre of water is most often used, increasing to 12 drops if *Giardia* is suspected. It is always best to assume that *Giardia* is present and add 12 drops to 1 litre when treating small amounts of water, or measure out 0.3–0.4ml/l when treating large tanks. The longer the treated water is left to stand – the contact time – the better, 30 minutes being the minimum.

An alternative to the tincture is to use water-sterilising iodine tablets, but these are expensive and lose their potency after the bottle has been opened. Iodine tablets should always be crushed into the water; they can take time to break down if left whole, which can seriously effect the contact time. Another method is to use iodine crystals (the Kahnn–Visscher method), but it is rather fiddly and not suitable for

TABLE 11.1 **REMOVAL OF SEDIMENT AND ORGANIC MATERIAL**

Filter/purifier	*Litres*	*Filtration time/litre (minutes)*	*Purification time (minutes)*	*Chemical/filter employed*
Pocket Travelwell	25	10	2	Filter/iodine
Millbank bag	Unlimited	5	n/a	Cloth filtration
First Need Microlite	100	2	Instant	Microfilter
Aqua Pure bottle	350	2	15	Filter/iodine
Trekker Travelwell	100	10	2	Filter/iodine
First Need Original	400	2	n/a	Microfilter
P U R traveller	400	2	3	Filter/iodine
The Pure Cup	500	25	5	Filter/iodine
P U R Scout	1,000	2	3	Filter/iodine
P U R Explorer	2,000	1	3	Filter/iodine
Katadyne Mini Filter	7,000	2	Instant	Ceramic filter/silver
Katadyne Pocket Filter	10,000	1.5	Instant	Ceramic filter/silver

Note: purifying water using a pump filter can be fast, but organic matter may cause frequent blockages, making the process labour intensive.

Figure 11.1 *A Millbank bag in use (Nomad Traveller's Store)*

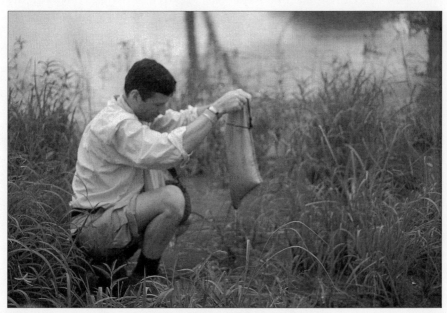

preparing large amounts of water.

The horrible taste of iodine-treated water can be reduced by adding small amounts of ascorbic acid (vitamin C) to neutralise the iodine. Clearly this should be done only at the point of use.

Chlorine

This is effective against a wide range of organisms, except for amoebic cysts, *Giardia* and *Cryptosporidium*. The effectiveness of chlorine is reduced by a number of factors which may not be easy to control, such as alkaline water, very cold water or the presence of organic matter – hence the need for prior filtration.

Puritabs tablets are the most widely available method of chlorination and one tablet of the maxi size will treat 25 litres. For very large tanks some expeditions prefer to use a substance called chloramine T, where 5mg is added to each litre of water. Treated water should be left for at least half an hour before drinking and longer if it is very cold.

Taste can be removed with sodium thiosulphate. This will inactivate the chlorine so it should be added by individuals only at the point of use, i.e. to a drinking cup. It should never be added to a storage receptacle such as a canteen or jerry can.

Silver compounds

Micropure tablets contain a compound called Katadyne silver which is not effective against *Amoeba*, *Giardia* or viruses. It does not impart a bad taste and it is claimed to be able to prevent recontamination of water for many weeks. Micropure tablets should not be added to water previously treated with chlorine or iodine.

Filters and pumps

There are now many devices available for purifying water (see Table 11.1), but care must be taken in choosing the right one for your expedition. Some devices employ a simple filtration method, whereby water is pumped through tiny holes through which organisms are unable to pass. Be careful to look at the pore size (measured in microns), as anything greater than 1 micron will not remove all organisms. Other devices employ both a filter and chemical treatment which strains and sterilises in one go. Choosing the right device is important, so here are some tips:

- Manufacturers often say how many litres of pure water a device will produce. However, this can be drastically reduced if the water is silty.
- If heavy use is expected, make sure that the purifier can be taken apart, cleaned and reassembled in the field to prevent blockages.
- Check the pump rate as some can take a lot of effort to produce a small amount of water.
- Many manufacturers of pumps go to great lengths to state what they will

remove, while keeping quiet about what is not removed. For example, pumps will not remove chemical effluent, such as mercury in the tributaries of the Amazon, without the addition of a carbon filter. For those visiting areas where there is mining or factories up-river this may be important.
- Water storage time is also important; ideally after sterilisation the water should be used within 24 hours.

CHOICE OF SYSTEM

This will depend on the size and circumstances of the expedition. If practicable a large pot should be put on to boil at the end of an evening meal to allow preparation of water for the following morning. In addition, all members should have some method of sterilising their own drinking water. As a rough guide the choice of methods is as follows:

- Large groups could consider chlorination, where the condition of the treatment tanks can be carefully monitored.
- Smaller groups might use iodine, provided that everyone in the group can tolerate it.
- For smaller groups, particularly if on the move, it would be acceptable to prepare water that has been strained through a Millbank bag and provide members with their own small bottle of iodine or chlorination tablets to treat water after drawing it off in their own canteens. The strained water could be used for boiling water, e.g. for beverages.
- A new generation of water bottles with a filtration/purification method attached (e.g. Aqua Pure – see below) can be used to improve fluid intake (the ease of use helps the user to keep up a constant intake of water). However, there is a question of the contact time and it is suggested that the water be squeezed through and left to stand.

All field parties should be provided with small Millbank bags and some method of chemical sterilisation, or alternatively a portable filtration system.

Drinking bottle filters

These are bottles with filters attached to the top. The most well known is the Aqua Pure traveller (99,000g, 24cm diameter). The bottle is filled with the water to be treated then squeezed into a drinking cup for purification. Drinking bottle filters are slightly misleading as they make it look as though you should be able to drink safe water straight from the bottle. By the addition of an iodine sleeve to the carbon micro-filter, the Aqua Pure can be turned into a purifier so long as the water is left to stand for 15 minutes once it has passed through the system.

Camp arrangements

Providing enough treated water, from a natural source, for a camp of 20 is time-consuming but exceedingly important. The best approach is to incorporate a strict regime from the start by appointing one person as "water chief" to supervise the sterilisation, safe storage and use of the water. The appointed person should also make sure that every member of the expedition is capable of sterilising his or her own drinking water.

Rigid plastic containers with a tap and handle are the best for water. These come in 10- or 25-litre sizes, but the latter is heavy when full of water so keep in mind distances to water source and terrain. If you do not have a method of removing the taste of chemicals, water will taste better when cold. Storing water in special canvas bags will keep it cool through evaporation from the small pores of the canvas. If they can be obtained, army surplus ones are excellent and come in sizes suitable for storage of large volumes in camp or for tying to the back of a vehicle.

If a daily average of 6 litres per person is required for drinking and 4 litres for cooking/washing up, containers holding 10 litres per person per day will be required. Water treatment could be split into sessions if it is necessary to reduce the number of containers in use. To avoid confusion, have a good system of marking containers for the three different types of water treatment:

- untreated for storage, sedimentation or settling process;
- strained ready for treatment;
- fit for drinking.

Field parties

Always make sure that field workers carry their own water bottles, with a metal cup. Avoid plastic beakers as these often break. Each member should also have personal equipment for sterilising water; if a filter system is used, a small Travelwell might be a good choice.

If travelling by vehicle, do not use one large container for storing water; a single puncture may have disastrous consequences. Jerry cans or the canvas bags previously mentioned are the best option, but try to adopt the same system of markings as employed in base camp.

12 ASSESSMENT OF THE INJURED OR ILL PATIENT

Charles Siderfin

This chapter aims to cover the assessment of the injured or ill patient in a way that is easily understood by non-medical people. It can also be used as basic revision for people who are medically qualified. When reading this chapter please refer to the Medical Assessment Questionnaire (MAQ) in Appendix 3.

The assessment of a patient involves establishing what the problem is and monitoring the patient's progress. There are four components to assessment:

- History – the patient's account of events
- Examination of the patient
- Investigations
- Monitoring the patient's condition.

INITIAL ASSESSMENT OF THE INJURED CASUALTY

In the injured casualty the initial priorities are:

- **A**irway
- **B**reathing
- **C**irculation
- Head-to-toe assessment.

Airway, breathing and circulatory (ABC) assessment is covered in Chapter 13.

Head-to-toe assessment

The objective of the head-to-toe assessment is to make a quick, thorough examination of the casualty to gain an overview and plan the priorities for treatment. Mentally reconstruct the sequence of events to alert yourself to possible injuries. Start your examination at the head and work down to the toes. The three basic tenets of examination are *look, feel* and *listen*. You may need to remove clothing, but do not move the casualty unless it is absolutely necessary. Comparison of each side of the body will help you to decide what is abnormal. While making the examination talk to the casualty, explaining what you are doing and giving reassurance, even if the person is unconscious.

The head

Observe the colour, temperature and state of the face for signs of shock. Look at the face and head for deformity or bruising. Bruising just behind and below the ears may indicate a skull fracture, as does blood or clear fluid draining from the ears or nose. Blood in the whites of the eyes (subconjunctival haemorrhage) suggests a significant head injury. Check the pupils are equal in size and that there are no foreign bodies in the eyes. Run your fingers through the hair feeling the skull for blood, swellings, depressions or areas of tenderness.

The neck

Loosen any tight clothing around the neck. Look for bruising, bleeding or swelling and feel the back of the neck for swelling or steps between the spinal vertebrae. The line of the neck should be straight; any deviation from this should arouse suspicion of an injury such as a dislocation or fracture.

The chest

Look for regular chest movements and whether both sides are moving equally. Firmly feel the chest for wetness (blood), swelling, deformity, tenderness and chest movement. Remember to feel around the sides and back of the chest as far as possible without moving the patient. Listen to the breathing.

The abdomen

Feel the abdomen (Figure 12.5, page 123) for muscle tensing (guarding) or tenderness. With a hand on either side of the pelvis gently rock it (Figure 12.1). You are feeling for any movement or grating that would indicate a fracture. Place your hand in the small of the back and feel along the spine, as far as possible, for any irregularities.

The limbs

Lastly, examine the legs and arms; these are your lowest priority. Injuries to the head, spine, chest and abdomen can kill. Limb injuries, with the exception of severe bleeding, are rarely life threatening. Look for deformity and bleeding. Feel each leg and arm and compare, starting at the top and working down. If the patient is conscious ask if he can feel you touching him and ask him to move the limbs. Any inability may indicate a spinal injury.

You now have a good idea of the patient's state and are in a position to plan his or

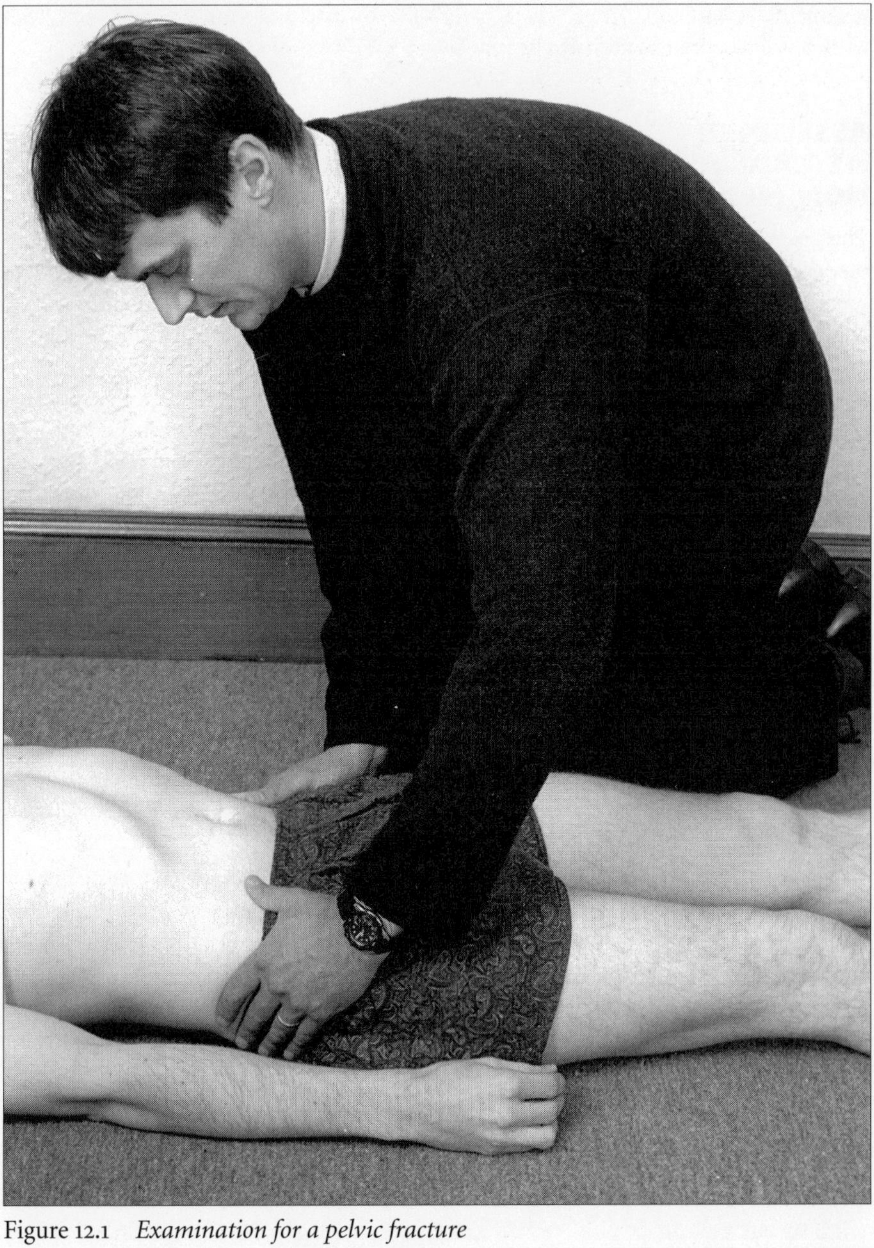

Figure 12.1 *Examination for a pelvic fracture*

her further treatment. Once the casualty's life-threatening injuries have been dealt with, a full assessment needs to be made.

ASSESSMENT OF AN INJURED OR ILL PATIENT USING THE MEDICAL ASSESSMENT QUESTIONNAIRE (MAQ) FOR NON-MEDICAL PERSONNEL

The degree of assessment required depends on the circumstances. A sore throat with no other features requires little attention. A sore throat accompanied by fever, cough, breathlessness and chest pain requires more detailed assessment. Making an accurate diagnosis is not essential. Many medical conditions have similar features, especially early on, and it is not until later that specific features emerge.

An accurate and thorough description of a medical disorder is necessary to establish a comprehensive care plan . The MAQ was developed to help non-medical personnel achieve this. The MAQ leads you through a history and examination, ensuring that relevant information is not missed. It was originally developed to transfer information to a remote doctor via radio or fax so that medical advice could be given. For expeditions with medical back-up the MAQ may be a valuable additional tool for communication when the doctor and patient are separated. For expeditions without medical back-up the MAQ will help ensure that a full history and examination are performed.

This section guides you through an assessment using the MAQ. Remember that symptoms are the patient's description of how he or she feels; a sign is what you observe during the examination.

It is important to explain to the patient what you are about to do during the assessment.

The history

The history must give a clear picture of events. Time taken to gain an accurate history is always time well spent. The history is about the events that led up to the illness and what the *patient* feels. It is not about what the examiner observes. *Listen to the patient and other eyewitnesses.*

To make full sense of this chapter, please refer to the Medical Assessment Questionnaire in Appendix 3. The alphabetical sections that follow correspond to the alphabetical subsections in the MAQ.

(A) PATIENT DETAILS

Make a note of the patient's personal details, including name, address, date of birth, age, sex, occupation plus time, date and location of where the form was completed.

(B) PATIENT'S MAIN COMPLAINT/COMPLAINTS

This identifies the central problems. Later components of the history build upon this initial description. For example, a patient's main complaint might be:

1 abdominal pain
2 vomiting.

(C) A SHORT DESCRIPTIVE HISTORY

Describe briefly the main features of the illness or injury. It is often useful to start with the question "When were you last completely well?", followed by "What was the first thing that you noticed was wrong?" and "What happened next?" Specify the nature, location and duration of symptoms. Identify changes or additional symptoms that occur and factors that worsen or improve the symptoms. The information should be related to time. Do not use technical medical terms, as they cause confusion unless their precise definition is known to the users; statements should be in the patient's own words. For example: "Last completely well 2 days ago. Yesterday had no appetite, ate nothing and only small amount to drink. Woke at 4.00am today with pain in centre of abdomen, gripping in nature. Unable to sleep. About 8.00am pain more in the right, lower side of abdomen. Vomited twice at 9.00am and 9.40am."

SECTIONS (D) TO (K)

Apparently unrelated symptoms can help you to reach a diagnosis. It is therefore necessary to ask the patient all the questions from Section D onwards. The questions systematically cover the systems of the body and ensure that relevant information is not missed.

The examination

The examination questions need to be answered from your own observations. They are not questions to ask the patient. For example, "Is there pain on moving?" requires the patient to move and for the examiner to decide if this causes pain. Information is gained in three ways during the examination.

1. Look

Start by taking a good look at the patient and observing his or her general well-being and attitude. It may seem subjective to ask whether the patient looks well or unwell, but your gut feelings are valuable. When examining a part of the body it should be fully exposed. Stand back and look. Remember to compare both sides.

2. Feel

A number of questions ask whether an area is tender and to answer you need to feel that area. You must watch the patient's face when examining as even small twinges of pain are usually registered on the face. Similarly, if an area is painful the patient usually tenses when it is touched.

To minimise discomfort be *gentle but firm* with your hands. Do not prod and poke, or be so cautious that you tickle the patient. Firmly apply pressure; you will learn nothing from prodding, poking and tickling.

3. Listen

Listen to the breath or bowel sounds either with a stethoscope or by putting your ear to the part you are examining.

SECTION (N)

The thirteen questions in section N are important because they provide a lot of information about the patient's overall condition. Each one must be answered.

Taking the temperature

The temperature can be taken from three places.

1. The mouth

Place the thermometer under the tongue and close the mouth. Leave for 3 minutes before reading. This method is unreliable if the patient has recently eaten, drunk or been exposed to cold, or is breathing heavily through an open mouth.

2. The armpit

The thermometer is placed in the armpit and held in position for 3 minutes. This temperature is usually about 1°C lower than the oral temperature.

3. The rectum

This is the most accurate place to record the temperature and, despite its obvious disadvantages, is the best site. In a patient suspected of being hypothermic, the temperature must be taken with a low-reading thermometer in the rectum.

Lie the patient on his or her or her side and gently insert a lubricated thermometer no more than 6cm into the rectum. Hold it in position for 3 minutes and do not let go. After taking the reading, clean the thermometer with gauze and an alcohol swab and identify it for rectal use only.

A normal temperature ranges between 36.5°C and 37.5°C
Hypothermia is defined as 35°C or less
A temperature greater than 37.5°C is elevated

Taking the pulse

Blood is pumped from the heart to the arteries. The arteries transport the blood to the cells of the body. With each heart beat blood is ejected into the arteries causing them to expand. This expansion is transmitted along the arteries, and can be felt as the pulse. The pulse rate is the number of pulses (or number of heart beats) per minute.

Normal adult pulse rate at rest is 60–90 per minute

The pulse is easily felt, but it requires practice. Feel for it with the pulp at the end of your middle finger. The pulse can be felt at one of four sites.

1. The wrist

Press gently in the groove that runs between the lump on the thumb side of the wrist and the tendons.

2. The neck

The neck (carotid) pulse is sometimes the only pulse that can be felt in a very ill patient. Locate the Adam's apple (larynx) with two fingertips. (The Adam's apple is the lump at the front of the windpipe that moves up and down when swallowing.) Run the fingers down the side of the neck towards you, until you reach an easily felt

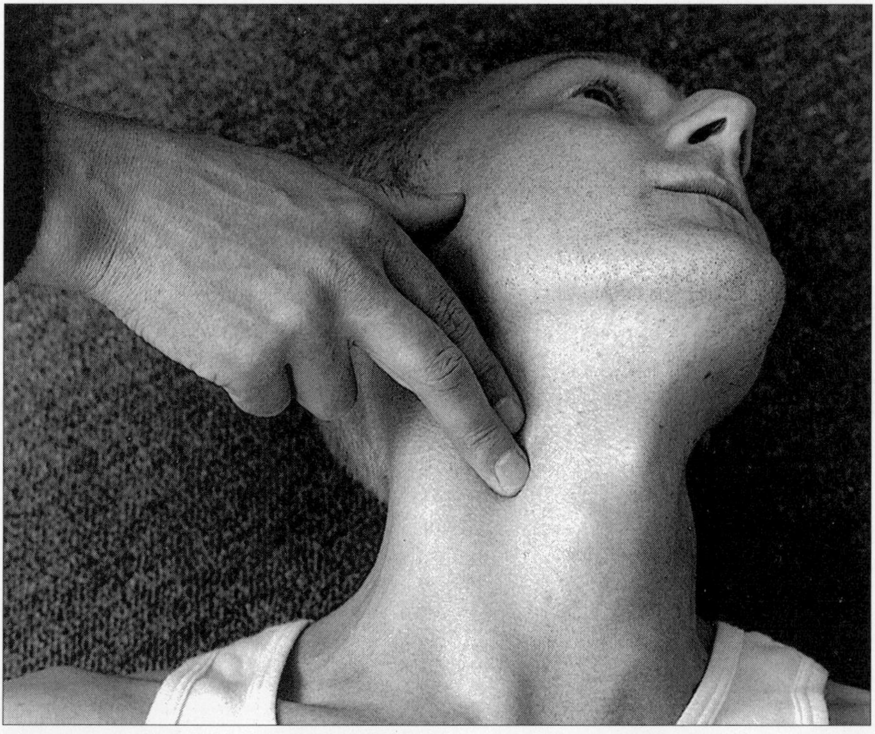

Figure 12.2 *Examination for a carotid pulse*

groove. This is the junction between the windpipe and the neck muscles. The carotid pulse can be felt with the fingertips in this groove (Figure 12.2). Press gently into the groove. Do not press hard as this will compress the artery, and do not press both sides simultaneously as this will reduce the circulation to the brain.

3. The groin

Press firmly into the skin crease at the top of the leg, at a point half-way between the mid-line and the prominent bony lump of the pelvis.

4. The antecubital fossa

This is the hollow in the bend of the arm, in front of the elbow where blood is usually taken by venepuncture. Straighten the arm at the elbow and feel the brachial pulse in the hollow between the muscles.

Once you have located a pulse, count the number of beats during a timed minute. This is the pulse rate. Exertion, fever, shock, pain, excitement and anxiety raise the pulse rate; it is slowed by hypothermia and fainting. You may also be able to evaluate the pulse strength and whether it is regular or irregular.

Taking the blood pressure

The blood pressure is the measurement of two pressures. The systolic pressure is the pressure of blood in the artery caused by the heart contracting. The diastolic pressure, which is lower, is the resting pressure in the artery when the heart is relaxed.

Blood pressure varies enormously between individuals. Interpretation needs to be made in conjunction with the clinical situation and other measurements such as pulse and breathing rate. Because of the wide variability, a normal range for blood pressure is not given. The blood pressure is extremely important in monitoring, as much can be learnt from whether it is stable, falling or rising.

- Take the blood pressure with a sphygmomanometer.
- Ease any constricting clothing from the upper arm and firmly wrap the cuff above the elbow.
- With the palm upwards, straighten the patient's arm and locate the brachial pulse which lies just below the elbow, about one third of the way across from the inner side. Continue to press gently on the pulse.
- Inflate the cuff and note the reading when the pulse disappears. Inflate the cuff a further 20–30mm of mercury.
- Place the diaphragm of the stethoscope over the pulse and press gently to ensure good contact (Figure 12.3).
- Release the pressure in the cuff at a rate of 3–5mm of mercury per second by easing open the screw valve.

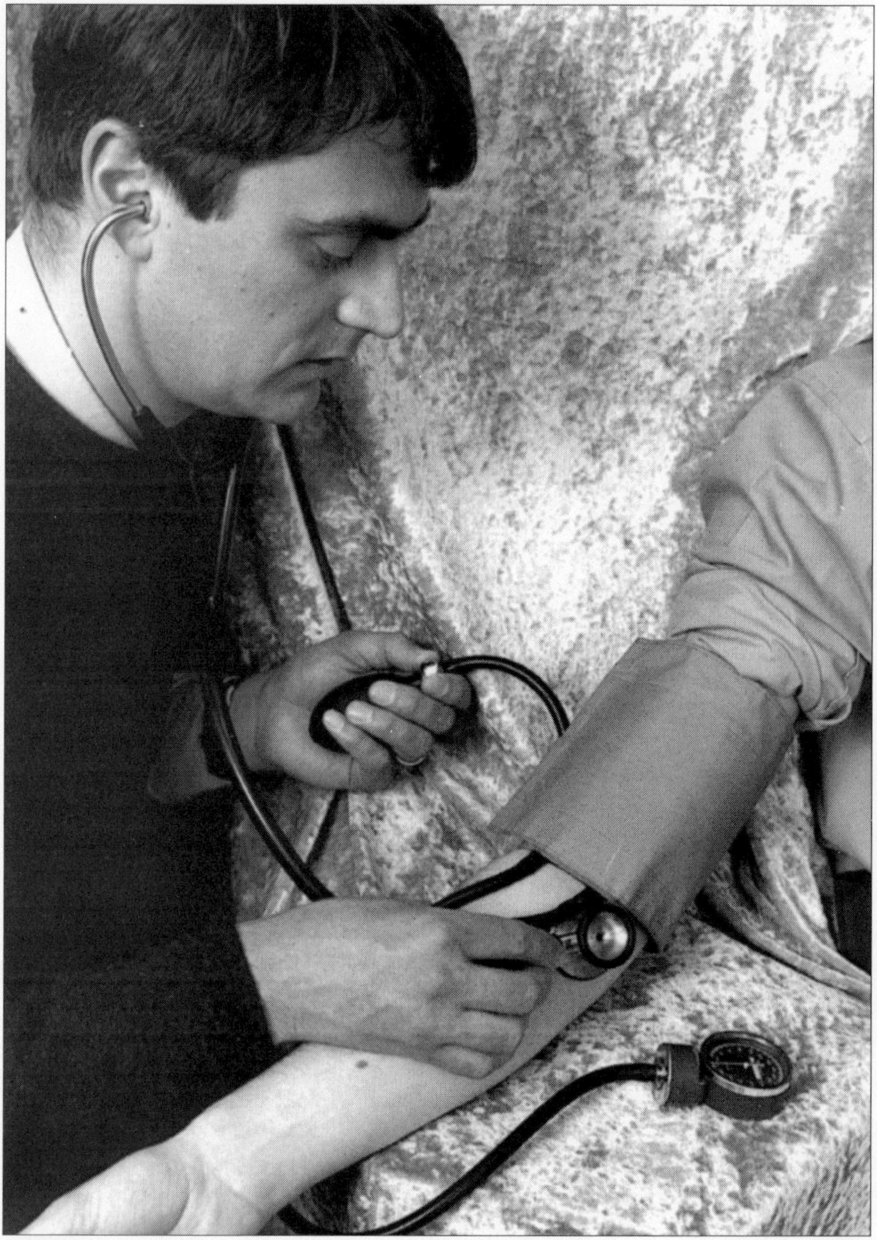

Figure 12.3 *Taking the blood pressure*

- Listen for the first pulse beat while watching the pressure fall. The pressure at which you hear the first thumping sound is the systolic pressure. (This is about the same level at which the pulse was felt to disappear during inflation.)
- Continue to listen. The sounds will suddenly muffle and then disappear. The disappearance marks the diastolic pressure.

Mercury thermometers and sphygmomanometers should not be carried on aircraft as spilled mercury can form an amalgam and weaken the integrity of the aircraft fuselage

The blanching test (capillary refill time)

This can be a useful additional test of the circulation. It is unreliable if the patient is cold and needs to be interpreted in the context of other findings. There are two sites to perform the test:

1. Press your thumb on a fingernail or toenail for 5 seconds. The nail bed will blanch immediately and the colour should return as soon as the thumb is removed. If the nail does not begin to return to normal after 2 seconds, then circulation is poor.
2. Press your thumb on the patient's chest or any bony prominence for 5 seconds. This causes a white (blanched) area where the blood has been squeezed out of the capillaries. The colour should begin to return in 2 seconds. If the circulation is poor it will take longer.

Measuring the breathing rate

Do this while pretending to count the pulse as the breathing may alter when the patient becomes aware of what you are doing.

Normal adult breathing rate at rest is 12–18 per minute. The breaths should be quiet, regular, effortless and painless

Use of the stethoscope

There are two points about using the stethoscope:

1. The earpieces are angled and should be placed in your ears angled forwards – the ear canal runs downwards and forwards
2. Most stethoscopes have a bell and diaphragm. They can be switched by spinning the end piece of the stethoscope. You should use the diaphragm.

(O) EXAMINATION OF THE CHEST

Much can be gained from looking at the chest as the patient breathes normally, but remember that the chest has a front and a back. When examining the back, get the patient to sit forward with the arms crossed to pull the shoulder blades apart.

If one of the lungs collapses, the windpipe (trachea) may either be pulled towards or pushed away from the collapsed lung (tension pneumothorax). The position of the windpipe can be assessed by feeling with two fingers in the mid-line at the base of the neck. You will feel a notch immediately above the breast bone, and by pushing your fingers gently into it you will feel the windpipe as it disappears into the chest cavity (Figure 12.4). It should be positioned centrally. Listen under the collarbones and just outside the nipples. Breath sounds may be normal, absent or there may be added sounds. (If you are unsure what is normal listen to your own chest with a stethoscope first and compare this with your patient.)

(P) EXAMINATION OF THE ABDOMEN

The patient should be as relaxed as possible, lying on the back, head supported by one or two pillows. The whole of the abdomen needs to be exposed. The male genitals are considered part of the abdomen, including the groin, but keep the genitalia covered (to minimise embarrassment) except when you examine them.

Look

Look at the abdomen and separately at the male genitals. If there is any suggestion of a genital disorder, gently feel for the abnormality.

Feel

Ensure your hands are warm before touching the patient. Ask first if there is pain or tenderness and start feeling the abdomen away from the region of maximum pain, gradually working towards it. The following technique for feeling the abdomen is simple but essential to follow.

The flat of the hand is placed on the abdomen (Figure 12.5). Gentle pressure is then applied with the whole of the flat of the whole hand. Repeat this process over the entire abdomen. The abdomen is normally quite soft.

You are feeling for tenderness or resistance (guarding) to your hand, caused by contraction of the abdominal wall muscles. You need to know whether guarding is local or over the entire abdomen. At its most extreme the whole abdominal wall will be rigid, like a board. This results from peritonitis, general inflammation in the abdomen. An additional and useful sign is the "rebound sign", whereby gentle pressure from the flat of the fingers into the abdomen, followed by quick release of the fingers, causes more severe pain *on release* than on pressure. This procedure should be performed only once. This again is used to detect peritonitis or evidence of abdominal irritation, for example from a perforated bowel or blood in the abdominal cavity.

The signs of guarding and tenderness are important. The technique described is the only way they can be elicited accurately. Some patients have a sensitive abdomen

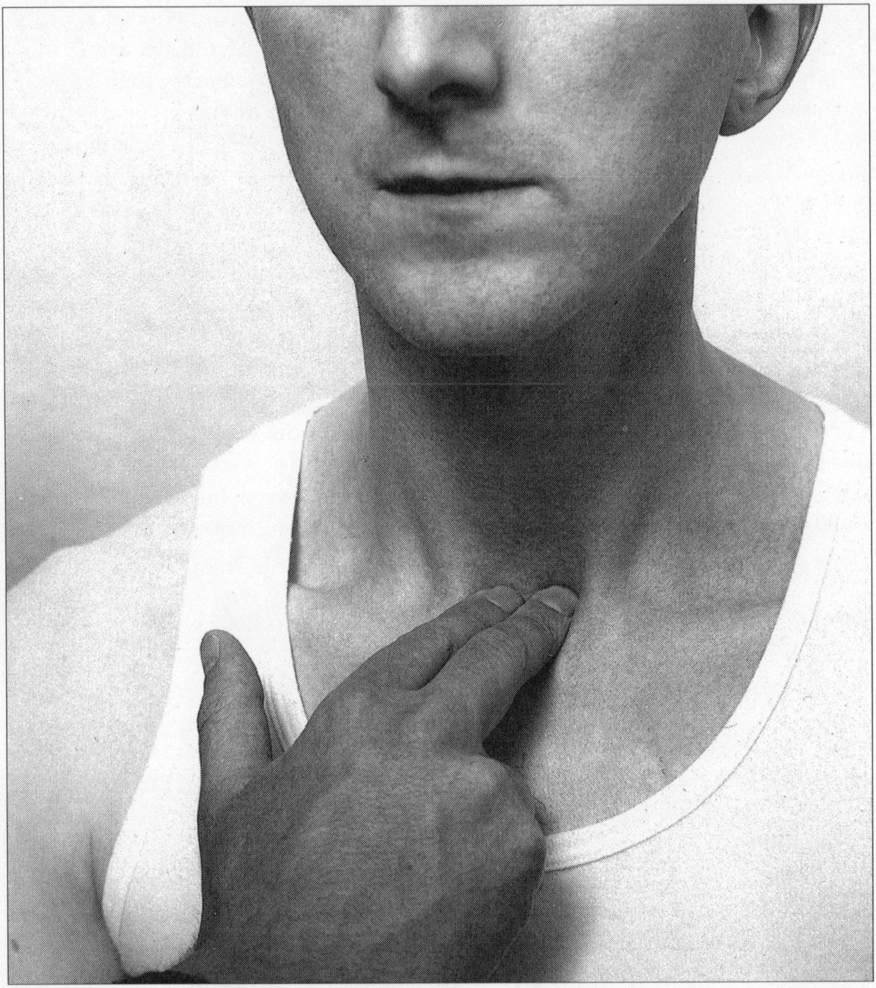

Figure 12.4 *Examining for the position of the trachea*

which demonstrates guarding at the first touch, especially if your hand is cold. Under these circumstances your examination can be helped by asking the patient to bend the knees and rest the heels on the ground. This helps relax the abdomen.

Listen for bowel sounds by placing the ear on the abdomen or placing a stethoscope firmly an inch below the belly button. The normal gut is moving all the time, which is heard as quiet gurgles, a few times a minute. Sounds are increased when the bowel is overactive, as in diarrhoea, or if the bowel is obstructed. Bowel sounds are absent in peritonitis, when the bowel is paralysed due to inflammation.

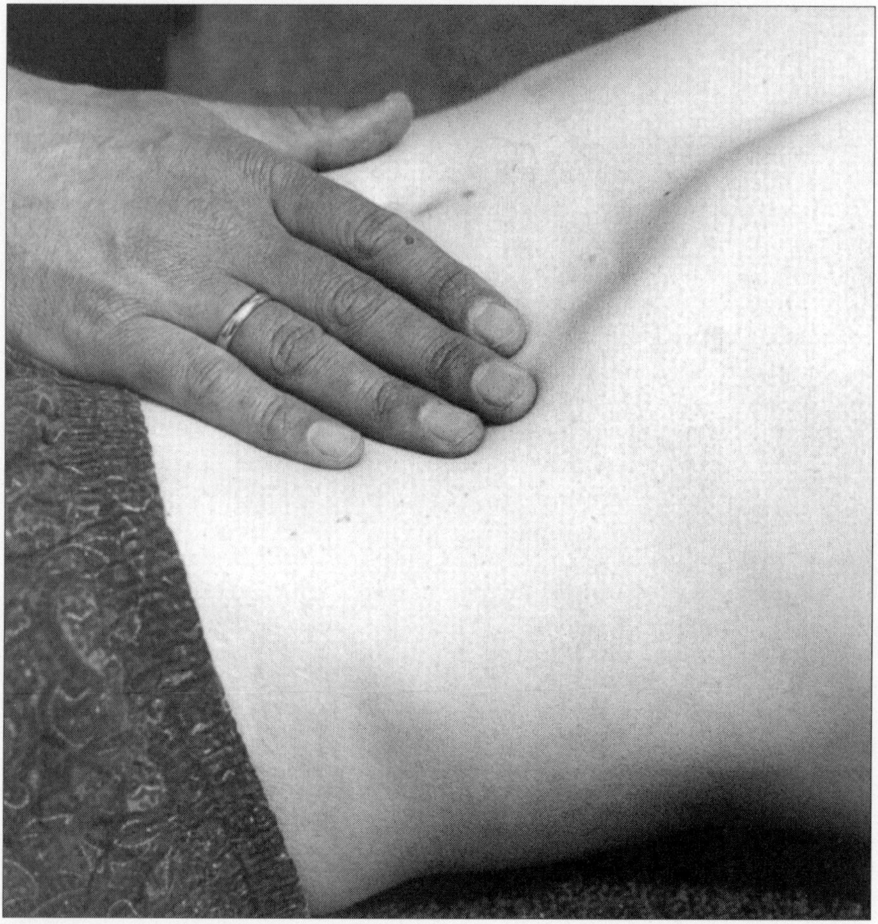

Figure 12.5 *Abdominal examination*

(Q) GENERAL EXAMINATION

Lymph glands are found in the neck, the armpits and the groin. The patient can often direct you to enlarged tender glands. If there is an infection in the area that the glands serve, they will become enlarged. They will also be tender and can be felt with the fingertips. Normally glands cannot be felt (except in the groin) and they are not tender. The tonsils can be seen at the back of the throat and are an example of a lymph gland. It is worth looking at the back of a friend's throat with a torch so that you are familiar with what a normal throat looks like.

In order to perform a good examination it is necessary to know what a normal body looks, feels and sounds like. To gain this knowledge you need to practise examining fit individuals and yourself. The skills are readily learnt and guidance from a doctor will be a great advantage

Investigations

One useful investigation is the testing of urine using a Dipstix, a multicoloured strip. The strip is dipped into the urine and examined for colour changes against a range of standard colours on the side of the container. Changes indicate the presence of substances in the urine such as blood, sugar and protein.

Monitoring of progress

It is important that you should be able to determine whether a patient is getting better, deteriorating or remaining much the same. This information is gained by relating the initial assessment to ongoing assessments.

Always monitor the patient and record your findings

Take notes on the patient's condition, remembering to include the date and time. If the patient is seriously unwell monitor them every 15 minutes. Use a vital signs chart (Figure 12.6) to record the pulse rate, temperature, breathing rate and blood pressure. The trends in these measurements are more important than isolated readings in determining how the patient is progressing.

THE ASSESSMENT OF THE UNCONSCIOUS PATIENT

Hourly head injury observations are needed if the patient:

- is unconscious, even for a short time;
- develops headache, vomiting, dizziness or visual disturbance.

Observations should be made for a minimum of 24 hours after regaining consciousness or from the resolution of all symptoms and signs.

Head injury observations

The depth of unconsciousness can quickly be determined using the mnemonic AVPU:

- **A**wake and alert
- **V**erbal – responds to voice
- **P**ain – responds to pain
- **U**nresponsive – no response to a painful stimulus

A more sensitive assessment can be made by examining three areas of basic brain function: eye opening, speech and movement. This is the basis of the **Glasgow Coma Scale** (GCS).

- **Eye opening** is assessed by the question: "When does the patient open his eyes?" Scores are: spontaneously (4), when spoken to (3), when pain is applied (2) or not at all (1).
- **Speech** is assessed by how the patient responds to the stimulus. Scores are: orientated speech (5), confused speech (4), use of inappropriate words (3), incomprehensible sounds (2) and no vocalisation (1).
- **Movement** is assessed by the patient's response to an external stimulus. Scores are: patient obeys commands to move limb (6), attempts to push away a

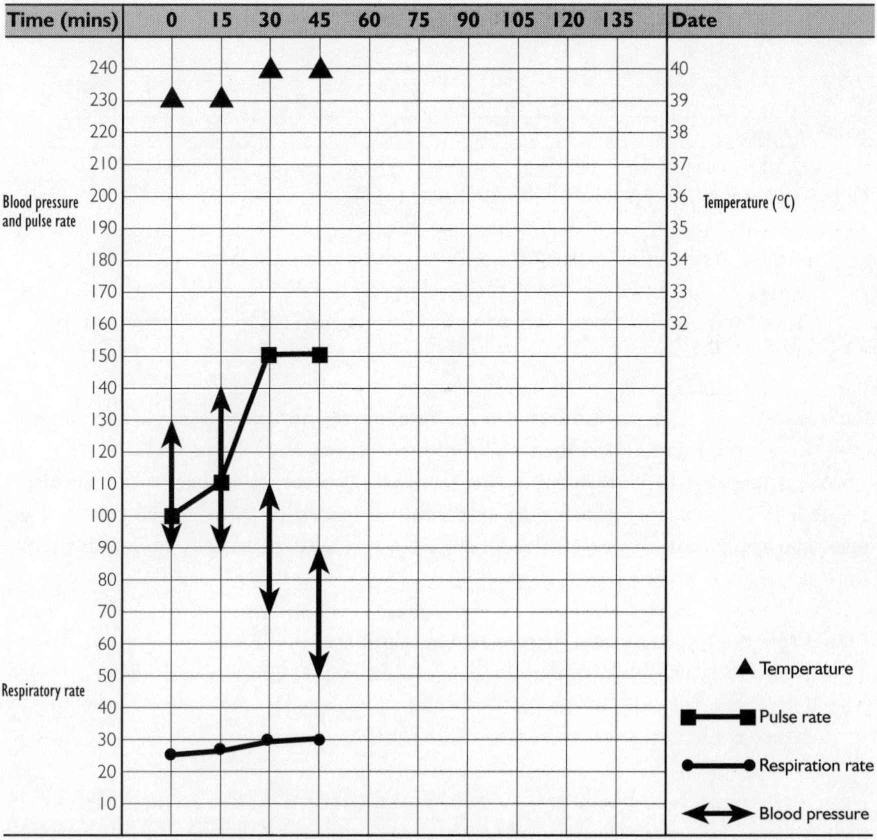

Figure 12.6 *Vital signs chart (with example data)*

Basic brain function	Level of response		Time (min) 0	15	30	45	60				
Eyes opening	4	Spontaneous									
	3	To speech									
	2	To pain	✔	✔							
	1	None									
Verbal response	5	Orientated									
	4	Confused		✔							
	3	Inappropriate words									
	2	Incomprehensible sounds	✔								
	1	None									
Motor response	6	Obeys commands									
	5	Localises to pain		✔							
	4	Flexion	✔								
	3	Abnormal flexion									
	2	Extension									
	1	None									
GCS SCORE			**8**	**11**							

Figure 12.7 *The Glasgow Coma Scale (GCS) chart*

painful stimulus (localises) (5), moves away from pain (withdraws) (4), the arms flex and the back bends forward in response to pain (flexion) (3), limbs straighten and the back arches to pain (extension) (2), no movement to pain (1).

Each response is given a number and the total score (out of 15) reflects the patient's conscious level. Figure 12.7 shows a chart for recording these responses.

When assessing these basic brain functions increase the stimulus until a response is elicited. If there is no response to speaking, squeeze the shoulder. If this gets no response apply pain in one of the following ways, taking care not to aggravate any injury:

- Press the flat of a pencil firmly against a fingernail.
- Pinch the ear lobe between finger and thumb.
- Grind the knuckles on the breast bone.
- Squeeze the tendon at the back of the heel.

Deterioration is caused by bleeding, swelling or infection of the brain, and it will be picked up early only if regular observations are made. Deterioration is indicated by the following:

1. Deepening level of unconsciousness (a decreasing total score) on the Glasgow Coma Scale.
2. One pupil, possibly followed by the other, may become large and non-reactive to light (does not constrict). Fixed, dilated pupils are a characteristic and serious sign of the brain under pressure. The pupils should be round, equal in size and react with a brisk contraction when light is shone into the eye.
3. A slowing of the pulse rate, which follows a deepening unconscious level.
4. There is little change in the breathing pattern or blood pressure until very late. Deep rattling breathing and elevation of blood pressure are grave signs.
5. Rarely the temperature may become raised above 40°C.

Any decrease in the GCS (Glasgow Coma Scale) requires rapid evacuation and medical attention

Acknowledgements
This chapter is based on a similar chapter in Milne, A. H. and Siderfin, C. D., *Kurafid: The British Antarctic Survey Medical Handbook.* It is reproduced here in a modified form with the kind permission of the British Antarctic Survey, High Cross, Madingley Road, Cambridge CB3 0ET.

13 FIRST AID AND MANAGEMENT OF MINOR INJURIES

Jon Dallimore

Serious accidents and injuries on expeditions are rare. However, minor injuries of one kind or another are encountered on most expeditions. In some cases injured expedition members need to be evacuated to medical care, but most injuries can be managed adequately in the field. First aid books are of limited use to expeditions going overseas as they place great emphasis on getting medical help which in many parts of the world may be many days' travel away. This chapter covers the following topics:

- Approach to the injured casualty
- Resuscitation
- Disorders of consciousness
- Wound care
- Wound infections
- Burns
- Bone and joint problems
- Pain management.

APPROACH TO THE INJURED CASUALTY

When approaching any injured patient, stop and think. After an accident it is vital to avoid producing other casualties. Ask yourself the question: "Am I safe?" If it is safe to approach try to avoid moving the casualty. Occasionally you will need to "scoop and run", for example if there is a danger of rock fall or avalanche. In these cases move the casualty to a safe place as carefully and quickly as possible. Particular care will be required if you suspect a back or neck injury. Using the principles of first aid assess the casualty.

TABLE 13.1 **PRINCIPLES OF FIRST AID**
• Assess the situation • Make the area safe • Assess the casualty – starting with the ABC of resuscitation – identify the injury or illness • Give easy, appropriate and adequate treatment in a sensible order of priority • Make and pass on a report • Organise removal of casualty to secondary care where appropriate

First aiders will be familiar with the following system for assessing and examining any casualties: ABCDE (Table 13.2).

TABLE 13.2 **PRINCIPLES OF RESUSCITATION**	
A	**A**ssessment of the scene
A	**A**irway with neck control
B	**B**reathing
C	**C**irculation with control of bleeding
D	**D**isability
E	**E**xposure with environment control

BASIC RESUSCITATION

Basic life support is the maintenance of breathing and circulation without the use of equipment apart from a simple airway device or a shield to protect the person being resuscitated from possible infection. The combination of (mouth-to-mouth) expired air resuscitation and chest compression is known as cardiopulmonary resuscitation (CPR). The best way to learn about CPR is to go on a first aid course (see Chapter 4). The main points are summarised here as a reminder.

Outcome of cardiopulmonary resuscitation

Survival from cardiac arrest is most likely when the collapse is witnessed, when early cardiopulmonary resuscitation is started and defibrillation (electric shock treatment of the heart) and advanced life support are started at an early stage. On an expedition, it is unlikely that advanced life support will be available. If attempts at resuscitation are not successful after 30 minutes, the chances of success are extremely low.

There are two important exceptions: where a victim has been struck by lightning or has been immersed in cold water. In these cases successful resuscitation has occurred after 2 hours or more.

Important note. If the pulse is absent (cardiac arrest) it is unlikely that the casualty will recover as a result of cardiopulmonary resuscitation alone. Once the heart has stopped beating the casualty is dead, and if your attempts to resuscitate are unsuccessful the casualty remains dead. It is important to remember this if the casualty does not recover.

Outline of resuscitation (revised guidelines 2000)

At the scene of an incident on an expedition where there appears to be an unresponsive patient:

- Stop and think.
- Do NOT put yourself in danger – ask the question "Am I safe?"
- Approach the casualty and assess the situation.
- Assess the casualty's response; say loudly: "Are you OK?" *Gently* shake the shoulders.

If the casualty responds:

- Assess and treat any injuries or medical conditions (see Chapter 12).
- Consider placing the casualty in the recovery position (Figure 13.1), but always remember that a spinal injury may be present.

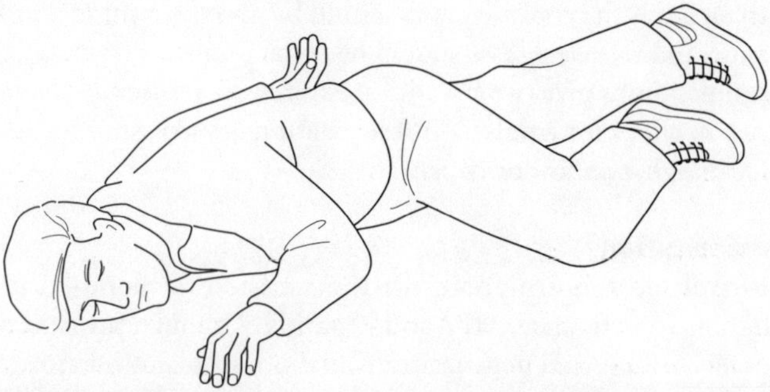

Figure 13.1 *The recovery position*

If there is no response:

- Shout for help.
- Open the airway by lifting the jaw upwards (chin lift), but avoid extending the neck more than necessary (head tilt).
- Remove any obvious obstructions in the mouth but do not poke fingers blindly into the mouth.
- Look at the chest, listen and feel if the casualty is breathing out against your cheek for 10 seconds.

If there is no breathing:

- Give two breaths of expired air resuscitation. Pinch the casualty's nostrils, take a breath, place lips over the casualty's lips and breath out steadily into the casualty's chest. This should take about 2 seconds. Watch to ensure that the chest rises. Use a protective shield if available.
- After two breaths check the carotid pulse (if trained to do so) in the neck for 10 seconds and look for other signs of circulation: choking, coughing, return of colour.

If there is no pulse or sign of circulation commence chest compressions.

- First identify the site for chest compressions: run fingers along the rib margin to the breast bone.
- Place your index and middle fingers together at this point then slide the heel of the other hand to touch above your fingers. Ensure that only the heel of the hand is in contact with the casualty.
- Interlock the fingers and leaning well over the casualty with your arms straight, press down vertically at a rate of approximately 100 compressions per minute. In an adult the compressions should be about 4–5cm in depth. Compression and release phases should be equal in time.
- After 15 compressions give two breaths of expired air resuscitation and repeat. Do not stop to check for a pulse – if resuscitation is successful the casualty will start to cough, swallow or choke.

Dangers of resuscitation

There is understandable concern about the transmission of blood-borne diseases during resuscitation – particularly HIV and hepatitis. Although viruses can be isolated from the saliva of infected persons, transmission is rare and there are only fifteen documented cases of CPR-related infection in the literature. Three cases of HIV have been reported and were acquired during resuscitation of infected patients – on two occasions from a needle-stick injury and in the third after heavy contamination of broken skin.

To minimise the risk of acquiring infection rescuers should wear gloves and use barriers whenever possible. Great care must be taken with sharp objects.

DISORDERS OF CONSCIOUSNESS

It is very worrying if someone cannot respond normally on an expedition because of an accident or illness. There are many reasons why someone may not be fully conscious; some of the commoner causes are:

- Head injuries
- Fainting
- Convulsions
- Death.

Head injuries

Head injuries are a significant risk on expeditions, particularly in mountaineering accidents, motor vehicle accidents and on building project sites. Head injuries can result in changes in conscious level, bleeding, infection and disability.

It is very important to avoid injuring the neck when moving patients after head injuries as about 10% of individuals who receive a head injury that causes unconsciousness will have an associated neck injury. Be suspicious of a neck injury in anyone who has a significant injury above the collarbones.

Minor head injuries may cause a transient loss of consciousness, but serious open head injuries are usually rapidly fatal. It is helpful to know a little more about head injuries so that decisions about the need for evacuation can be made. The following types of head injuries will be discussed:

- Closed head injuries
- Closed head injuries
  – with internal bleeding
  – with brain swelling
- Open head injuries
- Base of skull fractures.

Closed head injuries

In closed head injuries the skull remains intact and there is no communication between the brain and the outside world. Bleeding or brain swelling may complicate closed head injuries.

Closed head injuries with internal bleeding

Any head injury may result in loss of consciousness. If the head injury is serious a patient may never regain consciousness; conversely, a minor injury may result in a brief loss of consciousness with mild concussion (a temporary loss of brain function). Where bleeding inside the skull complicates a head injury, the patient may be knocked out at the time of the injury, regain consciousness (the lucid interval) and then lose consciousness again. As blood collects inside the skull it exerts pressure on the brain tissue. Increasing pressure inside the skull results in increasing coma and eventually death. The Glasgow Coma Scale describes the changes as a patient becomes more deeply unconscious (see pages 125–7).

Closed head injuries with brain swelling

During a head injury, the brain moves inside the skull and may be damaged against the bony ridges inside the base of the skull or by the impact against the inside of the skull. The greater the degree of swelling, the deeper and longer the coma is likely to be.

Open head injuries

These injuries are usually serious because there is communication between the inside of the skull and the outside world and hence the main danger is the risk of infection. A common scenario might be a large scalp laceration with an underlying skull fracture. If available, antibiotics should be given during evacuation. In severe open head injuries the skull is open with brain substance exposed. Great force is required to produce these injuries and the outcome is usually severe disability or death, even if the injury occurs near a properly equipped hospital.

Fractures of the base of the skull

These are open head injuries, because in fractures of the base of the skull infection may spread from the nose, ears or sinuses. Features of base-of-skull fractures are as follows:

- Racoon eyes – bruising around both eyes following a blow to the head
- Battle's sign – bruising behind the ear
- Cerebrospinal fluid leaking from the ears or nose.

Cerebrospinal fluid (CSF) is the straw-coloured fluid that bathes the brain and spinal cord and helps to protect them from injury. Bloodstained fluid from the ears or nose may contain blood and CSF. If the fluid is dripped onto a sheet or handkerchief, two concentric rings are formed if both blood and CSF are present. Because of the risk of infection, antibiotics should be given during evacuation.

Treatment of head injuries

All head injuries should be treated according to first aid principles:

A Assessment of the scene. Ensure that you do not endanger yourself.

A Airway with neck control. An unconscious casualty's airway is at risk as many people vomit following a head injury. The gag and cough reflexes may not function normally to clear the airway, depending on the level of unconsciousness, so it is important to place the casualty carefully in the recovery position (see Figure 13.1). A chin lift and head tilt will normally open the airway. Remember the possibility of an associated neck injury, but always give the airway priority. Try to avoid overextending the neck and stabilise the neck in a neutral position.

B Breathing. Once the airway is secure, check that breathing is adequate and measure the breathing rate.

C Circulation with control of bleeding. Look for any obvious external haemorrhage and control bleeding with direct pressure. Measure the pulse rate.

D Disability. Assess the response level using AVPU:

- **A**wake and **A**lert
- **V**oice – responds to voice
- **P**ain – responds to pain
- **U**nresponsive.

Look at the pupils and check that they constrict when a light is shone into the eye. Rising pressure inside the skull may mean that one or both pupils fail to respond to light and are fixed and dilated. This is a serious sign and means evacuation should be arranged immediately.

The Glasgow Coma Scale (see Chapter 12) allows a more comprehensive assessment of unconsciousness.

E Exposure with environment control. Examine the casualty carefully from head to toe by undressing but always be aware of the risk of hypothermia. Do not move the casualty unnecessarily.

Head injuries and the need for evacuation

When a head injury occurs in a remote place, it is often difficult to know whether you should cancel your expedition plans and head off to the nearest hospital or whether it is safe to observe a casualty in a base camp or similar.

Three groups of patients always need to be evacuated for expert medical assessment:

1. Patients who remain unconscious.
2. Patients who have open or base-of-skull fractures.
3. Patients who have had a convulsion or fit.

It is more difficult to decide whether to evacuate a conscious patient following a head injury. The following pointers may be helpful in deciding who to evacuate:

- Worsening headache
- Vomiting
- Drowsiness
- Confusion
- A dilated, unresponsive pupil on one or both sides
- Convulsions
- Blood or fluid seeping from the ears or nose
- Deep scalp lacerations
- Worsening Glasgow Coma Scale score.

It is always better to be overcautious where head injuries are concerned. If in doubt, make arrangements to evacuate the patient for assessment in a hospital.

Glasgow Coma Scale

This Scale (see Figure 12.7, page 126) helps to assess the severity of a head injury when monitoring a casualty during evacuation. The patient's GCS score is assessed in terms of eye opening and their verbal and motor responses.

Any patient should be closely observed on a regular basis, at least every hour, following a significant head injury. A decrease in the GCS score should alert you to the need for immediate evacuation.

Fainting

Fainting is not usually a serious condition and may follow severe pain, exhaustion, dehydration (for example, following a bout of diarrhoea), lack of food or an emotional upset. Faints are caused by a temporary decrease in the flow of blood to the brain. The pulse becomes very slow during a faint, unlike in shock where the pulse is rapid.

Someone who is about to faint usually becomes very pale, starts to sweat and may feel nauseated. At the first signs, encourage the patient to sit down with their head between their legs or to lie flat. If the patient loses consciousness, lay him or her flat, loosen tight clothing and elevate the legs. Usually, unconsciousness lasts only a few minutes; sometimes there are convulsive movements during the faint. After regaining consciousness the casualty should be reassured and checked for any injury that may have been sustained during the fall to the ground.

Convulsions

A fit or a seizure is caused by abnormal electrical activity in one or more parts of the brain. Fits are most commonly seen in people with epilepsy but can occur with brain infections (meningitis and encephalitis) or following head injuries. People with diabetes may fit when their blood sugar level becomes low. People with alcohol and drug problems may fit during withdrawal. If there are people with epilepsy in your expedition team it would be wise to learn more about the management of their disease.

If a fit does occur it is important to note the following:

- How long did the fit last?
- Was there loss of consciousness?
- Were all limbs involved in the convulsion?
- Was there eye rolling, salivation and incontinence?
- Was there a period of sleepiness after the fit?

During a fit, teeth may be broken and the tongue may be bitten. Sometimes vomit is breathed into the lungs leading to pneumonia or asphyxia. Injuries may occur as a result of falling at the beginning of a seizure. Prolonged fits may deprive the brain of oxygen and result in brain damage, although this is rare.

Treatment of a fit (see also Chapter 15, page 173)

- Do not restrain the person unless injury is likely.
- Open the airway with head tilt and chin lift.
- Do NOT force things between the teeth – you may break teeth or get bitten.
- Place the casualty in the recovery position (see Figure 13.1).
- If a fit occurs following a head injury, evacuate immediately.
- If meningitis appears likely treat with antibiotics and arrange evacuation. Meningitis should be suspected if a patient has a high fever, severe headache, vomiting or a stiff neck, is very sensitive to light and has a rash.

The diagnosis of death

Unfortunately, death is always a risk in a remote wilderness setting. It is therefore essential to diagnose death with certainty, particularly if a body is to be buried at sea or cremated in the mountains. Victims of hypothermia and cold water immersion injury should not be considered dead until they are warm and dead. In some cases where a body must be left behind it may be important to take photographs to establish the facts.

The signs of death are as follows:

- Unresponsiveness
- Absent heart sounds (listen with a stethoscope or your ear against the chest for 2 minutes)
- No breathing effort
- Pupils are fixed and dilated when a light is shone into them

- Later signs include rigor mortis (stiffness) and clouding of the cornea of the eyes.

WOUND CARE

Minor cuts and grazes are common on expeditions. All wounds may be managed using the following principles:

- Stop the bleeding.
- Decrease the risk of infection by cleaning.
- Dress the injury for comfort and to maintain cleanliness.
- Promote healing and restore function.

Stopping bleeding

All wounds bleed to a greater or lesser extent. In some cases, bleeding may be life threatening. As always, use first aid principles:

- Apply *direct pressure* over the wound with any available clean material or dressing.
- Lay the casualty down.
- Raise the limb above the level of the heart.
- Apply further dressings to control the bleeding on top of any original pad.
- Bandage firmly to hold dressing in place.

When there are very deep wounds it may not be possible to control bleeding by applying pressure on the surface of the skin. The only way to stop severe, persistent bleeding from deep inside a wound may be to remove the dressings, open the wound, remove clots and debris, and pack the wound open with sterile gauze. The use of artery forceps should be avoided as they may damage important structures such as tendons and nerves.

Tourniquets should be reserved for injuries where a limb has been amputated or for uncontrollable bleeding. The tourniquet should be released every 20–30 minutes otherwise tissues beyond the tourniquet will die.

Preventing infection

- Clean all wounds with an antiseptic solution.
- Remove any foreign material.
- Cover wound with a non-stick dressing.
- Bandage to hold the dressing in place.

If foreign bodies are deeply embedded and cannot be removed easily, they should be left in place for removal by a surgeon. If an object remains embedded, the surrounding wound should still be cleaned carefully and then dressed. In the UK wounds are quickly seen by a doctor or nurse; however, during an expedition it may be necessary to care for wounds for days or even weeks. Every wound should be inspected at least daily and clean dressings applied. Any pus or exudate should be gently removed but damage to healing tissues must be avoided. If dressings do stick, soaking may allow easier removal. Infection with tetanus should not be a risk for expedition wounds if all expedition members are immunised correctly prior to travel (see Chapter 2), but always check on a casualty's tetanus immunisation status.

Dressings and bandaging

The principle of wound dressing is to apply layers to the wound:

1. Non-stick sterile dressing against the wound (such as Melolin or Jelonet).
2. Sterile gauze swabs to absorb any pus or exudate from the wound.
3. Crepe bandage, Tubinet or Tubigrip to hold the dressing in place.

The bandage should hold the dressing in place without producing pressure or constriction. Bandaging techniques are taught on all first aid courses.

Promoting healing and restoration of function

Wound healing is aided by a healthy diet and rest. Any significant wound will heal more quickly with an increase in oxygen at altitudes below 3,000m. Rest is needed initially but prolonged splinting leads to stiffness and muscle wasting. Joints adjacent to a wound or burn should be kept mobile.

Methods of wound closure

A gaping wound will heal better if the skin edges are brought together. This may be accomplished with Steri-strips or sutures.

Steri-strips

Steri-strips are paper stitches which come in a variety of lengths and widths. They are placed across a laceration and, if left in place for a week or so, result in a clean, neat scar. Steri-strips are not as effective near joints, on the palms of the hands and soles of the feet, or on the scalp. However, they are excellent for finger lacerations and facial wounds. Steri-strips stick less effectively in humid or wet environments, such as the jungle or at sea. Applying Friar's Balsam to the skin may help to keep the Steri-strips in place.

Suturing (Figure 13.2)

Steri-strips should be used where possible. If Steri-strips will not close the wound, sutures will be necessary. Only clean wounds that are less than 12 hours old are suitable for suturing. Deep wounds may need to be closed in layers by a qualified surgeon. This is outside the skill of an expedition paramedic; in this case the wound should be cleaned, packed open and redressed daily. This may allow the wound to heal from the bottom upwards. Sutures should never be applied to animal or human bites, deep wounds or contaminated wounds.

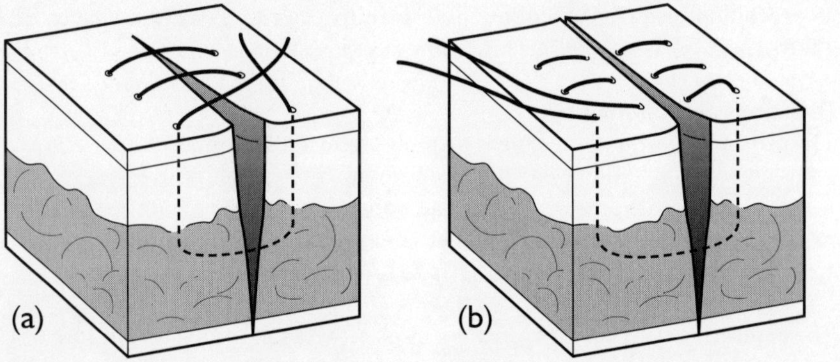

Figure 13.2 *Suturing of wounds: (a) ordinary suturing; (b) eversion suturing*

Types of wounds

Abrasions

These are grazing injuries where the top surface of the skin is removed. Abrasions should be cleaned and a non-stick dressing applied. Ingrained dirt, if not removed, will result in tattooing and makes wound infection more likely. Dressings may need to be changed once or twice daily depending on the environment. Dressings may stick and can be soaked off with clean water or saline.

Puncture wounds

Infection may occur at the base of deep, penetrating wounds. Tetanus is a risk, particularly with puncture wounds, and all expedition team members should be immunised. The skin surface should be prevented from sealing over by placing a small wick into the wound. This allows healing to occur from the bottom of a puncture wound upwards, otherwise abscess formation may occur.

Blisters

Blisters are best prevented. All group members should be encouraged to stop walking and to cover "hot spots" before they develop into blisters. If a blister does develop, the fluid should be drained using a clean (sterile) needle and then the area covered with an adhesive plaster or Moleskin. Compeed and Spenco are alternative dressings. Blisters may become de-roofed; in this case treat as a graze with a non-adherent dressing. A thin application of Friar's Balsam at the edge of a blister may help the dressing to stay in place. Healing is rapid if friction at the blister site can be eliminated. Leaving the blister uncovered, where possible, will assist healing by allowing the area to dry out.

Bruises

Contusions or bruises are usually caused by a direct blow to the skin surface. Bleeding under the skin gives the bruise its characteristic appearance. Rest, ice, compression and elevation (RICE) all help to reduce swelling and pain. Compression may be achieved by applying a crepe bandage firmly around the affected area. Anti-inflammatory drugs such as ibuprofen or aspirin may also help. After a day or two the affected part should be mobilised to reduce stiffness. A subungual haematoma (a blood blister beneath the finger nail) can be easily treated by melting a hole through the nail using an opened paper clip heated to red heat in a flame. This is surprisingly painless and gives immediate relief.

Crush injuries

Large amounts of tissue may be damaged in crushing injuries and the potential for infection is high. The crushed part should be carefully cleaned and then elevated. Swelling in the affected part may cut off the blood supply to the limb beyond the injury. If the injury is severe there may be a risk of losing the limb and it is important to evacuate the casualty for medical assessment.

Amputation

A digit or limb may be replaced by microsurgery if the patient and the amputated part can be delivered to a surgeon in less than 6 hours. The amputated part should be kept cool, preferably in a container with ice, but not in direct contact with the ice. In an expedition setting it is highly unlikely that such surgical facilities will be available; in this case, treat the bleeding with direct pressure and elevation. The stump should be cleaned gently and then covered with a non-adherent dressing such as paraffin gauze. People with these injuries need to be evacuated to allow surgical treatment to shorten any bone ends and cover the stump with a flap of skin so that healing can take place.

Impalement

An impaled object protruding from a wound should be left in place. Removing an impaled object may cause further damage and therefore should be done in a suitably equipped hospital. Large objects, such as arrows or fence posts, may need to be stabilised and carefully cut to allow evacuation. Pain relief will be required.

Wounds causing particular problems

Deep wounds

In a deep wound underlying structures, for example arteries, nerves, tendons and muscles, may be damaged. It is important to assess:

- Movement: the patient should be asked to move the affected part through the full normal range.
- Circulation: check by feeling for pulses and look for capillary refill (see below).
- Sensation: check beyond the level of the injury.

To check for capillary refill press firmly over a fingernail or bony prominence for 5 seconds to produce blanching. When the pressure is released the colour should begin to return quickly (in less than 2 seconds), otherwise indicating the patient to be extremely cold or shocked, or that the blood supply to the limb is interrupted. If the blood supply to a limb is completely interrupted it will be painful, pulseless, pale and cold. Surgical treatment is required within a few hours to salvage the limb. Deep wounds are also prone to infection. They should be cleaned carefully and packed open so that the wound can heal from the bottom upwards. Dressings should be changed daily until the wound can be dealt with surgically.

Neck wounds

Injuries to the neck may be associated with damage to important underlying structures such as blood vessels, nerves and the airway. Neck wounds should be cleaned carefully but never probed. Unless the wound is clearly superficial it should be assessed medically. Bandages should never be placed around the neck as subsequent swelling may compromise the airway.

Flaps

Flap wounds are caused by slicing injuries, for example with machetes on expeditions. Proximal structures are those near to the trunk; distal structures are those further away. In a proximal flap the point of attachment of the flap of skin is towards the trunk. Since arteries travel away from the heart, proximal flaps have a reasonable blood supply. Conversely, in a distal flap the point of attachment of the skin lies distal to the rest of the wound. The blood supply is therefore poor and so the skin overlying distal flaps often becomes infected and dies.

When managing a flap wound:

- Turn the skin flap back and clean underneath.
- Snip away small pieces of dead tissue with sterile scissors.
- Apply a non-stick dressing around the edges of the wound, under the flap. This stops the wound from sealing and allows exudate to drain away.

It is important to let a flap wound heal from its base to its tip. Distal flaps usually become dusky and either dry out and go black or become infected. Patients with such flaps need to be evacuated for surgical treatment and usually require skin grafting. Treated properly, however, proximal flaps often heal well without infection. Flap wounds need to be re-dressed daily and a little less non-stick dressing applied each day so as to allow the flap to heal. Flap wounds should not be closed with sutures.

Contaminated wounds

Wounds are very likely to become contaminated in some environments such as the jungle. Wounds should be cleaned carefully to remove any foreign material that might form a focus for infection. Painkillers given half an hour before scrubbing out a wound may decrease pain during the procedure; alternatively, an injection of local anaesthetic may make the task of cleaning the wound easier if someone is available to administer it. Debris can be flushed out of the wound using sterile saline. Contaminated wounds should not be sutured closed. It is better to let the wound heal from the bottom upwards by packing the wound open and changing dressings daily. Oral antibiotics may be necessary if wounds are very deep or contaminated, particularly if there are signs of infection (see below). These wounds should heal but there may be scarring.

Hand and foot wounds

Wound complications in the hands or feet may result in crippling deformity. Any significant foot wound will not heal while an expedition member continues to walk around, so rest is imperative. Wounds should be treated by cleaning, careful assessment of movement, circulation and sensation, and then rest in the position of function. In the case of the hand, this means bandaging the hand with a sock or a crepe bandage initially, followed by gentle mobilisation. It should never be splinted with the hand and fingers straight, since if there is any stiffness after the injury the hand will be useless. Infections in the hands or feet can be devastating. If there is any suspicion of infection antibiotics should be started sooner rather than later (flucloxacillin or erythromycin).

Facial wounds

Facial wounds usually heal quickly and with little infection. They should be cleaned, closed using Steri-strips rather than sutures where possible, and dressed as usual.

Eye abrasions

Corneal abrasions can be caused by the removal of part or all of the top surface of the transparent cornea. This may be caused by a foreign body such as a contact lens, which may or may not leave a remnant in the eye. These abrasions can be extremely painful and visually debilitating. Immediate relief and some restoration of vision can be achieved with a drop of amethocaine, which can be repeated but should not be used in excess. If the patient is in safe surroundings, a drop of tropicamide and chloramphenicol ointment can be applied and the eye should then be firmly padded, taking care that the lids are closed beneath the pad. Even a total removal of the corneal top layer should heal within 36 hours. If not, further specialised attention should be sought to exclude an infection or retained foreign body.

Bites

Animal and human bites almost invariably become infected. Wounds should be cleaned very carefully and any dead tissue snipped away with a pair of sterile scissors. As these wounds are likely to become infected it is sensible to use antibiotics (co-amoxiclav or Augmentin) prophylactically (see also Chapter 20).

Scalp wounds

The scalp has a very good blood supply and lacerations usually bleed copiously. Bleeding should be stopped with direct pressure. The skin edges may be brought together by tying the hair together, by using surgical "superglue" (for example Histoacryl) or by suturing the skin edges.

Foreign bodies

Foreign bodies in the eye

The patient is usually sure that something has gone into the eye. Check the surface of the eye carefully by asking the casualty to look in all directions. It may be possible to see the offending object and to remove it with a moistened cotton bud. However, often the foreign body is under the upper lid or there is too much spasm of the eyelid muscle to allow a good view. A couple of drops of local anaesthetic (amethocaine drops) will produce numbness after momentary stinging. It should then be possible to examine the eye more easily and evert the cartilagenous tarsal plate of the upper lid to check for a foreign body. To evert the lid ask the patient to look downwards. Grasp the upper eye lashes firmly while applying a cotton bud or match-stick to the skin crease of the upper lid. Push down with the cotton bud while lifting the eyelashes upwards with the other hand. This should provide a good view of the underside of the upper lid. Any foreign body can then be removed. If the foreign body cannot be removed easily the patient should be assessed by a doctor or nurse. Relief is usually instant and dramatic but the foreign body may have left an abrasion that can feel like a persistent foreign body. The treatment of an abrasion is described on page 143.

Foreign bodies in the ear

Insects and ticks may crawl into the ear on expeditions. This may be very frightening for the individual. Water or oil should be poured into the ear. This will kill the insect and may allow it to float out. Avoid using instruments to try to remove foreign bodies in the ear as they may cause damage.

Splinters

Splinters can usually be removed using a fine pair of tweezers (the ones on Swiss Army knives are good) or a sterile needle. For more stubborn splinters, soaking may help. Spines from sea urchins are easier to remove after a couple of days when the wound becomes inflamed, or after softening the skin by soaking or applying salicylic acid ointment.

Wound infections

Any wound can become infected. However, certain wounds, particularly bites, contaminated wounds and deep wounds, are more likely to become infected. Signs and symptoms of wound infection are pain, redness, heat, swelling and loss of function. In the later stages, red lines may be seen running from a limb wound up towards the body. Lymph nodes in the armpit, groin or neck may become enlarged and fever may develop.

Abscesses

An abscess is a collection of pus. Even small collections of pus around the fingernails or toenails (whitlows) are extremely painful and debilitating. As pus accumulates, the skin over the abscess thins; this is referred to as pointing. Once the pus discharges through a breach in the thinned skin the pain, which is usually described as throbbing, rapidly resolves. If an abscess develops during an expedition, local heat and oral antibiotics (for example, flucloxacillin) may help. However, once pus is present it may be quicker and kinder to drain it. The skin may be numbed by applying ice, and then a swift crescent-shaped cut in the skin will produce a large enough hole to let the pus drain. A small piece of gauze soaked in saline inserted into the incision will act as a wick and stop the roof of the abscess healing over before all the pus has drained. In this way the abscess cavity will heal from the bottom upwards. The wick should be changed daily until the abscess has healed.

Cellulitis

Cellulitis means infection of the skin. There may not be an obvious source of infection but the signs are the same as for a wound infection, i.e. redness, heat, pain and swelling. Treatment with antibiotics for streptococci or staphylococci will be necessary (amoxicillin plus high-dose flucloxacillin, or erythromycin).

BURNS

Burns may be caused by dry heat, chemicals, friction or hot liquids. On expeditions open fires and fuel stoves commonly cause injuries, particularly when people refuel lighted stoves or burn rubbish with petrol.

Classification of burns

Burns may be divided into superficial, partial-thickness and full-thickness burns.

- Superficial burns: characterised by redness, swelling and tenderness; for example, mild sunburn or a scald from hot water.
- Partial-thickness burns: characterised by painful, red, raw skin and blisters.
- Full-thickness burns: characterised by pale, waxy and sometimes charred skin with a loss of sensation.

On an expedition it is important to differentiate between partial-thickness and full-thickness burns. Full-thickness burns need skin grafting so evacuation to medical help will be necessary.

Extent of burns

The "rule of nines", which divides the surface area of the body into areas of approximately 9%, is used to calculate the proportion of the body that is burned and so helps determine treatment (Figure 13.3). It may be easier to remember that the patient's palm and outstretched fingers constitute approximately 1% of the body surface area. The severity of burns is often underestimated, even by doctors and nurses, and extensive burns need specialist assessment and treatment.

Treatment of burns and scalds on an expedition

The usual first aid aims of caring for a burned patient are to:

- halt the burning process and relieve pain;
- resuscitate if necessary;
- treat associated injuries;
- minimise the risk of infection;
- arrange urgent removal to hospital.

In practical terms, to treat a burned patient:

- Resuscitate as appropriate, following ABC guidelines.
- Lie the casualty down.
- Douse the burn with copious amounts of cold water.
- Clean the burn carefully, leaving any adherent burnt clothing, etc., on the skin.
- Drain large blisters, as appropriate, by inserting a sterile needle at the edge of the blister, although the skin should not be removed.

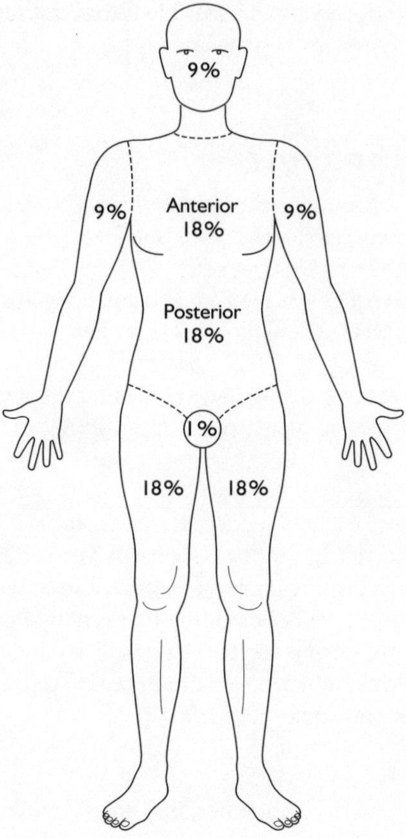

Figure 13.3 *"Rule of nines", a method to help assess the percentage of body surface burnt (a patient's palm is approximately 1% of body surface area)*

- Apply Flamazine cream (silver sulphadiazine) or Bactroban cream as an antiseptic.
- Dress with a protective layer, such as plastic kitchen Clingfilm or a polythene glove for a hand burn.

Dressings should be changed every one or two days as necessary, remembering that each dressing change increases the likelihood of infection.

Sunburn

Sunburn, like blisters, should be avoided. Young people particularly try to get a suntan on the first day of an expedition and thus end up with sunburn. Graded exposure to the sun, high-factor sun creams and sensible use of clothing should prevent sunburn. Once sunburn occurs, hydrocortisone cream or calamine lotion may relieve the discomfort of mild conditions.

BONE AND JOINT PROBLEMS

Fractures

Fractures may be classified as follows:

- Simple fractures, where there is a single, clean, bony break.
- Comminuted fractures, where the bone is broken into more than two fragments.
- Open or closed fractures, depending on whether the skin is breached.
- Complicated fractures, if other tissues are involved.

Diagnosis of fracture

A fracture is suggested by pain and tenderness at the site of injury, swelling, bruising or discoloration, deformity and grating (crepitus). The last sign usually confirms a fracture. Pain, tenderness, bruising and swelling can also be seen in sprains and other soft-tissue injuries. However, loss of limb function usually, but not always, suggests a fracture. In an expedition setting where X-ray facilities are not available, treat as a fracture if uncertain. Evacuation can sometimes be delayed until the exact nature of the injury becomes more obvious.

Treatment of fractures

Alignment of the bone ends at a fracture site to enable healing requires *immobilisation*, which prevents further damage, reduces pain and decreases the risk of shock. This cannot always be obtained in the field.

Many things can be used to improvise splints for immobilisation:

- Karrimat
- Sleeping bags
- Inflatable splints
- Trekking poles
- Skis
- Triangular bandages
- Canoe paddles
- Purpose-built splints such as Frakstraps.

When splinting any fracture, bony prominences must be padded and the joints above and below the fracture immobilised. It may be necessary to straighten the limb

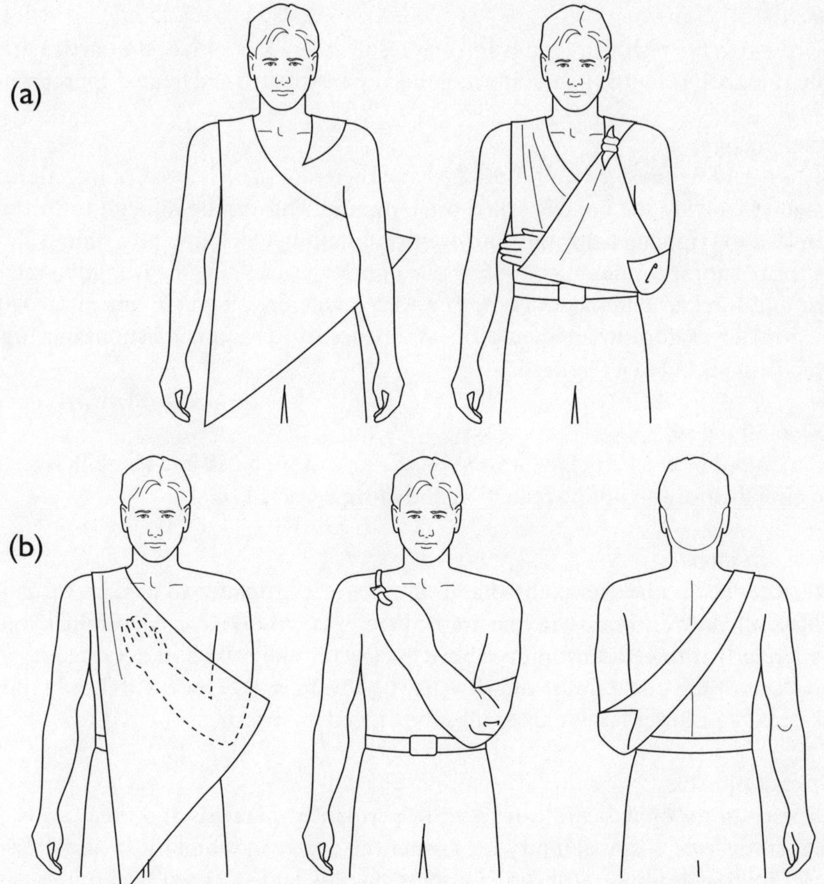

Figure 13.4 *(a) The broad arm sling for arm and forearm injuries. (b) The high arm sling for hand injuries, infections and dislocated shoulders*

in order to apply a splint, to relieve pressure on a blood vessel or to allow transfer on to a stretcher. Straightening the limb (reduction) is painful but rarely causes increased damage. Reduction requires strong traction/counter-traction in the long axis of the limb and is more readily done soon after the injury, before severe muscle spasm occurs. If there is no pulse beyond a fracture site the limb must be manipulated urgently into a position to restore the blood supply to the limb. Signs of an interrupted blood supply are absent pulses with pale, cold skin and severe pain. Movement, circulation and sensation should be checked both before and after any manipulation or movement.

Bleeding

Bleeding occurs with all fractures and may result in shock or even death, particularly in fractures of the thigh or pelvis. Shock should be anticipated and treated appropriately.

Open fractures

In an open fracture the skin is breached and therefore there is a risk of infection. Infection involving the bone is called osteomyelitis. This can be difficult to treat and can lead to crippling deformity and even amputation. Open fractures should always be treated as for contaminated soft-tissue injuries, by cleaning the wound to remove grit and foreign material and covering with sterile dressings. Co-amoxiclav (Augmentin) or erythromycin should be commenced to prevent infection and urgent evacuation should be arranged.

Pain relief

Pain caused by fractures is decreased by effective immobilisation. Painkillers should be given before attempting reduction and during evacuation.

Transportation

Fractures should be immobilised and other injuries attended to before evacuation, unless there are hazards in the immediate area. Always consider spinal injury, particularly if there is any injury above the level of the collarbones. Casualties with fractures of the upper limbs and ribs may be able to walk. Those with head injuries, back, neck or lower limb injuries must be carried by stretcher.

Spinal injuries

Damage to the spinal cord can result in permanent paralysis and even death. The higher the level of spinal injury the greater the degree of disability. In about 10% of head injuries leading to unconsciousness there is an associated neck injury so all casualties with significant head injuries should be treated as if they have an unstable neck fracture. Spinal injury should be suspected if there is neck or back pain or pain radiating around to the front of the body. On examining the casualty there may be a "step" or swelling along the vertebral column, or loss of sensation, weakness or paralysis. In males erection of the penis may occur (priapism). Remember the spinal cord may not be damaged initially even with a spinal fracture; however, moving an unstable spine may damage the spinal cord and result in permanent paralysis. All casualties at risk of spinal injury should therefore be moved with the spine "in line" as if they have an unstable spine. Movement, circulation and sensation should be assessed before moving the victim, unless the danger of further injury necessitates a scoop-and-run approach. For details on stabilising neck injuries and log-rolling patients see Chapter 14.

Patients with a suspected spinal injury should be evacuated by helicopter; how-

TABLE 13.3 MANAGEMENT OF SPECIFIC FRACTURES

Hand and fingers	Bandage in a fist around a rolled-up sock and elevate in a sling (i.e. splint the hand in the position of function)
Forearm	Splint the wrist straight and the elbow at 90°
Elbow/upper arm/ shoulder	Use a broad arm sling with a swathe around the body to reduce movement
Collar bone	Use a broad arm sling
Foot and toes	Often well-splinted in a boot. Watch for numbness and swelling. It may be necessary to cut the boot off if swelling occurs
Ankles	Immobilise the foot and knee. Assisted walking may be possible
Lower leg/knee	Immobilise foot, ankle and knee
Thigh/hip	Traction is desirable as the bone ends often override damaging the surrounding tissues. Splint both legs together or use a traction splint. In hip fractures there is characteristic shortening and external rotation on the affected side
Pelvis	Treat as for a fractured thigh. ***Pelvic fractures are associated with severe bleeding and damage to internal organs. Suspect if pressure on the pelvis leads to pain.*** Bind the legs together to prevent further movement of pelvic fragments

ever, if this is not possible every effort should be made to immobilise the neck and back completely. Patients who do not have normal sensation can quickly develop pressure sores so stretchers should be well padded. The patient will require regular and careful changes of position.

Dislocations and other injuries

A dislocation interrupts the normal relationships of a joint. The bone may be forced out of its socket (for example, shoulder, hip and elbow dislocations) or the joint surfaces may simply be displaced (for example, finger dislocations). Fractures, nerve and blood vessel injuries may be associated with dislocations.

Dislocations cause pain which is aggravated by movement, tenderness, swelling, discoloration, limitation of movement and deformity. The injured limb should be compared with the non-injured limb. Correction of dislocations can be technically

TABLE 13.4 SPECIFIC DISLOCATIONS

Fingers	Finger dislocations can usually be reduced easily Splint to the next finger, i.e. "buddy strapping", after reduction
Thumb	Often associated with a fracture, best management is immobilisation in the position of function
Elbow	Reduce elbow dislocations as quickly as possible As with all fractures and dislocations, check the pulse and sensation before and after reduction as nerves and blood vessels can easily be damaged. Considerable force may be required and, if the pulse is not restored, try again. Splint the elbow at 90°
Shoulder	Diagnosis is suggested by squaring of the shoulder joint, the arm is often rotated outwards and held away from the trunk. To reduce: – Bend the elbow to 90°. – Hold the elbow at the patient's side very gently and slowly move the arm outwards Immobilise the arm in a sling for 2 weeks
Knee	Major dislocations of the knee realign readily – because of severe damage to the ligaments Kneecap dislocations can be reduced by straightening the leg and pushing the kneecap back into position Immobilise as for a fracture
Jaw	If the jaw is locked open, it is dislocated Wear gloves and pad the thumbs to avoid injury as the person will bite involuntarily Place the thumbs over the victim's lower molars and press directly downwards Considerable force may be required

difficult as nerves and blood vessels can be damaged during reduction. However, attempts to correct the deformity are justified in certain circumstances, particularly in remote areas. For example, if the blood supply to the distal part of the limb is compromised by a dislocation, reduction must be attempted. This should be done as soon as possible after the injury because of increasing muscle spasm.

- Steady, firm traction along the limb's long axis should be applied to attempt to correct the deformity and to improve the blood supply. After reduction the limb should be splinted as for a fracture.

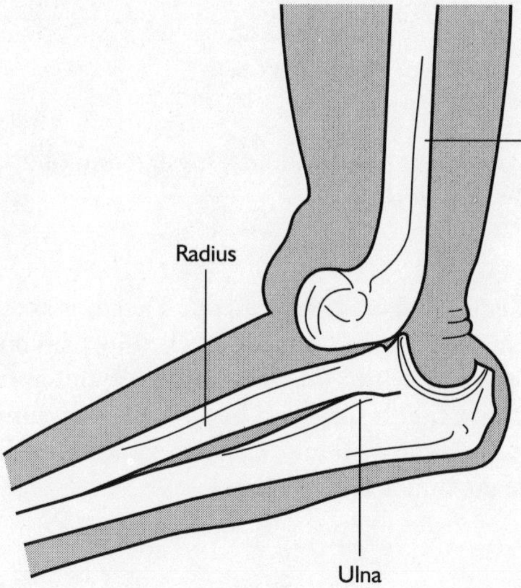

Figure 13.5 *Dislocation of the elbow*

Other injuries of bone and related injuries

Subperiosteal haematoma

A direct blow to a bone may damage the tissue, the periosteum, covering the bone. Bleeding underneath the periosteum produces a subperiosteal haematoma. This is a very painful injury, commonly seen on the shin; the area is often exquisitely tender with some swelling. Treatment consists of elevation, cold packs and anti-inflammatory drugs. If a fracture cannot be confidently excluded, treat the injury as a fracture.

Sprains and strains

These are tearing or stretching injuries of ligaments and tendons around a joint which can be associated with a great deal of swelling and bruising. The injury may impair function as seriously as a fracture or a dislocation. Treatment consists of **rest**, **ice**, **compression** and **elevation** (RICE – see Bruises, page 141). Immobilisation with a plaster of Paris backslab or splinting will improve pain.

Muscle and tendon tears

Muscles may be torn from their attachments by a sudden, strong force or by penetrating injuries. A complete tear will result in loss of muscle function and a partial tear will produce weakness.

Common sites of muscle/tendon tears are:

- Fingertip (mallet finger)

- Shoulder
- Achilles' tendon
- Thigh.

Treatment consists of rest, ice, compression, bandaging and immobilisation. Evacuation for surgical repair may be necessary.

Tenosynovitis

Tenosynovitis is inflammation of the sheaths that surround tendons and is caused by overuse or penetrating injury. The diagnosis is made by eliciting pain on movement of the involved tendon. If the cause is overuse, treat with rest and anti-inflammatories (such as ibuprofen). If infection is suggested by a history of trauma and there is painful movement with redness and swelling, antibiotics and immediate evacuation may be necessary to save the function of the limb.

Joint effusion

Swelling around joints, particularly the knee and elbow, occurs commonly following injury. Treatment consists of elevation, rest, support bandaging and anti-inflammatory drugs.

PAIN MANAGEMENT

A person's response to pain is subjective and is influenced by factors such as fear, anxiety, fatigue, extreme cold or heat, and the responses of those nearby. Since these factors are important in the perception of pain, much can be done to make a patient in pain more comfortable, even if an expedition is carrying very few drugs. Reassurance, shelter, warmth, splinting of fractures, relief of skin pressure by careful turning, adequate food and fluids, and rest will all help to relieve pain.

Severe pain may be associated with nausea. The control of associated symptoms such as nausea and vomiting with antisickness drugs (such as prochlorperazine, Stemetil) will, in itself, promote rest and improve pain.

The treatment of pain

The treatment of pain requires an assessment by taking a history and doing a physical examination to ascertain the likely cause of the pain. The best therapy for pain is to treat the underlying cause. Where this is not possible, a simple stepwise approach using a limited number of drugs should control pain in the majority of cases.

The following features of the pain may be helpful in reaching a diagnosis:

- When did the pain start? Was there an injury?
- Where is the main site of the pain and does it move anywhere else?

- What makes the pain worse or better?
- Is it constant or intermittent?
- What is the character of the pain, for example, burning, crushing, dull, sharp, etc?
- Are there any other associated symptoms, for example, nausea, diarrhoea or vomiting?

Painkilling drugs

Painkillers can be divided into three groups: simple painkillers, moderate-strength painkillers and strong painkillers. Expedition groups should have with them one or two simple painkillers, such as paracetamol or aspirin, and one or two moderate painkillers, such as dihydrocodeine or ibuprofen. Many groups choose not to carry strong painkillers, such as nalbuphine, tramadol and morphine.

Pain caused by an accident or injury should initially be treated with a simple painkiller given regularly, i.e. given by the clock rather than waiting until the pain returns. However, for a headache, it is sufficient to take a dose of a painkiller and then wait and see if the pain returns. If pain caused by an injury is not controlled by a regular, simple painkiller, then a moderate painkiller should be taken, again regularly and at the recommended dose. Pain caused by severe injury may require strong painkillers. The same principles of regular administration apply, but the dose may also need to be increased until pain is controlled.

Simple painkillers

Paracetamol

This can be taken for mild-to-moderate pain and fever. Side-effects are rare and the dose is two tablets (1g) 4–6 hourly (no more than eight tablets in 24 hours).

Aspirin

Aspirin is good for mild-to-moderate pain and fever. It is a good painkiller and an anti-inflammatory drug, but some people are allergic to it and it may cause stomach irritation. The dose is one to three tablets (300–900mg) 4–6 hourly (no more than 4g in 24 hours).

Ibuprofen (Nurofen, Brufen)

Ibuprofen is an anti-inflammatory drug that is useful in the treatment of muscle and joint pains, period pains and where pain is associated with inflammation. It can be taken in combination with paracetamol or weak or strong painkillers. However, it should not be given with aspirin or to patients with an aspirin allergy or a history of peptic ulcers. Side-effects are indigestion, heartburn and nausea. In some individuals asthma may be made worse. It should be taken with food and the dose is 400mg every 8 hours.

Minims Amethocaine (Amethocaine hydrochloride 0.5%)
One drop gives about 20 minutes of pain relief, suitable for the examination and management of a painful eye e.g. ocular abrasion, snowblindness or a foreign body in the eye. It is available in 10ml bottle or 0.5ml Minims.

Moderate-strength painkillers
Dihydrocodeine (DF118)
This can be taken for moderate pain. Side-effects are constipation, nausea and drowsiness. The dose is one tablet (30mg) three to four times a day.

Tramadol (Zydol)
Tramadol is used for moderate-to-severe pain. It can cause nausea, vomiting, dry mouth, drowsiness and a rash. It should not be taken with alcohol and should not be given after head injuries or to people with epilepsy as it may precipitate fitting. The dose is one to two tablets (50–100mg) 4–6 hourly, maximum eight tablets a day. It can also be given as an injection (50–100mg, 4–6 hourly).

Strong painkillers
Morphine
Morphine, an opiate, is a strong painkiller with potent sedative side-effects. Together these effects relieve pain and may help relieve anxiety following an accident or in serious illness. Morphine is a controlled drug and is difficult, but not impossible, to obtain and export for expedition use. As it causes sedation, it should not be given to any patient with a significant head injury. Morphine also depresses respiratory function and should be used with great caution in patients with chest injuries. It may cause nausea and vomiting and it is wise to give morphine with an antisickness drug, such as prochlorperazine, which can be given by mouth, by suppository or by injection. Morphine is very constipating. It should be given every 4 hours and the dose depends on the patient and the severity of the pain; however, a range of 5–15mg intramuscularly is usual. All opiates can cause drug dependence given over a prolonged period. This is not a problem for short-term use to relieve the pain of an injury. Morphine may also be given by mouth and by slow intravenous injection.

Nalbuphine (Nubain)
Nalbuphine is a strong painkiller but is not subject to the legal restrictions covering drugs such as morphine or pethidine. It is therefore more appropriate for most expeditions. Its side-effects are similar to morphine. Nalbuphine is given by injection subcutaneously, intramuscularly or intravenously. The dose is 10–20mg for a 70-kg patient every 3–6 hours.

Buprenorphine (Temgesic)

This drug is similar to morphine, although less potent, but is administered by placing a tablet under the tongue. It is also a controlled drug but the mode of administration may be easier in some cases. Other precautions and side-effects are as for morphine. Buprenorphine makes many individuals very nauseated and a drug such as prochlorperazine may need to be given with it. The dose is one to two tablets (200–400 micrograms) under the tongue 6–8 hourly.

If strong painkillers are necessary to relieve pain in an injured casualty, the doses used and the time they were given should be recorded and this information handed on when the patient is evacuated. If a group decides not to carry strong painkillers, a severely injured casualty can still be managed with weak painkillers and the comfort measures noted above; information and the presence of a competent, reassuring companion will be particularly helpful.

SUMMARY

Minor accidents and injuries do occur on expeditions, but with knowledge and a reasonable medical kit most should be treatable in the field and should not impair the enjoyment of the expedition. The expedition medical officer has a responsibility to consider when an accident or injury requires more expert help and to arrange for the patient's evacuation to a place of safety and competent care.

Acknowledgements

The author is indebted to Dr Karen Forbes, Macmillan Consultant Senior Lecturer in Palliative Medicine at Bristol University, for her advice on pain control.

14 MANAGEMENT OF THE SERIOUSLY INJURED CASUALTY

Stephen Hearns

Trauma is a leading cause of death and serious injury on expeditions. Major trauma is predominantly caused by road traffic accidents and falls. It is important to remember the limitations of medical care in a remote environment. One of the main factors that aids survival in victims of serious trauma is early access to definitive care, i.e. surgery and intensive care facilities. Once basic resuscitation and management of the casualty's airway, breathing and circulation are under way, rapid evacuation is essential. This chapter is largely intended for medically trained professionals.

THE APPROACH TO THE SERIOUSLY INJURED CASUALTY

When approaching a seriously injured casualty follow the principles of first aid as outlined in Chapter 13 (page 130, Table 13.1). Firstly, check that the incident scene is safe. This is especially important in the case of road traffic accidents, rock falls and avalanches. An injury sustained by a rescuer simply compounds the situation.

The casualty should be approached using the "ABC" principle. This is known as the *primary survey*. The **a**irway should be assessed and maintained with cervical spine immobilisation. Following this, the casualty's **b**reathing and **c**irculation should be assessed. Managing the casualty in this sequence ensures that the most life-threatening problems are addressed first. For example, casualties will die from an obstructed airway before they would from a collapsed lung. This ABC approach also ensures that the ultimate aim of resuscitation is achieved, i.e. the supply of oxygenated blood to the vital organs.

Primary survey

Airway

The airway can be obstructed in the trauma casualty for a number of reasons. These include facial fractures, swelling, blood and foreign bodies such as dislodged teeth. If the patient is unconscious, lack of muscle tone will cause the tongue to fall against the back of the throat, blocking the airway.

Assessment of the airway is relatively simple. If the patient is talking normally, the airway can be assumed to be normal. If the patient is not talking, ask them to stick their tongue out. Again, if they can do this, the airway will usually be clear. If they can't do this, the signs of airway obstruction should be looked for.

TABLE 14.1 SIGNS OF AIRWAY OBSTRUCTION

- Distress
- Cyanosis (blueness)
- Noisy breathing – gurgling
- Stridor – a rasping sound on inspiration

If the airway is obstructed, a jaw-thrust manoeuvre should be carried out. This pushes the jaw forwards and hence pushes the tongue away from the back of the throat. The jaw-thrust manoeuvre is carried out by placing both thumbs on the patient's cheekbones and the index fingers behind the angles of the jaw. The index fingers are then pushed forwards. The chin-lift technique is not appropriate for trauma situations as it involves moving the neck, which may cause a spinal cord injury.

Foreign bodies that can be clearly seen in the mouth should be removed. Blind finger sweeps should be avoided, as they tend to push the foreign body further down.

If the casualty carer has been trained to use oropharyngeal or nasopharyngeal airways, these may be used to aid airway maintenance. Remember that, although these devices may open the airway, they do not protect it from regurgitated stomach contents. Regurgitated stomach contents, if inhaled, can cause serious lung damage. If stomach contents are being regurgitated or if there is bleeding in the mouth, the patient should be rolled on to their side. This should be carried out with maintenance of in-line spinal immobilisation.

There is probably little role for endotracheal intubation for seriously injured casualties in the remote expedition environment. Casualties who can be intubated without the use of anaesthetic drugs have a very poor prognosis. Furthermore, blind insertion of devices such as laryngeal mask airways or Combitubes in the semiconscious casualty may cause laryngsospasm, vomiting and raised intracranial pressure.

Most airways can be maintained by a simple jaw thrust and a basic airway adjunct. Basic airway management is the most important skill for the casualty carer at all levels

Spinal immobilisation

Spinal injuries can occur in the neck, chest or lumbar area. Injuries to the thoracic and lumbar spine usually result from high-energy trauma such as high falls and road traffic accidents. Injuries to the neck (cervical spine), however, may occur following relatively minor trauma.

Assume that every trauma casualty has a spinal injury!

The danger associated with a spinal injury is damage to the spinal cord, which will cause paraplegia or tetraplegia. It should be understood that injured casualties may have spinal fractures with no damage to their spinal cord following the accident. However, inappropriate handling or movement by the casualty or casualty carer may cause damage to the cord at this stage. The aim of spinal immobilisation and appropriate casualty handling is to prevent spinal cord damage in casualties with spinal injuries.

There are many signs of spinal fractures and spinal cord damage. The presence of any of these signs indicates the presence of injury. Their absence, however, does not exclude a spinal injury, i.e. they can "rule in" but can't "rule out" injury. Spinal injuries can only be absolutely excluded in hospital following assessment and radiological imaging.

Signs of spinal fractures or dislocations may be indicated by tenderness, swelling, bruising or steps (abnormal knobs or depressions) felt when pressing on the spine. Spinal cord injury may be indicated by numbness, tingling or weakness in the limbs.

Cervical spine immobilisation should be initiated at the same time as the airway is assessed and managed. *The casualty carer should position themselves at the head of the casualty and place their hands on either side of the head to prevent head and neck movement.* This role can be taken by other members of the group when they arrive, to free up the main casualty carer for other tasks.

TABLE 14.2 **TO STABILISE NECK INJURIES**

- Reassure the casualty and tell them not to move
- Steady and support the head in the neutral position, placing your hands on the side of the head. Maintain this support
- Add a hard neck collar if available (to immobilise the neck) but always continue to hold the head and neck

If the head is lying to one side, it should be gently moved to its neutral position with the neck in line with the rest of the spine. Returning the neck to this position is extremely unlikely to cause any spinal cord injury.

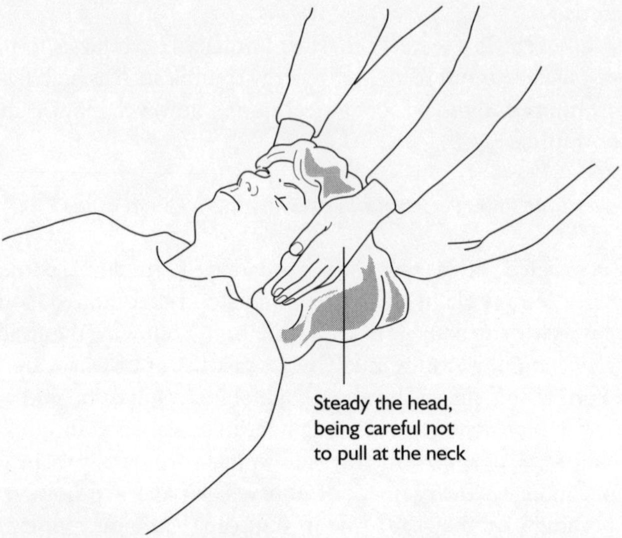
Steady the head,
being careful not
to pull at the neck

Figure 14.1 *Stabilisation of the neck*

If a cervical collar is available, this should be applied. Recently, a number of collars that are adjustable in size have become commercially available. These are ideal for remote travel as the number of collars that need to be carried is reduced from four to one. Appropriate training in their sizing and application should be undertaken before the expedition. The head should continue to be held even after application of the collar; 40% of the normal range of movement of the neck is still possible with a correctly sized collar in place.

The casualty should be log-rolled (see below) and placed onto a flat surface such as a rigid stretcher for evacuation. Placing casualties on hard surfaces such as rigid stretchers or spinal boards is uncomfortable and may rapidly cause serious pressure sores (these may occur within one hour). The stretcher should therefore be padded with a sleeping mat or Thermarest. Prolonged evacuations will require the patient to be turned frequently in order to prevent pressure sores developing.

TABLE 14.3 **TO TURN/ROLL A PATIENT WITH A SUSPECTED SPINAL INJURY**
• Stabilise the neck as in Figure 14.1 • While maintaining support at the neck, ask (ideally) four people to help log-roll the patient, keeping the head, trunk and legs in a straight line

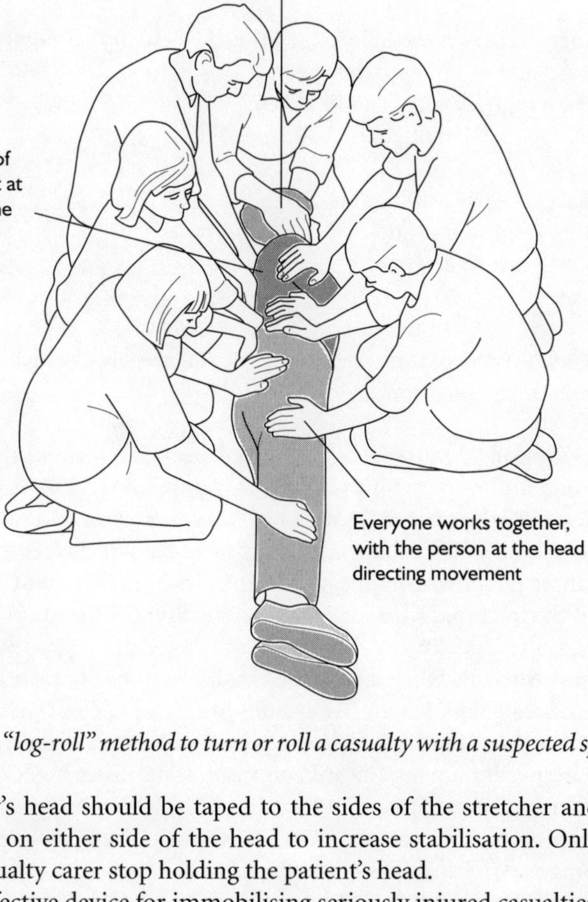
Never release support of the head
Plenty of support at the spine
Everyone works together, with the person at the head directing movement

Figure 14.2 *The "log-roll" method to turn or roll a casualty with a suspected spinal injury*

The casualty's head should be taped to the sides of the stretcher and rolled-up clothing placed on either side of the head to increase stabilisation. Only following this can the casualty carer stop holding the patient's head.

The most effective device for immobilising seriously injured casualties is the vacuum mattress. This is a hollow mattress, 5cm deep and filled with beads, which is moulded to the patient. The air is then removed from the mattress to form a rigid surface. This is more comfortable for prolonged transfers and reduces the incidence of pressure sores. This piece of kit is carried by almost all mountain rescue teams in the United Kingdom but is relatively expensive and bulky.

Spinal cord injuries in the neck may cause a condition known as neurogenic shock. Loss of nerve supply to blood vessels causes them to dilate, increasing their volume and hence reducing the blood pressure. In some cases, loss of nerve supply to the heart may cause a loss of the heart's drive to increase its rate to compensate for this low blood pressure. These patients, unlike those suffering shock from blood loss, may have a low blood pressure and a low or normal pulse rate.

Breathing

The respiratory status is assessed by examining the casualty's general appearance and respiratory rate, and listening to the chest.

Serious chest injuries may be indicated by:

- Distress
- Use of accessory breathing muscles in the arms and neck
- Increased respiratory rate
- Increased heart rate
- Cyanosis.

There are many types of injuries to the chest and chest wall which may cause compromised respiratory function.

1 **Fractured ribs** usually cause no serious problems. Movement of the fractured ribs with inspiration and movement causes sharp pain with local tenderness. This pain will be present until the fracture heals, which may take up to 6 weeks. Casualties will require good pain relief with ibuprofen or stronger painkillers (see Chapter 13, pages 155–7). The three potential complications of rib fractures are chest infection, pneumothorax (if the fractured rib ends puncture the lining of the lung) and flail chest.

2 A **flail segment** results when a number of adjacent ribs are each fractured at two separate places along their length. This results in an area of chest wall that is not fixed to the rest of the chest wall. This section of chest wall moves independently from the rest of the chest wall, moving inwards on inspiration instead of outwards. A large force is involved in these injuries and in all cases the lung underneath is damaged, causing a pulmonary contusion. These injuries are often also associated with a pneumothorax.

The pain associated with these injuries and the underlying pulmonary contusion often cause marked respiratory failure. Patients will show signs of respiratory distress and the paradoxical movement of the flail segment is often obvious.

Casualties should be given oxygen if available. They will require strong analgesia. Pain can also be reduced by splinting the flail segment to prevent its independent movement. This can be improvised by taping a rolled-up bandage or pair of socks over the flail segment. This is a very serious injury and casualties will require evacuation.

3 A **simple pneumothorax** or collapsed lung results from air collecting between the chest wall and the outer lining of the lung following puncture or rupture of the lung.

This can result from wounds penetrating the chest wall or fractured ribs damaging the lining of the lung. As most people can function adequately with only one lung, signs of respiratory distress are often minimal.

A simple pneumothorax is diagnosed clinically by listening to and percussing the chest. The side of the chest with the pneumothorax will have decreased air entry (reduced breath sounds) and will be more resonant to percussion than the normal side.

Patients with a simple pneumothorax should be given oxygen if available. All patients with a traumatic pneumothorax require the insertion of a chest drain and evacuation. The insertion of a Venflon into the chest is not indicated in a simple pneumothorax, even if traumatic in origin. The patient should be reassessed regularly for the development of a tension pneumothorax and this should be treated if it arises. Extreme care should be taken when considering evacuation of casualties with pneumothoraces by air (see Chapter 16).

4 A **tension pneumothorax** is an immediately life-threatening injury. It occurs in the same way as a simple pneumothorax. The complicating factor is that the source of the air filling the space between the chest wall and the lung, i.e. the hole in the chest wall or lung, acts as a one-way valve. This allows air into the cavity with inspiration but closes off with expiration, preventing air from escaping. As a result, the volume and pressure in the chest constantly increase. The volume increases so much that the heart and opposite lung are pushed over to the opposite side of the chest. This stops the other lung from functioning and stops blood flow to the heart.

The features of a tension pneumothorax include:

- Decreased air entry on side of pneumothorax
- Hyper-resonance to percussion on side of pneumothorax
- Trachea deviated away from side of pneumothorax
- Distended neck veins
- Marked signs of respiratory distress (cyanosis) and, eventually, shock.

Casualties with pneumothoraces deteriorate rapidly and will die in a matter of minutes if untreated. The treatment is decompression of the chest cavity. This is carried out by inserting a large-bore cannula into the side of the chest with the pneumothorax. The cannula should be inserted through the second intercostal space in the mid-clavicular line.

If available, oxygen should be administered and a chest drain inserted. Casualties with tension pneumothoraces require rapid evacuation.

5 A **haemothorax** is a collection of blood between the lung and the chest wall. Blunt or penetrating injuries cause bleeding from blood vessels in the chest wall or lung. It is often associated with a pneumothorax. A haemothorax is difficult to diagnose

without an X-ray but signs include decreased air entry and dullness to percussion over the haemothorax.

To manage a casualty with a haemothorax give oxygen, manage any associated shock, insert a chest drain (to drain the blood) and evacuate.

6 **"Sucking" chest wounds** are caused by holes in the chest wall from penetrating chest trauma. If the hole is sufficiently large, air passes into the chest cavity with inspiration through the hole rather than through the trachea. This rapidly results in respiratory failure. However, the wounds close off with expiration preventing air escaping. The result of this accumulation of air is a tension pneumothorax.

Sucking chest wounds should be covered with an occlusive dressing, which is taped down on three sides, with the fourth side left open. This type of dressing will close the wound during inspiration, stopping the flow of air into the chest.

Circulation

Trauma causes bleeding from wounds, blood vessels, internal organs and fractured bones. The body can compensate for a relatively large amount of blood loss in order to maintain the circulation to the vital organs. This compensation involves increasing the heart/pulse rate and the output of the heart, in addition to reducing blood flow to the skin and limbs.

Shock is the failure of perfusion of oxygenated blood to the body's tissues. Shock due to blood loss or dehydration is hypovolaemic shock.

TABLE 14.4 **SIGNS OF HYPOVOLAEMIC SHOCK**

- Increased heart rate
- Increased respiratory rate
- Pallor
- Cold peripheries
- Delayed capillary refill time
- Reduced urine output
- Reduced conscious level if severe
- Reduced blood pressure if severe

All of the above signs of shock can have causes other than blood loss, such as cold peripheries and delayed capillary refill in a cold environment. The heart rate may be increased by pain or anxiety rather than shock. It should also be noted that young, fit individuals can lose over 30% of their circulating blood volume before their blood pressure falls.

TABLE 14.5 MANAGEMENT OF HYPOVOLAEMIC SHOCK

- Manage any airway and breathing problems, maintaining spinal immobilisation
- Provide oxygen if available
- Lay the casualty down
- Raise the legs
- Stop external bleeding with localised pressure and elevation
- Reduce and splint fractures
- Administer intravenous fluids

The source of bleeding should be located for the shocked casualties. The sites of massive bleeding include:

- Fractures of femur or pelvis
- Abdomen
- Chest – haemothorax
- External bleeding from wounds and open fractures.

Bleeding from wounds can almost invariably be stopped with firm direct pressure and elevation. Tourniquets no longer have a place in the control of haemorrhage from wounds. They should be considered only as a last resort for life-threatening haemorrhage from an amputated limb in a remote setting.

Bleeding can be considerable from *long bone fractures*, especially the femur. Applying manual traction, followed by a femoral traction device, greatly reduces pain and bleeding into the thigh. Traction to a fractured femur with overlapping bone ends reduces soft-tissue damage and elongates the thigh. This reduces the volume of the thigh and hence reduces bleeding. Femoral nerve blocks are very effective in providing pain relief for femoral shaft fractures.

Open fractures in the remote environment should be cleaned and reduced. This again will reduce blood loss. Following this they should be covered with an iodine dressing and splinted. Broad-spectrum antibiotics should be given for open fractures as soon as possible.

A number of studies have looked at the effects of intravenous fluid administration in trauma casualties in urban environments. These have suggested that intravenous fluids may adversely affect outcome if the casualty is relatively near a hospital.

Two explanations are suggested for this. The first is that inserting a cannula and administering fluids pre-hospital may delay the time to definitive care in hospital. Secondly, the fall in blood pressure with severe haemorrhage may cause flow through injured vessels to decrease. This decreased flow of blood at reduced pressure creates a better environment for coagulation to occur. Giving intravenous fluids, which have no oxygen-carrying capacity, raises the blood pressure and hence the flow through the damaged vessels which may have "clotted off". As a result, it is suggested that bleeding may restart, causing further blood loss.

However, profound shock in the seriously injured casualty results in damage to the brain and other vital organs due to lack of perfusion. This perfusion may be improved, at least in the short term, by administration of intravenous fluids.

No studies have looked at the use of intravenous fluids in shocked trauma casualties in remote expedition environments far from definitive care. Therefore it is difficult to say whether the results of the above studies are applicable to expedition medicine.

Disability

It is important to assess the conscious level and the pupils in injured casualties as part of the primary survey.

The conscious level may be reduced as a result of head injury. Frequently, however, casualties with no head injury may be unconscious because their airway, breathing or circulation is compromised, causing impaired brain perfusion.

The conscious level can be assessed using one of two scoring systems, AVPU or the Glasgow Coma Scale. These allow accurate information about the state of the casualty to be passed to others via the radio or telephone and allow the progress of the patient to be precisely monitored and recorded.

The simplest method is to use the AVPU scoring system, which assesses the patient's response to verbal and then painful stimulus (see Chapters 12 and 13).

The most precise scoring system is the **Glasgow Coma Scale** (GCS) (see Figure 12.7, page 126). This scoring system is internationally recognised. The assessment is divided into three sections, examining eye movements, motor response and verbal response. A score is given for each of the sections and added together to give a score of between 3 and 15.

A score of 15 is normal and a score of 3 represents a casualty who is completely unresponsive. Coma is defined as a GCS score of less than 8.

Any casualty who is not "alert" on the AVPU scale or has a GCS score less than 15 following a head injury requires a formal medical assessment, usually necessitating evacuation.

The response of the pupils to light should also be examined following trauma. Normally the pupils are equal in size and reduce in diameter quickly when a light is shone into them. If, however, following a head injury the pupils are unequal or do not react quickly to light, this may indicate a serious head injury.

The ability to move all limbs spontaneously should also be checked and recorded following trauma.

Damage to the brain that occurs at the time of injury is called primary brain damage and, in the period following injury, secondary brain damage. Secondary brain damage has a number of causes including lack of oxygen, shock and infection. The pre-hospital management of serious head injuries aims to reduce secondary brain damage. Assessment and management of the casualty's airway, breathing and circulation will maximise the perfusion of the brain. Spinal immobilisation and careful handling will avoid any spinal cord damage occurring after injury. Rapid evacuation is essential for serious head injuries.

FURTHER MANAGEMENT OF A SERIOUSLY INJURED CASUALTY

Following the primary survey the casualty should be examined from head to toe for injuries. This is known as the **secondary survey**. A note should be made of the casualty's pre-existing medical illnesses, drug history and any allergies he or she may have.

Casualties who are immobile will rapidly become hypothermic and should be provided with adequate shelter and insulation.

During transfer their airway, breathing, circulation and disability should be continually reassessed. Similarly, if the casualty deteriorates in any way, the cause should be located and the primary survey restarted with A, B and C.

MULTIPLE CASUALTIES

A road traffic accident or avalanche may result in a number of people on an expedition being injured simultaneously.

A multiple casualty incident should be managed with the aim of identifying those most seriously injured and treating them first before moving on to those with non-life-threatening conditions. This is known as triage.

Triage was introduced during the Napoleonic wars and is now used in all accident and emergency departments in the UK.

Casualties are split into three groups according to their need for treatment:

- Immediate – e.g. airway compromised or shocked
- Urgent – e.g. isolated open femoral fracture
- Delayed – e.g. wrist fracture.

A casualty carer should be given the role of triage officer. It is the job of this person to perform a rapid assessment of all casualties and place them into each of the three categories. The carer should not stay and treat any casualty during this triage process, known as the triage sieve.

Following the triage sieve, the casualties should be assessed and treated in order of urgency.

The leader of the expedition should stand back from the immediate care of casualties and plan further management of the incident. This includes group safety, shelter, communications and evacuation.

A useful mnemonic for highlighting the priorities for management of a multiple casualty incident is that used in the Major Incident Medical Management and Support course – "CSCATTT".

Command and Control
Safety
Communications
Assessment of scene
Triage
Treatment
Transport

SUMMARY

Much can be done in the remote environment for the seriously injured casualty with an effective primary survey. Seriously injured casualties require definitive surgical care at the earliest opportunity.

The primary survey is a dynamic process and should be continually evaluated during evacuation.

Incidents involving multiple casualties require triage and effective incident management.

15 REMOTE MEDICAL EMERGENCIES

Stephen Hearns

Serious problems may arise during expeditions. Many will involve patients with pre-existing illnesses such as asthma, diabetes or epilepsy.

As with all aspects of expedition medicine the key is adequate pre-trip planning and preparation. Medical screening before the expedition will identify those with existing medical conditions and those with risk factors for the development of medical problems. This allows the medical officer to obtain specialist advice, equipment and medication. The chronic medical problems of expedition members should form an important part of the expedition risk assessment.

The management of all medical emergencies should focus on the assessment and management of the casualty's airway, breathing and circulation

Assessment and management of the casualty's **a**irway, **b**reathing and **c**irculation is often required before treatment of the specific condition is initiated. In an emergency, the ABC approach focuses the attention and facilitates the rapid identification and management of immediately life-threatening conditions.

Since equipment, investigations and assistance are limited in the expedition environment, it is essential rapidly to evacuate all casualties with medical emergencies to the most appropriate hospital for definitive care as soon as is possible.

PREVENTION

It is important that the medical officer (MO) and leader of the expedition are aware of all expeditioners' pre-existing medical conditions, medications and allergies. This should be carried in a written format. The medical officer should brief members of the expedition about signs of illness and immediate treatment for known conditions, especially asthma, diabetes and epilepsy. In addition, the medical officer should add to the expedition first aid kit relevant emergency medications for known pre-existing medical conditions of expedition participants. Expeditioners should take adequate supplies of their own medication with them.

Asthma

Asthma results from narrowing of the small airways in the lungs. It can be precipitated by cold, exercise, allergy or infection.

Signs and symptoms of asthma

- Shortness of breath with a feeling of chest tightness
- Expiratory wheeze
- Rapid respiratory (breathing) rate
- Rapid heart rate (pulse).

Signs of severe asthma

- Inability to complete sentences
- Heart rate > 110 beats per minute
- Respiratory rate > 25 breaths per minute
- Exhaustion from fighting for breath.

Management of asthma

The mainstays of pre-hospital care for asthma are branchodilator drugs such as salbutamol, oxygen and steroids.

Most people with asthma will have their own salbutamol (Ventolin) inhaler. They should be encouraged to use this. In severe cases they will be too breathless to use it effectively. In such cases it is possible to improvise a "spacer" device using a plastic bottle, inserting the inhaler through a hole cut in one end and inhaling through the bottle opening. Four to eight puffs of the inhaler should be given each time the spacer device is used. In severe cases this should be repeated frequently.

Steroids in the form of prednisolone tablets (adult dose 50mg) should be given in severe cases. It should be noted that these take 6 hours to be effective and that intravenous steroids (hydrocortisone) do not take effect more rapidly than oral tablets.

If the expedition has oxygen available, this should be provided for the casualty. If an expedition is carrying oxygen and has known people with asthma it should carry a nebuliser mask and salbutamol nebules.

In very severe asthma, salbutamol should be given parenterally. Ideally this should be in the form of a slow intravenous infusion. However, if this is not possible it can be given by subcutaneous or intramuscular injection.

It is important to be aware that in some severe cases movement of air in and out of the chest may be so reduced that a wheeze will not be produced. Therefore beware of the absence of wheeze or "silent chest". People with asthma often respond very well to initial treatment with salbutamol, but after a short period they may deteriorate again. Casualties with severe asthma should be evacuated to hospital urgently.

Summary of asthma management

- Oxygen (if available)
- Salbutamol inhaler via a spacer or nebulised
- Steroids – 50mg oral prednisolone or 200mg intravenous hydrocortisone
- Salbutamol by intravenous infusion in very severe attack.

Epilepsy

Seizures (fits) usually occur in patients with known epilepsy, but it is possible that first seizures may occur during an expedition in expeditioners with no previous history. Seizures can also occur in people who do not have epilepsy following head injury or alcohol withdrawal, as a result of hypoglycaemia (low blood sugar levels) or in severe brain infections (e.g. cerebral malaria).

It is important for people with epilepsy on expeditions to take their anticonvulsant medication as prescribed.

Signs of an epileptic seizure

- Collapse
- Unresponsiveness
- Jerking movements of arms and legs
- Tongue biting and jaw clenching
- Incontinence.

Seizures usually resolve spontaneously without treatment. Following a seizure a patient may be confused and sleepy and even weak or paralysed for a period of up to a few hours. This is known as the post-ictal phase.

Management of epileptic seizure

The main dangers during seizures are airway obstruction, injury caused by the fall or during uncontrolled movements, and aspiration pneumonia. As the casualty's teeth are normally clenched during seizures it is difficult to maintain the airway using an oropharyngeal airway. If the patient's airway becomes compromised a nasopharyngeal airway, inserted via the nose, is ideal and should be supplemented by a chin lift or jaw thrust.

Casualties should be placed in the recovery position (see Figure 13.1 on page 131) on their left side to help maintain their airway and reduce the risk of aspiration.

Other expedition members who are present during the seizure should attempt to reduce trauma to the head and body during seizures.

High-flow oxygen should be provided if available as the casualty's rate and depth of respiration are likely to be compromised. If the seizure continues for more than 5 minutes, diazepam should be administered. This can be done most simply using rectal preparations or it can be given by slow intravenous injection (dose 10mg by either route). If the seizure continues, a second dose of diazepam should be considered after a further 5 minutes. Be aware that intravenous diazepam may depress the breathing.

If hypoglycaemia is suspected this should be treated.

Seizures in people who are not epileptic and prolonged seizures in known people with epilepsy require that the patient be evacuated.

Summary of seizure management

- Maintain the airway
- Insert a nasopharyngeal airway (if trained to do so)
- Give oxygen
- Use intravenous or rectal diazepam (adult dose 10mg) if seizure continues for over 5 minutes
- Give a further dose of diazepam if seizure continues for another 5 minutes after the first dose.

Diabetic emergencies

With careful blood glucose control, there is usually no problem in taking people with diabetes on most expeditions. Diabetic expeditioners must have been trained to maintain their own diabetic control and fully understand how to adjust their insulin dosage according to exertion, food intake and blood glucose measurements.

Two types of emergency may befall people with diabetes:

1. Low blood sugar – hypoglycaemia (blood glucose less than 3.5mmol/l)
2. High blood sugar – ketoacidosis.

Hypoglycaemia

Hypoglycaemia, a blood glucose less than 3.5mmol/l, develops when food intake has been less than normal or physical exertion has been greater than normal. As these factors are regularly present in the expedition setting, people with diabetes must be able to adjust their insulin dose according to anticipated physical activities and environmental conditions.

Signs and symptoms of hypoglycaemia (low blood sugar)

- Confusion, anxiety or light-headedness
- Inappropriate behaviour
- Slurred speech
- Sweating
- Loss of consciousness (or failure to wake up in the morning!)
- Seizures.

Investigation

- Blood glucose measurement using a stick test (commonly known as a "BM").

Management of hypoglycaemia

- If casualty is conscious give sugary drink and something to eat
- If casualty is unconscious:
  – place in recovery position and maintain the airway
  – Hypostop to mucosa of mouth
  – give glucagon by intramuscular injection
  – administer intravenous 50% dextrose (50ml) if glucagon not effective
  – give casualty something to eat once they have regained consciousness.

Hypoglycaemic episodes in known people with diabetes who make a full recovery rarely require evacuation if a cause can be found.

Diabetic ketoacidosis

Diabetic ketoacidosis results from a blood sugar that is too high. A high level of glucose in the urine leads to water loss through passing excessive volumes of urine and dehydration. Excess glucose in the bloodstream leads to the formation of acidic ketones. Ketoacidosis is often precipitated by another illness such as a chest or urinary tract infection. It may, however, simply be due to a lack of insulin.

If people with diabetes develop an infection they should monitor their blood glucose more frequently than normal and usually need to increase their insulin dosage in order to prevent the development of ketoacidosis.

Symptoms and signs of diabetic ketoacidosis

- Thirst
- Passing excessive volumes of urine
- Vomiting

- Rapid breathing rate and unusually deep breathing
- Abdominal pain
- Reduced conscious level.

Management of diabetic ketoacidosis

- If unconscious, place in recovery position and maintain airway.
- Give oxygen if available.
- Measure blood sugar.
- Encourage oral fluids if casualty is conscious.
- Administer intravenous fluids if casualty is conscious. If diabetic ketoacidosis is confirmed commence an intravenous infusion of 0.9% saline giving 1000ml over ½–1 hour, followed by 500ml per hour for the next 2–3 hours. Persistent hypotension may require an increase in infusion rate and/or colloid administration. Avoid over-rapid infusion with the risks of pulmonary oedema and adult respiratory distress syndrome, especially in elderly people and patients with ischaemic heart disease. Once the blood glucose level is less than 15mmol/l, change the intravenous infusion fluid to 5% dextrose. This should be given at a rate of 500ml every 4 hours. If signs of hypovolaemia persist, a 0.9% saline infusion should be given concurrently with the dextrose.
- Give insulin according to a recognised protocol (e.g. "sliding scale") if high blood sugar is confirmed by stick testing. One such insulin "sliding scale" protocol is that recommended by the *Oxford Handbook of Accident and Emergency Medicine*, Wyatt et al. Oxford Medical Publications 1999. "Give 20 units of insulin (actrapid) IM immediately, than 6 units per hour IM. Check plasma glucose levels every hour initially and when the plasma glucose level is less than 14mmol/litre, reduce the amount of insulin to 4 units per hour IM."
- Treat any underlying infection with appropriate antibiotics.

Patients with diabetic ketoacidosis require intensive medical care and should be evacuated as quickly as possible.

Anaphylaxis

Anaphylaxis is a severe form of allergic reaction. This may result from ingestion of certain foods or drugs, or follow insect stings and bites.

Signs and symptoms of anaphylaxis

- Rash – red, itchy, raised, rapidly evolving
- Shortness of breath, chest tightness or feeling of obstruction in the throat
- Wheeze (like an asthma attack)

- Nausea, vomiting
- Colicky abdominal pain, diarrhoea
- Swelling of the lips, tongue, gums, throat and face
- Rapid heart rate
- Low blood pressure and shock (loss of consciousness, collapse).

Casualties with anaphylactic reactions deteriorate rapidly; this requires prompt assessment and treatment.

Many people with a history of anaphylaxis will carry their own adrenaline in the form of an EpiPen. The medical officer and fellow expeditioners accompanying such people should receive training in the appropriate use of this device.

Management of anaphylaxis

- If the casualty is unconscious, place him or her in the recovery position and maintain the airway.
- Give oxygen if available.
- Give adrenaline (1:1,000 or 0.1% solution) by intramuscular injection (adult dose 0.5mg of 0.1% solution). This may need to be repeated if ineffective or if the patient deteriorates following transient recovery. Adult EpiPen delivers only 0.3mg.
- Administer chlorpheniramine intravenously (adult dose 10mg). Give orally if intravenous administration not possible.
- Give salbutamol, either nebulised (adult dose 5mg) or 10 doses from a metered dose inhaler via a spacer if asthma, wheeze or respiratory distress is a feature of the reaction.
- Administer hydrocortisone intravenously (adult dose 200mg) or prednisolone orally (adult dose 50mg).
- Give intravenous fluids if shocked.

Steroids do not have an immediate effect but help to prevent the recurrence of anaphylaxis, which may occur a number of hours after the initial episode. This is known as the "rebound" phenomenon.

All casualties with anaphylaxis require evacuation to definitive care.

Chest pain

The possibility of angina or myocardial infarction (heart attack) should be considered in casualties with chest pain. In these cases chest pain results from a lack of blood flow to the heart muscle.

Signs and symptoms of angina and myocardial infarction

- Chest pain – heavy, tight
- Pain spreading to arms, neck or through to the back
- Sweating
- Shortness of breath
- Nausea, vomiting
- Collapse, shock.

Heart attacks, however, frequently occur with atypical symptoms or even with no chest pain.

Management of angina or suspected myocardial infarction

- Give oxygen if available.
- Give aspirin 300mg to chew.
- Spray glyceryl trinitrate under the tongue if blood pressure normal. Give one spray, then repeat after a few minutes if the blood pressure does not fall.
- Administer opiate analgesia intravenously if pain persists.
- Give prochlorperazine (Buccastem) or metoclopramide for nausea.

Aspirin helps to reduce clot formation in the blood vessels supplying the heart muscle. Glyceryl trinitrate makes the vessels supplying the heart muscle wider, improving blood flow, though it may lower the patient's blood pressure sharply or cause a headache.

Patients with suspected angina or myocardial infarction should be evacuated to hospital for further assessment.

Other causes of chest pain include indigestion, muscular strain, pulmonary embolism (special risk at high altitude and following long-haul flights), broken ribs, and infections causing pleurisy and pericarditis.

Septicaemia

Severe bacterial infections of any origin may rapidly spread throughout the body, causing damage to many organs. Toxins produced by the bacteria mean blood vessel walls become "leaky", causing the contents of blood vessels to leak out. This results in a depletion of fluid within the blood vessels, leading to shock (see page 179).

Patients will look unwell, have a rapid heart rate and rapid breathing rate. Unlike victims of shock from blood loss or dehydration, patients will be warm peripherally and may appear flushed.

Treatment is based on the administration of oxygen and intravenous fluids. If broad-spectrum antibiotics are available they should be given.

Alcohol intoxication

Excessive alcohol consumption can lead to a number of problems including trauma, aspiration, dehydration, hypothermia and hypoglycaemia.

The main form of treatment for alcohol intoxication is fluid replacement, given orally if conscious and intravenously if unconscious. Casualties should be nursed in the recovery position and their airway maintained to prevent aspiration of vomit. They should be kept warm to prevent hypothermia. If completely unconscious, they should be turned regularly to prevent the development of pressure sores.

Recreational drug ingestion

Recreational drugs can cause similar problems to alcohol intoxication. General supportive care, along similar lines to that described above, is required.

Substances such as *LSD* (acid) can result in psychosis which may require the administration of antipsychotic medication.

Stimulants such as *amphetamines* (speed) and LSD (acid) may cause agitation. Severely agitated patients may require sedation with a benzodiazepine.

MDMA (ecstasy) is a particularly harmful substance that may result in hyperthermia and is frequently fatal.

Opiate overdose causes reduced consciousness and breathing rate. The pupils will be very small. Opiate overdose can be reversed very effectively by the use of intramuscular or intravenous naloxone.

Shock

Shock is defined as a lack of tissue perfusion – basically, not enough blood is reaching the body's tissues. If shock is untreated, these tissues will rapidly die, causing irreversible organ failure.

Causes of shock

- Blood loss – trauma or bleeding into gut
- Dehydration
- Infection – septic shock
- Anaphylaxis
- Heart failure
- Spinal injury – neurogenic shock (see Chapter 14).

Signs of shock

- Rapid heart rate
- Rapid respiratory rate
- Weak pulse and low blood pressure

- Pallor
- Reduced conscious level if severe
- Reduced urine output.

In young people, almost 50% of the circulating blood volume must be lost before the blood pressure falls. This, therefore, is a late sign of shock.

Management of shock

- Maintain airway and provide oxygen
- Ensure casualty is lying down with legs raised
- Treat external bleeding with pressure and elevation
- Straighten and splint fractures
- Consider intravenous fluids.

The treatment for shock due to continuing blood loss is a surgical operation to stop the bleeding. Administration of intravenous fluids is a temporary measure only. Rapid evacuation is essential for shocked patients.

Dehydration

Severe dehydration results from lack of fluid intake and excessive loss from sweating, diarrhoea or vomiting. It has the same symptoms as shock, described above. Casualties will have dry mouths and will produce small amounts of dark, concentrated urine. Their core temperature (rectal) may be raised if they have heat stress or infection.

The cause of fluid loss should be addressed and fluid administered orally. If this is not possible intravenous fluids should be given. Oral fluids should have added salt and sugar to replace the large amount of salt loss in sweat, diarrhoea and vomiting. This can be in the form of commercially prepared oral rehydration salts (ORS) or by adding eight level teaspoonfuls of sugar and two teaspoonfuls of salt to a litre of clean/boiled water.

SUMMARY

Many potential medical problems can be anticipated and prepared for with adequate pre-trip planning. Casualties with medical emergencies should be assessed and treated using the ABC principle before specific treatment of the particular problem is initiated.

16 CASUALTY EVACUATION

Rod Stables

Thorough preparation and planning of all phases of an expedition are essential for a successful venture. This is particularly important in the handling of emergency evacuation. Casualty evacuation (casevac) procedures must be established and perhaps even rehearsed before deployment.

Expeditions vary in their destination, scale, complexity, duration, risk, isolation and levels of support. Beyond this each evacuation case will present its own problems, varying from the self-caring "walking wounded", to patients requiring continuous and intensive care.

The aim of this chapter is to provide a framework for sound planning. To do this the process of casualty evacuation has been broken down into several phases.

Preparation

⬇

Casualty event

⬇

Immediate rescue

⬇

Stabilisation

⬇

Call for help/move to help

⬇

In-county casevac

⬇

International recovery

Preparation

All aspects of the casualty evacuation process must be considered. An initial risk assessment should be undertaken to review expedition-specific factors. The aim and nature of an expedition often define key objective risks related to activities, terrain, climate and isolation. All expeditions must entertain the possibility that multiple casualties may be sustained either in a single incident or over the duration of the expedition. Other factors to consider are the size and composition of the team, and the age, physical capabilities, experience, training and specific medical needs of individual team members. All expeditions must strike a balance between the proposed level of intrinsic medical support and reliance upon external assistance. To some extent this dictates the requirements for medical specialists, rescue aids, medical supplies, communication systems and other equipment. For the 1992–3 Everest in Winter Expedition, the high level of objective danger and the isolation of the base camp location over the winter months demanded a high level of medical provision. In preparation, blood samples from all members were examined to identify opportunities for emergency transfusion between individuals.

Seek information from all available sources, paying particular attention to local agencies and those with recent experience of your expedition area. Reports from previous trips are often a useful reference. The Royal Geographical Society houses an extensive reference collection of past expedition reports. It has also published the results of a long-term survey of medical problems experienced by expeditions (*Journal of the Royal Society of Medicine* 2000;93:557–62).

When writing an outline casevac plan consider the evacuation chain. This usually involves a collaborative effort co-ordinated, in sequence, by key individuals or agencies (see Chapter 8).

Casualty event

⬇

Expedition base camp location

⬇

Local medical services/In-country support agency

⬇

UK medical services/Home base contact

Establish contact by telephone, email or fax with relevant external agencies and aim to involve them in your planning process. On arrival in the country allow time for personal visits to ensure close liaison with groups or individuals whom you may have to call on for support. Consular or other diplomatic officials have sometimes acted as local agents, but except in the case of a dire emergency their availability should not be assumed and alternative arrangements must be secured. Modern communications usually allow an effective link to be established between the home country contact and the local agent, but communications with the expedition group may be less secure and will vary from expedition to expedition (see "The call for (or move to) help", page 184).

Each element in this evacuation chain will require copies of key documentation. The basic requirements include (but are certainly not limited to) the following:

- A complete list of expedition members and their personal details, including nationality, passport number, full next-of-kin contact details, information about pre-existing medical problems and blood group information.
- Copies of all insurance policies relating to medical and evacuation cover.
- Contact details of involved travel and transport agencies, including international medical evacuation services.
- Contact details of local consulate or other diplomatic or home government officials for all nationalities represented on the expedition.
- Precise contact details of the other link agencies. This should include alternative contact individuals and fallback alternative telephone and fax numbers.

A similar but more personalised document pack should be produced for each expedition member. This should be kept readily available together with a passport and some cash, credit cards or other financial guarantee. An emergency casevac may separate an individual from the rest of the party and these documents should accompany the injured party. This "snatch bag" can be further enhanced by including a structured proforma to allow recording of the immediate medical history, clinical

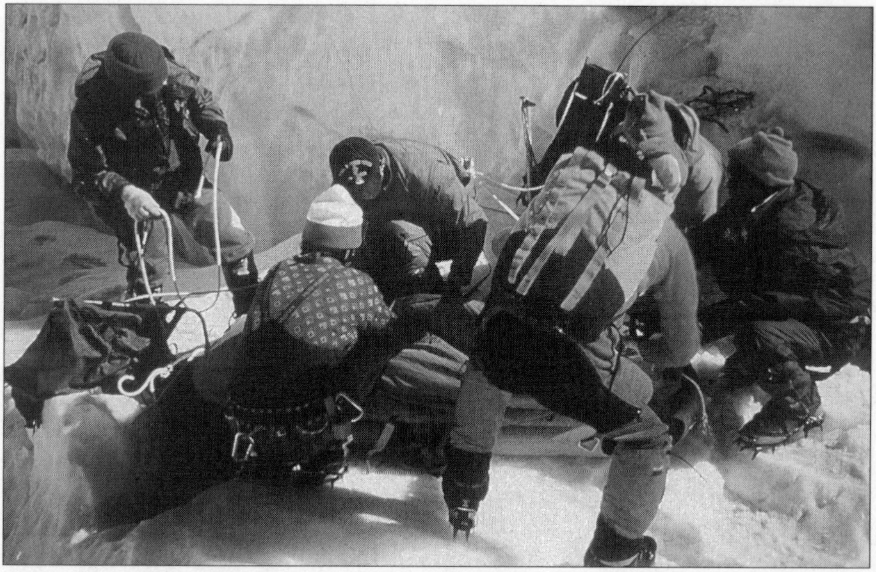

Figure 16.1 *Stretcher casevac in the Khumbu Icefall on Everest in winter. The victim had bilateral compound fractures of tibia and fibula from the fall (R. Stables)*

observations and treatment regimes and a copy of the patient's personal medical questionnaire.

Casualty event and immediate rescue

Expedition leaders and medical officers must consider the equipment that might be required in the immediate recovery of a casualty following an accident or sudden illness. Normal trauma packs are usually required, but steep rock, snow and ice, caves or the open sea may demand the procurement of specialist items. Improvisation and persistence can overcome most obstacles, but in difficult terrain there is no substitute for high-quality, purpose-built equipment.

Stabilisation

Once back at base camp an attempt can be made to stabilise the patient's condition. A decision on the need to evacuate and the timing of any such move must then be made. These can be difficult issues to resolve and involve a series of value judgements based on the patient's condition, the level of care immediately available and the complexities and rigour of the casevac chain. Good communications with the local agent and hence with specialist professional advice can be of great value in this setting.

It is important to document clearly the details of the case and to record key clinical observations and treatments administered. These data should be sent back with the patient.

Ideally, an expedition member should accompany the patient, taking all the patient's personal equipment with him or her. This is rarely possible but should be considered if personnel and other circumstances permit.

The call for (or move to) help

Expeditions with no means of summoning outside help will have to move their casualty to the nearest human habitation or aid post. The most appropriate means for this move should be considered in the planning phase. Pack animals or stretcher carriers can be slow and present great problems for a severely injured patient.

Even large and well-equipped expeditions may face this problem if they are operating in remote or high-altitude areas, beyond the range of helicopter operations. Everest Base Camp, for example, is inaccessible to helicopters in the winter months and casualties must be moved to lower altitudes down the valley. It is important to remember in planning helicopter tasks that there is a relationship between range and payload (or freight). When the aircraft is operating at the limits of its range or altitude ceiling payload limitations may mean that the casualty has to move alone with minimal equipment.

The most usual means of summoning help is by radio communication, although local runners can provide a remarkable service in some areas. Traditional HF or VHF radio links to a local agent have previously been the mainstay of expedition

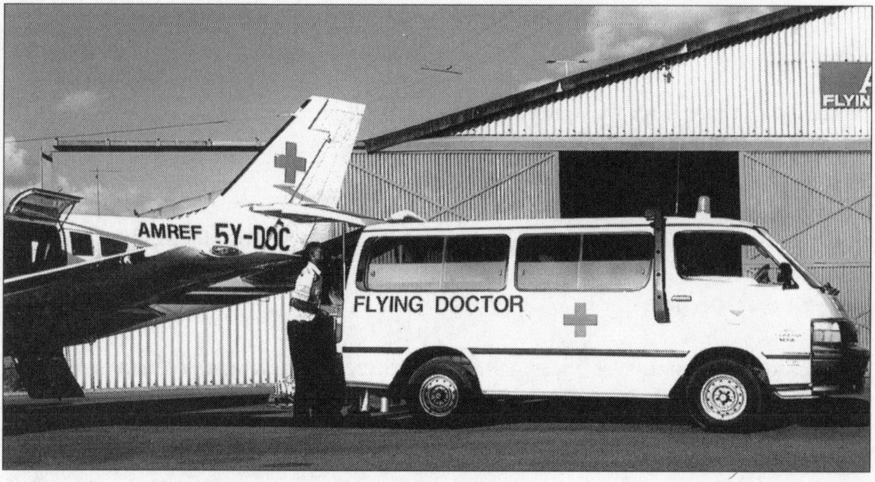

Figure 16.2 *Aeromedical evacuation (S. R. Anderson)*

communications, although in regions that are frequently overflown, such as the Denali National Park in Alaska, ground-to-air UHF systems can provide an effective alternative for emergency transmissions.

Satellite communication systems have revolutionised the potential for long-range communications. Secure voice and fax links across several continents are now readily available as are, increasingly, email links. This equipment is, however, expensive to hire or purchase and satellite air time is also charged at premium rates. For smaller expeditions, interested only in emergency communications, a number of companies now offer for hire a satellite emergency beacon transmitter device. This can be triggered to produce one of a number of coded signals to a central base. This central base will then notify the expedition's nominated agent that the expedition has, for example, transmitted "Message 2" logged as "Request immediate casevac at this location".

In-country casevac and international recovery

The involvement of established agencies usually makes this the least problematic part of the process. Aeromedical evacuation is expensive and appropriate insurance cover should be established for all expedition members. Most insurance companies insist on being involved from the earliest stages of a claim and should be contacted at the first opportunity.

Companies that provide air ambulance services

Europe and Africa

Cega Air Ambulance Ltd, Goodwood Airfield, Chichester, West Sussex PO18 0PH, UK
Tel. +44 1243 538888, fax +44 1243 773169

Compagnie Générale de Secours, Paris, France
Tel. +33 1 47 47 66 66

East Africa Flying Doctors Society (AMREF), 11 Old Queen Street, London SW1H 9JA, UK
Tel. +44 20 71233 0066, fax +44 20 7233 0099

Europ Assistance, Sussex House, Perrymount Road, Haywards Heath, West Sussex RH16 1DN, UK
Tel. +44 1444 411999, fax +44 1444 415775

International Assistance Services, 32–42 High Street, Purley, Surrey CR8 2PP, UK
Tel. +44 20 8763 1550, fax +44 20 8668 1262

Swiss Air Ambulance, Zurich, Switzerland
Tel. +41 1 3831 111

United States
Air Ambulance International, San Francisco, CA
Tel. +1 800 2279996, +1 415 7861592

Air Ambulance Network, Miami, FL
Tel. +1 800 327 1966, +1 305 447 0458

Air Response, Box 109, Fort Plain, NY 13339
Tel. +1 518 993 4153

International SOS, Box 11568, Philadelphia, PA 19116
Tel. +1 800 523 8930, +1 215 244 1500

Life Flight Hermann Hospital, Houston, TX
Tel. +1 800 231 4357

National Jets, Fort Lauderdale, FL
Tel. +1 305 359 9900, +1 800 327 3710

North American Air Ambulance, Blackwood, NJ
Tel. +1 800 257 8180

Nationwide/Worldwide Emergency Ambulance Return (NEAR), 450 Prairie Avenue, Calumet City, IL 60409 Tel. +1 800 654 6700

17 MEDICAL ASPECTS OF SURVIVAL

Rod Stables

Many readers will already be familiar with the demands of expedition travel to wild and unfamiliar places. Fatigue, hunger, pain, thirst and even a measure of fear are, to an extent, routine features of an expedition. It is probably these aspects of any venture that are the source of the best expedition anecdotes and the most enduring, if least accurately framed, memories.

Few people, however, will ever experience a true survival situation when life and death hang in a fine balance and all other concerns become secondary. Survival is the art of staying alive. The human body and, perhaps more importantly, the spirit have the capability to endure the most extreme hardship and deprivation under seemingly impossible conditions. Examples of this tenacity can be found in an extensive literature recounting survival situations.

Although a number of well-documented cases have involved a prolonged period of isolation, the "Robinson Crusoe" scenario is rare and most survival situations are played out in the course of hours and days rather than weeks and months. In all cases, however, it is usually possible to identify a number of core issues that determine the eventual outcome.

The pyramid of survival

Survival skills can be represented as a pyramid. The most important elements form the broad base and are the factors that distinguish the survivor from the victim. The relative importance of the other components varies in different situations and with different personalities.

The will to survive

Qualities of character and resolve usually dictate the chances of survival. Physically unprepared individuals with no equipment or specialist skills have survived against all the odds by refusing to surrender to death. The survivor will cling to the last threads of life, however desperate the circumstances. Escape or rescue, followed by

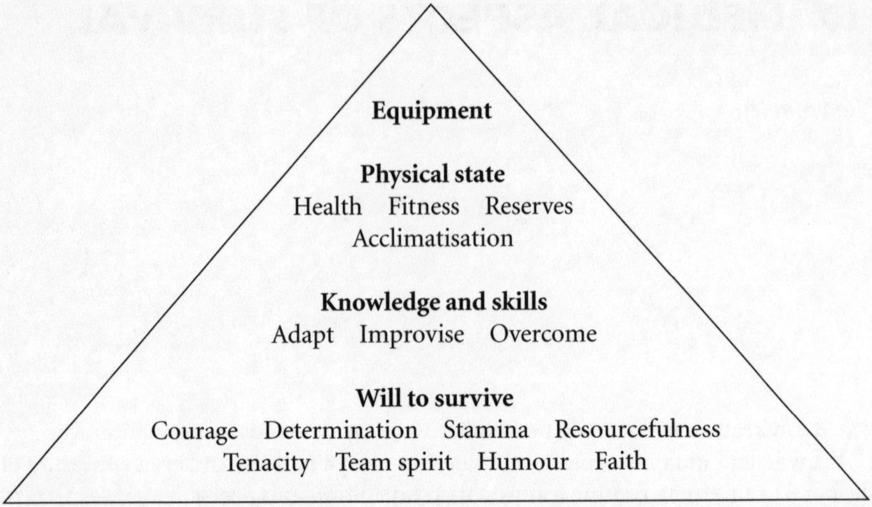

treatment and rehabilitation, allow a return to normal life in almost all cases, but once the threshold of death is crossed all is lost.

When disaster strikes, initial feelings of panic and self-pity must be controlled. Positive action even in a most rudimentary form will improve self-confidence. Courage, determination and tenacity are important qualities, but it is also important to maintain individual and group morale. Humour and faith (in all its forms) are important in this regard.

For groups, survival situations present new challenges for the leader or leaders. Often a very different style of leadership is required and the demands of the new circumstances can bring previously unrecognised strengths of certain individuals to the fore. The case of the Argentine rugby team isolated in the high Andes following an aircraft crash is an interesting example (see the film *Alive*, available on video).

Knowledge and skills

Self-confidence can be enhanced by good training and sound knowledge. Much of this will be of a general nature but basic skills in the essentials of survival should be practised by all who venture any distance off the beaten track. A number of books and training courses are available to provide an introduction to this subject.

For any specific trip or expedition, thorough research and planning are essential. The demands of the environment or other possible threats should be identified and studied. Contingency plans and reserves should be in place to cope with likely problems, and a means of summoning help or evacuation should be established. Throughout the venture all team members should be kept fully informed of key data, such as local terrain, key locations, personnel distribution, weather patterns and communication plans.

Knowledge dispels fear and is an important weapon in the fight for survival. This must be coupled with resourcefulness and a will to adapt, improvise and overcome.

Figure 17.1 *High-frequency radio communication between Everest Base Camp and Kathmandu (R. Stables)*

Physical preparation

Medical and dental health should be checked before departure on any venture. Personal health issues, such as the need for medication (even the contraceptive pill), should be considered and an emergency stock carried on the person at all times.

Physical fitness is a key factor in a survival situation and will allow the individual to cope better with not only physical exertion but also sleep deprivation and climatic extremes. In some environments and for prolonged expeditions it can, however, be a mistake to be too lean. Adipose (fat) tissue is laid down to act as a food reserve in times of need and can provide important thermal insulation.

A period of thorough acclimatisation to extremes of temperature, altitude or other environmental factors should be allowed before expedition members are subjected to the risks of isolation from support.

Equipment

Well-chosen equipment is obviously important but it is critical to ensure that key

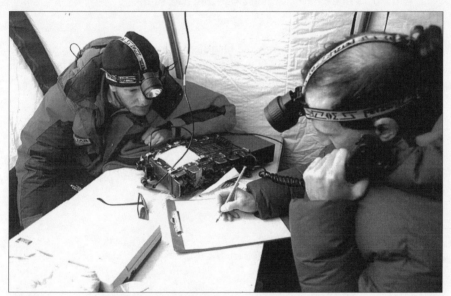

items are available when needed. Each expedition or individual should have a clear concept of what should be carried:

- on the person;
- in the pack or on the belt when away from base camp;
- at the base camp.

Survival situations often start with the loss of equipment. Key items such as map, compass, torch and whistle should be carried on the person and secured by lanyards at all times. Other equipment choices and standard procedures will be governed by the nature of the trip and personal preferences.

Summary

It is impossible in this short chapter to offer anything more than basic guidelines. More detailed information, perhaps specific to the expedition aims, will have to be sought in appropriate texts and appropriate skills acquired and practised.

18 COMMON INFECTIONS

Matthew Dryden

Minor infections are among the most common health problems likely to be experienced by a traveller. The usual infections seen at home such as colds and the myriad of minor and self-limiting viral infections are also common abroad. However, it is important not to assume that a fever can be ignored when it could be a sign of a much more serious and potentially lethal infection such as malaria (see Chapter 19). By and large exotic tropical infections are comparatively rare.

Diarrhoea (gastroenteritis), also common at home, is more common on expeditions because standards of food hygiene are frequently less good. Judging by the variety and richness of the terminology – Delhi belly, Monteczuma's revenge, Hottentot runs, Saddam's secret weapon, to name but a few – there can be few travellers who have not had personal experience of traveller's diarrhoea.

Diseases like HIV or hepatitis B that occur at home are much more common in certain parts of the world, but can be avoided by preventing exposure, or by vaccination in the case of hepatitis B. Many infections, some of which are serious and occasionally lethal, can be prevented by vaccination prior to departure (see Chapter 2). These include hepatitis A and B, polio, diphtheria, tetanus, typhoid, yellow fever, Japanese encephalitis, tick-borne encephalitis, rabies and meningococcal meningitis.

DIARRHOEA

Traveller's diarrhoea is extremely common and is likely to afflict the majority of longer-term travellers to developing and tropical countries. In a study of over 17,000 Swiss tourists on two-week holidays the attack rate ranged from 4% to 51%, depending on where they went. One report in British tourists recorded an attack rate of 26% in Africa and 8% in North America.

Diarrhoea = more than three stools per day of increased volume
Dysentery = blood mixed with stool
Cholera and other serious diarrhoeas kill by dehydration, fluid replacement saves lives

A change in bowel habit may be caused by a change in diet or the stresses of travel but infective diarrhoea is caused by consuming food or water contaminated with a pathogenic organism. If it were possible to have immaculate hand hygiene and adequately to cook, boil or peel everything that was consumed, traveller's diarrhoea could be avoided. In reality such high standards are difficult to achieve and it is impossible to have control over food preparation by others while travelling. Since to refuse new and interesting foods would greatly diminish the experience of travel, most travellers must accept diarrhoea (gastroenteritis) as a calculated risk. Most traveller's diarrhoea is caused by strains of *Escherichia coli* (a normal commensal of the bowel) which produce a toxin. This toxin upsets the normal passage of electrolytes and water across the bowel wall and thus causes watery diarrhoea. The locals are probably immune to the infection. *E. coli* causes abdominal cramps and pain, diarrhoea, loss of appetite, and sometimes nausea and vomiting. It is self-limiting which means that it will get better without treatment after 24–48 hours. Gastric viral infections cause similar signs and have much the same duration. Other infections can cause a longer duration of symptoms and although usually self-limiting can on occasions cause more serious and persistent infection.

Causes and mechanisms

The following is a brief guide to the common causes of diarrhoea.

Prevention

Almost all of these organisms are transmitted in the same way: by contaminated food and water. Infective material must be swallowed in order to contract the illness. One result is that all causes of diarrhoea can be prevented by devoting rigorous attention to hygienic food preparation and handling, and to water sterilisation. Preparing one's own food is the best way to prevent gastroenteritis.

The following pose a potential risk to health, and are best avoided:

- *Shellfish and seafood.* Molluscs and crustaceans are filter feeders, and accumulate whichever organisms happen to be present in the local sewage system. They need a minimum of 8 minutes' vigorous boiling to be rendered safe.
- *Salads, raw fruit and vegetables.* These have the reputation of being healthy and nutritious at home, but human and animal excreta are widely used as fertiliser in most developing countries. They require careful sterilisation and preparation.
- *Rare meat (including undercooked chicken), raw fish.* There may be a high risk of parasitic contamination.
- *Buffets, food left out in warm temperatures.* Bacteria multiply fast at warm temperatures, and trivial contamination can rapidly turn into a serious risk.

TABLE 18.1 CAUSES OF DIARRHOEA

Cause	*Usual duration of illness*	*Symptoms*	*Antibiotic treatment (if required)*
E. coli	24–48 hours	Diarrhoea, abdominal pain, loss of appetite	Ciprofloxacin
Virus	24–48 hours	Diarrhoea, abdominal pain, loss of appetite	No antibiotics
Campylobacter	2–10 days	Diarrhoea, abdominal pain, loss of appetite, occasionally blood in faeces	Ciprofloxacin or erythromycin
Salmonella	2–7 days	Diarrhoea, abdominal pain, loss of appetite, occasionally fever	Ciprofloxacin
Shigella	2–10 days	Explosive diarrhoea, abdominal pain, fever, listlessness, loss of appetite, blood in faeces (severe cases)	Ciprofloxacin
Giardia	3–14 days	Diarrhoea, abdominal pain, loss of appetite, flatulence, bloatedness	Metronidazole or tinidazole
Entamoeba (amoebic dysentery)	3–14 days	Diarrhoea of gradual onset, blood in faeces	Metronidazole or tinidazole

TABLE 18.2 THE WORLD HEALTH ORGANIZATION'S "TEN GOLDEN RULES FOR SAFE FOOD PREPARATION"

1. Choose foods processed for safety
2. Cook food thoroughly
3. Eat cooked foods immediately
4. Store cooked foods carefully
5. Reheat cooked foods thoroughly
6. Avoid contact between raw food and cooked food
7. Wash hands repeatedly
8. Keep all food preparation surfaces meticulously clean
9. Protect food from insects, rodents and other animals
10. Use safe water

- *Food on which flies have settled.*
- *Food stored and reheated after cooking.*
- *Spicy sauces and salsa, left out on the table.*
- *Food handled by other people's dirty fingers.*
- *Milk products and ice cream.*
- *Foods containing raw egg* (e.g. mayonnaise).
- *Fruit juices from street vendors.*
- *Ice.*
- *Tap water*, even for brushing teeth.
- *Hospitality.* If you are offered unsafe food make an excuse and refuse it.

The following foods are usually safe:

- Freshly, thoroughly cooked food, served hot.
- Fruit peeled or sliced open by yourself (bananas, melons, papaya, avocado).
- Freshly baked bread (find the bakery).
- Packaged or canned food.
- Bottled drinks opened in your presence; the safest are carbonated.
- Boiled water, tea.
- If nothing else looks safe, ask for chips, omelettes, boiled eggs or other dishes that must be cooked to order.

Drugs for prevention

For practical purposes there are no effective drugs for prevention
Prevention is only possible by rigorous hygiene

Many drugs have been proposed for prevention, but none is entirely suitable. Advocates of such treatment argue that precautions can be difficult to follow, and do not always work. The contrary view is that drugs can cause harm without offering complete protection, and make travellers more likely to expose themselves to risk in the mistaken belief that they are protected against all ills.

Bismuth subsalicylate (Pepto-Bismol) is one drug that is believed to reduce the incidence of traveller's diarrhoea, and has some popularity in the United States. It needs to be taken in substantial doses, and may cause a black, furred tongue and black stools.

Another approach is to use the quinolone group of antibiotics (e.g. ciprofloxacin). However, these drugs are expensive, not without risk, and may make it more difficult to diagnose and treat any illness that does occur despite the treatment. Prophylactic drugs are not recommended.

Treatment

Most cases of diarrhoea improve without treatment, but rehydration is always important.

Rehydration

The most important aspect of treatment is to correct dehydration, particularly in a tropical environment, and particularly if the sufferer has not yet acclimatised to the heat; in such circumstances, fluid losses can be considerable. Children and elderly people are most at risk from the consequences of dehydration; for them rehydration must be an urgent priority. Healthy adults only rarely become severely dehydrated due to diarrhoea, but rehydration is none the less worthwhile, making sufferers feel rapidly better.

The fastest and most effective way to replace fluid is to use oral rehydration solutions. These are available as sachets of powder to be made up in clean water. Well-known brands include:

- Boots Diareze Oral rehydration powder (Boots)
- Oralyte (UNICEF)
- Dioralyte (Rhône-Poulenc Rorer)
- Rehidrat (Searle)
- Electrolade (Eastern).

Alternatively, add eight level or four heaped teaspoons of sugar (white, brown) or honey, plus two teaspoons of salt, to 1 litre of boiled water. Adding a little citrus juice adds potassium and makes the drink more palatable. A further alternative is to use the water in which rice has been cooked. Rehydration should occur at a dose of 200–400ml of solution after every loose motion.

Drugs for the treatment of diarrhoeal symptoms

Anti-motility drugs, such as loperamide (Imodium) or codeine phosphate, are widely promoted and used to treat traveller's diarrhoea. These drugs treat the symptoms of diarrhoea by reducing the frequent bowel motions, but they do not necessarily make you feel better and do not treat the infection. The author does not recommend the use of anti-motility drugs routinely. These drugs are useful if there is irregular access to toilet facilities; if you have to sit on a bus for 4 hours they are indispensable.

The most effective and fast-acting drug for controlling the symptoms of diarrhoea is loperamide (Imodium, Arret). It should be remembered, however, that this does not treat the underlying infection. Loperamide should not be used in children; it is otherwise widely considered to be a safe drug. Concern has been expressed on theoretical grounds that such medication might have the effect of prolonging infection, but several studies have shown such fears to be unfounded. The dose of loperamide is two 2mg capsules at once, followed by one capsule with each loose stool.

Other drugs used in the treatment of diarrhoeal symptoms include: Lomotil, which is a combination of diphenoxylate (a morphine-like drug) and atropine (the atropine component of this combination is included only to prevent Lomotil from being abused and results in symptoms such as a dry mouth and headache); and codeine phosphate. Both of these drugs have constipating effects. None has any advantage over loperamide.

Drugs for the treatment of infection

Traveller's diarrhoea caused by *E. coli* is self-limiting and usually resolves in 24–48 hours. Salmonella, shigella and campylobacter infection can be more severe and prolonged. The problem is that, in the absence of accessible and immediate laboratory diagnosis, it is impossible to know whether you have an illness that is almost certain to get better after a couple of days or one that will persist for some time. Largely for this reason, and for the fact that even 24 hours spent lying prostrate and feeling miserable is best avoided if possible, it is usually worth taking 500mg of the antibiotic ciprofloxacin as soon as the first symptoms of impending gastroenteritis are felt, in other words the first griping abdominal pain closely followed by the first really watery bowel motion, and a feeling of not wanting to eat the next meal. Ciprofloxacin should be used with caution in patients with a history of epilepsy, with liver or kidney impairment, in pregnancy, when dehydrated and in children. Often a single dose will bring the infection to an immediate halt. If necessary continue the ciprofloxacin (500mg) twice daily for 3 days. Do not forget the importance of rehydration at all times.

If amoebic dysentery (diarrhoea with blood) is suspected, the drug of choice is tinidazole (500mg, four tablets every morning for 3 days) followed by diloxanide furoate (Furamide 500mg, three times a day for 10 days). If *Giardia* is suspected (abdominal pain, bloatedness, wind, diarrhoea) take a single 2g dose of tinidazole. If tinidazole is not available, metronidazole (Flagyl 400mg, two tablets three times a day for 5 days) is also an effective alternative for both amoebic dysentery and giardiasis. Note that no alcohol should be drunk while tinidazole or metronidazole is being taken.

When to seek medical attention

Symptoms that justify seeking further medical assessment and support are: a temperature above 40°C; significant fever lasting longer than 48 hours; diarrhoea lasting longer than 4 days; severe diarrhoea with difficulty keeping down fluid and salt replacement; and diarrhoea with blood. Laboratory tests may also be necessary.

Persistent diarrhoea

The commonest cause of diarrhoea persisting after returning home is giardiasis.

Other causes are cryptosporidiosis and cyclospora. Laboratory tests are worthwhile and essential to exclude other possible causes. However, a negative laboratory result may not completely rule out the possibility of giardiasis and, if the symptoms are convincing, presumptive treatment such as with tinidazole, as described above, preferably taken under medical supervision, may be worthwhile.

Another important cause of persistent diarrhoea is lactose intolerance. This is not an infection, but a problem that frequently follows damage to the lining of the small intestine after one or more episodes of severe gastroenteritis. In this condition, lactose – the sugar present in milk and all milk products (yoghurt, cheese and so on) – is poorly digested and instead undergoes a fermentation process. This results in symptoms that are similar to those of giardiasis. There is no easy way of confirming the diagnosis, other than by excluding infective causes and completely eliminating lactose from the diet. It is usually necessary to avoid lactose for about 6 months.

TABLE 18.3 **GASTROENTERITIS – A SIMPLE PLAN OF MANAGEMENT**

SYMPTOMS
Diarrhoea
Often with crampy abdominal pain
Nausea, loss of appetite

↓

Ensure good oral fluid and electrolyte replacement
Dioralyte, rice water

↓

Most traveller's diarrhoea will settle of its own accord in about 48 hours
Single dose of ciprofloxacin 500mg taken at onset of symptoms may settle symptoms
If symptoms persist continue ciprofloxacin 12 hourly for 3 days and rehydration

↓

Loperamide for symptomatic relief
Useful to reduce frequency of bowel motions (especially while travelling) and rehydration

↓

If diarrhoea persists this may be a protozoal infection – *Giardia* or *Entamoeba* (amoebic dysentery)
Take metronidazole 2g once a day for 3 days and rehydration

OTHER COMMON INFECTIONS

Respiratory infections

Viral **upper respiratory tract infections** are more common in travellers, partly because of increased exposure to other people in crowded airports, aircraft, buses and so on, and partly because of exposure to new strains of viruses to which the traveller has not previously developed immunity. Coughs, colds and flu are unpleasant but rarely life threatening. These infections are self-limiting but symptomatic treatment with paracetamol or aspirin may help. Most sore throats are viral in origin and also get better with time. However, some may be bacterial, caused by bacteria such as *Streptococcus pyogenes.* If there is evidence of pus (white spots) on the tonsils (**tonsillitis**) or at the back of the throat, it may be prudent to take antibiotics. Phenoxymethylpenicillin or erythromycin (500mg, four times a day for a week) would be reasonable choices. Ampicillin/amoxycillin should be avoided in these circumstances as it may lead to a severe rash if the sore throat is due to glandular fever (infectious mononucleosis).

If an expedition member develops a cough with a fever and brings up purulent (yellow/green) sputum, he or she may have **bronchitis** or **pneumonia** caused by *Streptococcus pneumoniae* or "atypicals" such as *Mycoplasma pneumoniae.* Pneumonia is more serious and is often accompanied by breathlessness and chest pain that is made worse by deep breathing. In these circumstances, antibiotic therapy with erythromycin (500mg, four times a day for a week) is appropriate, but patients with severe pneumonia will need evacuation and hospital care.

Sinus infections can sometimes be a problem, presenting with nasal stuffiness, pain and tenderness over the sinuses, and sometimes a fever and headache. Although usually caused by viruses, some are bacterial in origin and complicate viral colds and flu. If flu or cold symptoms persist for longer than a week with new symptoms suggestive of **sinusitis**, an antibiotic such as co-amoxiclav (Augmentin 375mg, three times a day for a week) should be considered.

Ear infections

These may be a particular problem for expeditions involving diving or caving. Sometimes the lining of the ear canal becomes infected (**otitis externa**) and is red and painful. This can usually be treated with antibiotic ear drops, such as hydrocortisone (Otosporin, two drops, three times a day), and careful attention to keeping the ears as dry as possible. Rarely in adults the middle ear can become infected (**otitis media**). Again, pain in only one ear is the main symptom and, if observed, the eardrum appears red. Oral antibiotics should settle this down, co-amoxiclav (Augmentin 375mg, three times a day for 5 days) being first choice.

Eye infections

Sometimes the small glands in the eyelash follicles in the eyelids become blocked and infected, producing a painful swelling called a **stye**. This will usually settle with topical antibiotics, such as chloramphenicol ointment. Warm compresses help the symptoms.

Conjunctivitis is not uncommon and is normally bacterial in origin. The best treatment is usually chloramphenicol ointment or drops (drops are easier to insert without a mirror). Put a little snake of cream on the turned down lower eyelid. Pull the upper eyelid over it and massage gently. This should clear the infection in the course of a couple of days. It should be remembered that this condition is highly contagious so an affected person should not share face flannels or towels with others. Other eye infections are rare in otherwise healthy people, but trauma to the eye may lead to secondary infection. If trauma does occur urgent help should be sought, but if none is readily available it is appropriate to use chloramphenicol eye ointment prophylactically.

People who wear contact lenses, especially soft ones, are at increased risk of infection and need to be scrupulous with their hygiene. A widely present amoeba can occasionally infect the cornea, which can lead to serious scarring. It is important to discuss the situation with a contact lens practitioner before leaving home. If it is not possible to guarantee good hygiene, contact lens wearers should revert to spectacles.

Orbital cellulitis is extensive redness, pain and swelling around the eye. It can result from spread of infection from the eye or spread from an infected sinus. This needs urgent medical attention and intravenous antibiotics. Start co-amoxiclav (Augmentin 375mg 8 hourly) and ampicillin (500mg 8 hourly) initially while evacuating.

Management of eye infections

For conjunctivitis use chloramphenicol ointment. For a stye – usually staphylococcal – if severe use flucloxacillin 500mg orally 6 hourly as well as chloramphenicol ointment. If the infection is more severe, particularly if associated with contact lenses or orbital cellulites, evacuate and seek medical attention but initially start co-amoxiclav (Augmentin 375mg 8 hourly) and ampicillin (500mg 8 hourly).

Urinary tract/genital tract infections

Women are more at risk of urinary infections than men, mainly because of their comparatively short urethra. However, men over the age of 40 have an increasing chance of infection, often originating in the prostate gland. Infections of the urinary tract are usually limited to the bladder and produce a variety of possible symptoms including urinary frequency, pain or discomfort when passing urine, and urgency. Sometimes the urine appears cloudy or smells offensive. If the infection ascends the urinary tract to the kidneys, the patient is usually more unwell with the above symptoms and in addition loin pain, fever and, sometimes, rigors (shivering). Most simple urinary tract infections can be treated with oral antibiotics. Co-amoxiclav (Augmentin 375mg,

TABLE 18.4 **MANAGEMENT OF RESPIRATORY AND EAR INFECTIONS**

Diagnosis	*Symptoms*	*Treatment*	*Other*
Colds or flu (viral)	Runny nose, dry cough, mild sore throat	Paracetamol or aspirin every 6 hours	Antibiotics do not help
Sinusitis	Pain over sinuses/headache.	Paracetamol or aspirin	If severe persisting pain consider Augmentin 375mg three times a day for a week. Steam inhalations help ease the symptoms
Ear problems	Inflamed (red) ear canal	Otosporin ear drops (two drops, three times a day)	Use antibiotics if there is increasing pain, redness, discharge or if the ear drum is red (Augmentin 375mg, three times a day for 5 days)
Sore throat		Most are viral – paracetamol or aspirin, gargle with soluble preparations if available	If very red throat, swollen tonsils with pus, sometimes with swollen tender lymph glands in the neck give phenoxymethylpenicillin or erythromycin (500mg, four times a day for a week)
Acute bronchitis/ chest infection	Cough and sputum, if persistent purulent (thick yellow/green) sputum	Augmentin 375mg, three times a day for 5 days. If penicillin allergic use erythromycin	May follow a bad cold
Pneumonia	If dry cough ± chest pain, fever, breathlessness	Erythromycin 500mg, four times a day for a week	If same plus productive cough with purulent sputum give Augmentin 375mg, three times a day for 5 days. Consider evacuation

three times a day for 3 days) or ciprofloxacin (250mg, twice a day for 3 days) are all reasonable choices for empirical therapy. A good fluid intake is also important. Proper hydration is a good prophylaxis against urinary infection.

Women may sometimes be troubled by thrush, a vaginal yeast infection (*Candida*), often causing a thick white discharge. Thrush occurs more commonly in tropical climates and may also be triggered by taking antibiotics. Thrush can be treated using local clotrimazole (Canesten) cream and pessaries. Frequent sufferers should discuss the problem with their doctor before leaving home and ensure that they travel with a suitable supply of medication.

Sexually transmitted diseases may present as a discharge from the penis or vagina. This may be chlamydia or gonorrhoea. The medical officer should establish how this was acquired, treat the case, and treat any accessible sexual contacts with ciprofloxacin 500mg as a single dose plus erythromycin 500mg four times a day for 10 days or doxycycline 100mg twice a day (if available). Give health advice regarding risks of HIV, herpes, hepatitis B and syphilis, all of which can be acquired by unprotected sexual contact.

Management of urinary/genital tract infection

1. For cystitis (bladder infection) in young woman – stinging when passing urine, urgency, frequency – give co-amoxiclav (Augmentin 375mg, three times a day for 3 days) or ciprofloxacin (250mg, twice a day for 3 days). Increase fluid intake.
2. For sexually transmitted infection give ciprofloxacin 500mg as a single dose plus erythromycin 500mg four times a day for 10 days. If HIV contact is a strong possibility, consider evacuation for assessment for anti-HIV drugs immediately.
3. For thrush give local clotrimazole (Canesten) cream or pessaries. For other types of discharge (such as anaerobic vaginosis) give metronidazole 2g as a single dose.
4. For prostatitis – burning when passing urine, frequency, urgency and pain give ciprofloxacin 500mg twice a day for 10 days.

Skin and soft-tissue infections

Small cuts and wounds and insect bites easily become infected on expeditions, particularly in the tropics. Most of these infections are caused by staphylococcal or streptococcal bacteria. Any cuts, however small, should receive first aid treatment and be cleaned with an antiseptic solution and covered with a plaster. Wounds that are infected are red, painful and inflamed, and pus may be present. Boils are abscesses of the skin and are usually caused by staphylococci. Soft-tissue infections respond to antibiotics such as flucloxacillin (250–500mg tablets, four times a day for 5 days). Larger abscesses may require incision and drainage of the pus.

Sometimes large areas of skin on the legs develop a rapidly spreading infection, usually caused by streptococci, and cause the leg to become painful, red and usually swollen. Sometimes blisters appear in the skin and the lymph glands above the affected area may be swollen and tender. This condition is called **cellulitis** and requires antibiotics. If not treated quickly, the infection may spread further, necessitating intravenous or intramuscular antibiotics. Initially, large oral doses of ampicillin/amoxicillin (500mg–1g three times a day) are the most effective treatment.

Animal bites need urgent attention. Clean thoroughly with antiseptic solution (Savlon, chlorhexidine) or failing that soap and water. Give co-amoxiclav (Augmentin 375mg, three times a day for 5 days). Consider the risk of rabies (see Chapter 19).

Athlete's foot, or **tinea pedis**, is a fungal infection of the skin between the toes. This can be particularly tiresome for people with sweaty feet. Wash the feet thoroughly, and dust the feet and socks with Mycil or some similar antifungal dusting powder, or apply cream, such as Canesten.

Antihistamines can be used to suppress **allergic reactions** of various sorts and are useful in suppressing nettle rash, itchy skin conditions, hay fever and the itch associated with insect bites. Remember that all antihistamines, to a varying extent, cause drowsiness. People who are at all drowsy should not drive. Loratadine (Clarityn), available over the counter, is very effective and only needs to be taken once a day at a dose of 10mg. Chlorpheniramine (Piriton) is a slightly sedating antihistamine but again is very effective taken as 4mg up to six times a day. People who are driving should not use the latter.

Bites by insects, mites, fleas, ticks, etc. may introduce important infections (e.g. malaria, dengue, Lyme disease, scrub typhus, African tick typhus, plague, etc.) and often become secondarily infected, especially if the mouth parts (ticks) are left *in situ* or the itchy bite is scratched.

Cutaneous larva migrans

This is a travelling "worm" track, usually red and itchy, and commonly on the foot or any other part of the body that has come into contact with the ground. It is quite a common problem in many parts of the world, particularly the Caribbean and Africa, and results from infestation with animal parasite worm larvae, usually dog hookworm. It is harmless and self-limiting, because the animal parasite larvae cannot mature in human tissue. It is often irritating and itchy and for that reason those with it want something done about it.

Myiasis

This is maggot infestation. The African variety is caused by the Tumbu fly and is particularly prevalent in West Africa. The fly lays its eggs in clothes hanging up to dry or on the ground near human habitation. The young larvae hatch when they come into contact with warm skin and burrow into the skin and grow. Kill the eggs by ironing clothes (if at all possible) or dry them in the direct sunshine until they become crisp. This kills the eggs. As the maggot grows a lump develops under the skin (usually painless and not red). Cover the little hole at the top of the lump with Vaseline and the maggot will emerge to breathe. Catch it with tweezers and pull out.

The Central/South American variety is caused by the fly *Dermatobia hominis.* It lays its eggs on mosquitoes or ticks which transmit the maggot when they bite a host. Treatment is the same as for the Tumbu fly larva.

Tick bites and Lyme disease

Tick bites can transmit many infections from tick typhus in Africa (see Chapter 2) to Rocky Mountain spotted fever, ehrlichiosis in North America, and tick-borne encephalitis in Europe. Lyme disease is a common infection transmitted by ticks across the northern hemisphere.

Ticks should be removed as soon as they are noticed. There are many patent methods for tick removal. Avoid burning them off as it will hurt you more than the tick. Pulling them off tends to leave the tick mouth parts in the skin. Noxious substances such as insect spray and alcohol will remove the tick but probably not before it has vomited into the wound and this may potentiate the transmission of any infection. Two methods work well. The first is to use a dog tick remover available from pet shops. It is a metal strip with a V groove at one end. This slips under the tick mouth parts and levers the tick out. The second is to cover the tick with Vaseline or sun protector. The tick cannot breathe and releases its hold.

Lyme disease is a bacterial infection transmitted by ixodes ticks. It is characterised by a spreading red rash, often with a red leading edge and pale centre, at the site of a tick bite. If this is present, treat with 10 days' worth of ampicillin/amoxicillin (500mg three times a day) or doxycycline (100mg two times a day). Untreated Lyme disease may lead to spread of the bacteria in the body and cause later complications, lasting from several weeks to months after the initial infection. The most common complication in North American Lyme disease is arthritis. In European Lyme, nervous system complications such as a Bell's palsy (weak face), peripheral neuropathy (weakness or tingling in the limbs) or radiculopathy (pain in a skin area served by a spinal nerve root) can result. If this is suspected the diagnosis should be confirmed with a serological blood test and appropriate treatment should be given by a doctor.

Management of skin and soft-tissue infection

Clean all minor wounds with antiseptic and keep covered and dry.

1. Where skin is infected skin/soft tissue is red, inflamed and tender ±pus give flucloxacillin 500mg 6 hourly for 5 days.
   For spreading cellulitis give ampicillin/amoxicillin 500mg–1g three times a day for 5 days.
   For bites – clean, give co-amoxiclav (Augmentin 375mg, three times a day for 5 days) and consider the risk of rabies.
   For patients allergic to penicillin treat with a course of erythromycin (500mg, three times a day for 5 days).
2. Chronic (unhealing) ulcer at the site of a sandfly bite. In several parts of the world but especially Central America this may be cutaneous leishmaniasis (a protozoal infection). Not immediately dangerous. Seek medical attention on return.

3. Myiasis: abscess swelling which may be tense but is not usually too painful. It has a central punctum (hole)and no pus. This may be maggot infestation, especially in West Africa (Tumbu fly) or Central America (*Dermatobia*). If suspected cover the hole with Vaseline. Wait several minutes and the maggot will emerge slightly to breathe. Grasp firmly with tweezers and pull out!
4. A circular raised spreading rash, sometimes scaly or damp and oozing, may be fungal "ringworm" infection. Use miconazole (Canesten) cream.
5. Cutaneous larva migrans is a spreading itchy red track travelling just beneath the skin surface, usually found on the foot, leg or buttock. This is the larval stage of an animal parasite. It is not dangerous, merely irritating and will resolve without treatment after 2–3 months. Apply topical thiabendazole liberally over the tracks daily for 5 days (grind up a 500mg tablet with 5g petroleum jelly).
6. For tick bites, remove the tick. If suspected Lyme disease rash develops treat with 10 days' worth of ampicillin/amoxicillin (500mg three times a day) or doxycycline (100mg twice a day)

HIV and AIDS

HIV and AIDS are increasingly prevalent throughout the developing world, particularly in sub-Saharan Africa, south Asia and Latin America. In these areas HIV is spread mainly through heterosexual activity. In many African cities more than 80% of prostitutes are infected with HIV. There has been a steep increase in the incidence of HIV infection in south-east Asian countries, such as Thailand and the Philippines, and in India.

HIV infection is essentially a sexually transmitted disease. **Unprotected sexual activity carries a risk of HIV infection**. HIV can also be transmitted by transfusion of blood and blood products that have not been properly screened; by intravenous drug abuse when needles or syringes are shared with infected people; by needlestick injuries with contaminated needles (percutaneous exposure); and across the placenta from an infected mother to her fetus. However, the virus is delicate and does not survive for long unless it is in blood or body fluids. It is not spread through the air and is not transmitted by biting insects, handshakes or lavatory seats.

Prevention

For expedition members the message is simple: do not have unprotected sexual intercourse. If having sex a good-quality condom must be worn by the male partner or a female condom by the female. Oral sex is not safe sex. Unprotected sex also carries the risk of acquiring potentially severe hepatitis B infection as well as a wide range of familiar and more exotic sexually transmitted diseases, such as gonorrhoea, chancroid, non-specific urethritis and syphilis.

Unfortunately rape and assault are not uncommon. Try to avoid getting into situations where you are at risk of an assault. If the unthinkable happens, then do not forget HIV in the aftermath and seek early reliable medical attention. If there is a serious risk of HIV infection then expensive and not always available anti-HIV drugs can be given to prevent infection. Established HIV infection remains incurable, but anti-HIV drugs may prevent infection becoming established if they are given rapidly, within a few hours of exposure if possible or within a few days if not. Specialist advice should be sought after sexual assault and it is best to evacuate the victim to their home country as soon as possible. There is no vaccine against HIV infection and no immediate prospect of one being developed.

Avoiding contaminated needles and blood transfusion in developing countries

Many infectious diseases can be spread in infected blood from person to person through the use of non-sterile needles and unscreened transfused blood. Some of the most important are HIV, hepatitis B and other hepatitis viruses, malaria, relapsing fevers, South American trypanosomiasis (Chagas' disease) and haemorrhagic fever viruses. Intravenous drug abusers (mainliners) are at particularly high risk through contaminated needles. Of course, drugs of addiction have no place on an expedition for, apart from any long-term damaging effects on health, they will dangerously impair the competence and judgement of expedition members.

Earlier in this book it was pointed out that an accident is a common hazard facing all expeditions. It can be small, such as a cut that needs suturing or a cut that has become infected and needs injection of an antibiotic. Lone travellers and small expeditions must take with them a small kit of sterile medical equipment (see Chapter 3, page 32) and insist that the contents be used for any injections or suturing that may be necessary. For larger expeditions a more elaborate kit, containing "giving sets", plasma expanders and so on, is now essential (see Chapter 3, page 32). It is wise for every traveller to have his or her blood group determined before departure. It may be that two or more members of an expedition have compatible blood. If it has been screened in a blood transfusion centre in the UK, it will automatically have been screened for HIV. Find out in advance where you can get access to screened blood supplies in the host country. It may also be possible to obtain cover from Blood Care Foundation, a registered charity that couriers and transfuses compatible blood in the event of an emergency, in return for a nominal fee paid in advance. Cover can be arranged through most travel clinics.

Managing HIV

Practice safe sex (use a condom at all times) – oral sex is not safe sex
Avoid sex with high-risk partners
Avoid contaminated needles and blood products
If raped or assaulted seek urgent medical attention.
If risk of HIV is high, early antiviral prophylaxis may well prevent infection

TABLE 18.5 A SELECTED LIST OF ANTIBIOTICS SUITABLE FOR TREATING MOST COMMON INFECTIONS FOR A LARGE EXPEDITION

Antibiotic	*Common uses*
Penicillin	Streptococcal sore throat, cellulitis
Ampicillin/amoxycillin	Chest infection, spreading infection on skin (cellulitis)
Co-amoxiclav (Augmentin)	Chest infection, skin infection, bites, urinary tract infection
Flucloxacillin	Staphylococcal skin infections, boils, impetigo
Doxycycline/tetracycline	Chlamydia infection, tick typhus, Lyme disease, atypical pneumonia
Erythromycin	Skin infection, pneumonia and for penicillin-allergic patients
Metronidazole or tinidazole	*Giardia*/amoebic bowel infection, some genital tract infection
Ciprofloxacin	Urinary tract infection, severe bacterial gastroenteritis
Chloramphenicol eye ointment	Conjunctivitis

TABLE 18.6 A SHORT SELECTION OF ANTIBIOTICS FOR A SMALL EXPEDITION

Antibiotic	*Common uses*
Co-amoxiclav (Augmentin)	Chest infection, skin infection, bites, urinary tract infection
Ciprofloxacin	Urinary tract infection, severe bacterial gastroenteritis
Metronidazole	*Giardia*/amoebic bowel infection, some genital tract infection
Chloramphenicol eye ointment	Conjunctivitis
Erythromycin	For penicillin-allergic patients

TABLE 18.7 MANAGEMENT OF A HIGH FEVER

Management of a high fever > 38°C

↓

Is there an obvious site of infection (i.e. throat, chest, skin, gut, urine)?

YES	NO
1 Red painful throat ±lymph glands enlarged. Glandular fever or streptococcal throat. Treat with penicillin or erythromycin 2 Chest infection/cough. If productive sputum is purulent (mucky) give Augmentin. If dry cough give erythromycin 3 Severe abdominal pain. This may be a surgical problem, e.g. appendicitis. Emergency – get to hospital Give Augmentin initially 4 Diarrhoea as main feature: – give ciprofloxacin and rehydrate 5 Skin and soft tissue: – spreading redness, swelling and pain (cellulitis), give Augmentin – localised infection/abscess/pus present, give flucloxacillin 6 Pain passing urine or loin pain, i.e. over kidney, give ciprofloxacin or Augmentin	1 Is this heat exhaustion/dehydration? If so treat appropriately, i.e. cool and rehydrate 2 In a malarious country fever, shakes (rigors), muscle aches, headache = likely malaria. Give quinine 600mg three times a day and evacuate. Emergency 3 Rash that does not blanch when pressed, cool peripheries – hands, feet; with or without stiff neck, headache, aversion to bright light = meningococcal sepsis. Emergency – evacuate. Give intravenous antibiotics (penicillin, ceftriaxone) if available. If not give oral ciprofloxacin + penicillin 4 Tick bites that look inflamed (±black scab). Raised red rash elsewhere. May be tick typhus. Give doxycycline 100mg twice a day

19 MALARIA AND OTHER TROPICAL DISEASES

David Warrell

MALARIA

Malaria is endemic in almost all parts of the tropical world as far north as southern Turkey, as far south as north-eastern South Africa, as far west as Mexico and as far east as Vanuatu in the western Pacific (see Figure 19.2). The females of certain species of mosquito (genus *Anopheles*), which nearly always bite between dusk and dawn, transmit malaria (Figure 19.1). Four different species of malarial parasites commonly infect humans: life-threatening *Plasmodium falciparum* and the three so-called benign malarias, *P. vivax, P. ovale* and *P. malariae. P. falciparum* malaria kills 1 to 2 million people each year and is particularly dangerous to those who have not acquired immunity to it by growing up in a malarious part of the world. About 2,000 cases of imported malaria are reported in the UK each year, but over the last few years the proportion of dangerous *P. falciparum* cases has increased to over 60%. Each year, a few people die of imported malaria in the UK and an unknown number die abroad. Most of these deaths could have been prevented by better education of the travellers, use of approved methods of prevention and prompt medical attention when a person falls ill.

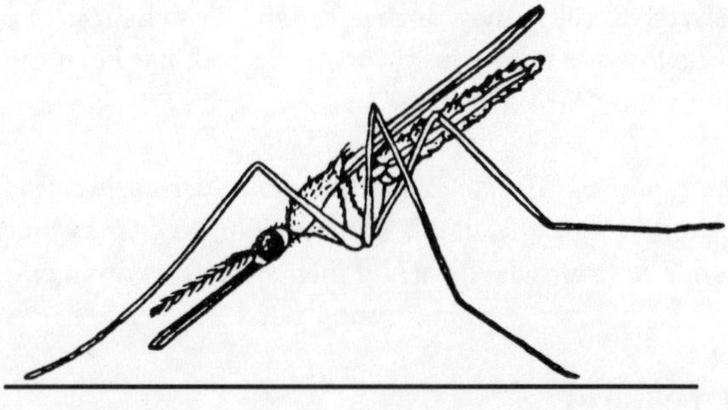

Figure 19.1 *An anopheles mosquito*

Prevention

TABLE 19.1 PRINCIPLES OF PERSONAL PROTECTION AGAINST MALARIA

1. **Awareness of risk:** vulnerable individuals, such as pregnant women, infants or immunocompromised people, should avoid entering a malarious area
2. **Anti-mosquito measures:** kill, exclude, repel and avoid mosquitoes
   - Sensible clothing (long sleeves, long trousers) between dusk and dawn
   - Diethyltoluamide (DEET) – containing insect repellent applied to exposed skin
   - Insecticide (pyrethroid) – impregnated mosquito bed net or screened accommodation sprayed with insecticide each evening
   - Vaporising insecticide in the sleeping quarters (electrical, mosquito coil, knock-down insecticide)
3. **Chemoprophylaxis:** mefloquine (Lariam) or other drugs, depending on the particular geographical area
4. **Standby treatment:** Fansidar, mefloquine, quinine, Malarone
5. **In case of feverish illness within a few months of return: see a doctor and mention malaria specifically!**

Assessing the risk

Within malarious countries, the areas of malaria transmission may be patchy, depending on environmental factors such as temperature, altitude and vegetation as well as the season. Thus there is no malaria transmission in some African capital cities that are at a comparatively high altitude, such as Addis Ababa and Nairobi, and in other areas malaria transmission occurs only during a brief rainy season. If possible, reliable local advice should be obtained about the status of malaria transmission in the area where, and at the time when, the expedition is to take place. Even within a transmission area, the risk of being bitten by an infected mosquito can vary from less than once per year to more than once per night. The chances of catching malaria during a 2-week visit, while taking no protection at all, has been estimated at about 0.2% in Kenya and 1% in West Africa.

People who are especially vulnerable to malaria should seriously consider whether they need to enter the malarious area at all. These include pregnant women, infants and young children, and those who have had their spleens removed or are otherwise immunosuppressed

Anti-mosquito measures

Since most malaria-transmitting mosquitoes bite in or near human dwellings during

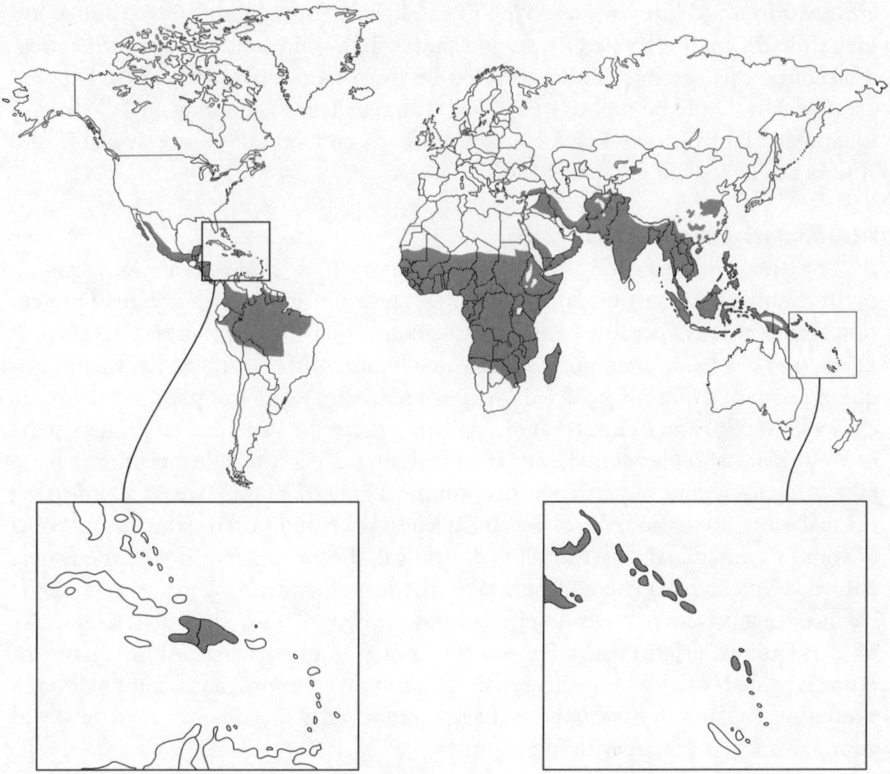

Figure 19.2 *Malaria is endemic in almost all parts of the tropical world as far north as southern Turkey, as far south as north-eastern South Africa, as far west as Mexico and as far east as Vanuatu in the western Pacific*

the hours of darkness, the risk of infection can be reduced by insect-proofing sleeping quarters or by sleeping under a mosquito net. Individual, lightweight, self-supporting mosquito nets are available. Protection against mosquitoes and other biting invertebrates (sandflies, lice, fleas, bed bugs and so on) is greatly enhanced by soaking the net in a pyrethroid insecticide such as permethrin (0.2g per m^2 of material every 6 months). Screens and curtains can also be impregnated with insecticide. In addition, bedrooms should be sprayed in the evening with a knock-down insecticide to kill any mosquitoes that may have entered the room during the day. Mosquitoes may also be killed or repelled by vaporising synthetic pyrethroids (Bioallethrin 4.2% w/w) on electrical heating devices (such as No Bite and Buzz Off) where electricity is available or over a methylated spirit burner (Travel Accessories UK Ltd, PO Box 10, Lutterworth, Leicester LE17 4FB). Burning cones or coils of mosquito repellent "incense" may also be effective. To avoid bites by any flying insect, light-coloured long-sleeved shirts and long trousers are preferable to vests and shorts. To avoid malaria-transmitting mosquito bites, this sensible clothing should be worn particularly after dark. Exposed areas of skin should be rubbed or sprayed with repellents containing *NN*-diethyl-*m*-toluamide (DEET). Insecticide-containing soaps and suntan oil are available and clothes can be soaked in repellent solution.

Anti-malarial chemoprophylaxis

At one time comparatively harmless drugs, such as chloroquine (Nivaquine), pyrimethamine (Daraprim) and proguanil (Paludrine), gave a high degree of protection against malaria parasites. However, the rapid emergence of resistant strains of *P. falciparum* has made chemoprophylaxis much more difficult. In particular, chloroquine-resistant strains of *P. falciparum* now predominate in most parts of the tropics except in Mexico and Central America, north-west of the Panama Canal, Haiti, parts of West Africa and the Middle East. The failure of travellers to take their antimalarial tablets regularly, and in particular to continue taking them for 4 weeks after leaving the malarious area, also reduces the effectiveness of chemoprophylaxis. During bouts of vomiting and diarrhoea (traveller's diarrhoea), these drugs may not be adequately absorbed. In choosing chemoprophylaxis, the risk of contracting malaria should be balanced against the risk of side-effects from the drug. This is illustrated by the case of mefloquine (Lariam) which has recently excited a heated debate. Although mefloquine is probably twice as effective as the chloroquine plus proguanil combination in preventing malaria in Africa, the incidence and severity of side-effects, especially in young women, is greater with mefloquine.

Chemoprophylactic drugs and combinations

Mefloquine (Lariam)

This drug is effective against most multiresistant *P. falciparum* strains. It has some unpleasant side-effects: nausea, stomachache and diarrhoea in 10–15% of people who take it; insomnia and nightmares; giddiness and ataxia (unsteadiness and incoordination) in some; and, much more serious, a rare "acute brain syndrome" consisting of psychological changes and in very rare cases generalised convulsions (epileptic attacks). For these reasons it is recommended for use only in areas with a high risk of resistant malaria (such as Africa, the Amazon region and south-east Asia). The dose is one tablet (of 250mg) a week.

Proguanil (Paludrine) and chloroquine (Nivaquine)

The combination of proguanil – two tablets (each of 100mg) every day – and chloroquine – two tablets (each of 150mg base) once a week – was the standard recommended and most widely used prophylactic regime in areas where *P. falciparum* is chloroquine resistant. Unfortunately, its efficacy has now declined, so that it is no longer recommended for Africa, the Amazon region or south-east Asia and Oceania. It is safe in pregnancy and (in a lower dose) in children. The only side-effects are rare mouth ulcers, mild indigestion and hair loss. Since this combination is no longer effective, it should be pointed out to travellers that despite taking antimalarials they may still develop malaria. However, if they are on antimalarials they are unlikely to become seriously ill with malaria, but *they must seek medical treatment if they get a fever, especially during the first few months after returning from the malarious area.*

There is no evidence that chloroquine, taken in the doses recommended for prophylaxis against malaria, ever causes damage to the eyes in people who take the drug continuously for 5–6 years. Checks after chloroquine prophylaxis are therefore unnecessary, unless the individual has taken the drug for a very long time (more than 6 years continuously) and the total cumulative dose approaches 100g.

Atovaquone–proguanil (Malarone)

This safe, effective but expensive drug needs to be continued for only 7 days after leaving the malarious area. The dose is one tablet each day for adults.

Doxycycline (Vibramycin)

This tetracycline antibiotic has proved useful for prophylaxis in areas where mefloquine resistance is prevalent, such as the Thai–Cambodian border region. It gives some protection against other traveller's diseases such as typhus, leptospirosis and some types of traveller's diarrhoea. One 100mg tablet a day should be taken. Side-effects include photosensitive rashes, skin irritation, diarrhoea, and oral/oesophageal or vaginal thrush. It should not be used by pregnant women and young children.

Maloprim, Deltaprim

This is a combination of dapsone 100mg and pyrimethamine 12.5mg which, unlike mefloquine and chloroquine, is safe for sufferers from epilepsy. Its manufacture may soon be stopped. When used, one tablet a week (for example every Sunday), no more, no less, should be taken.

Choice of prophylactic drug/combination in different geographical areas

- Middle East, West Asia, Indian subcontinent, parts of South America (except Amazon region of Brazil), China: use proguanil plus chloroquine.
- Mexico, Central America, Haiti, Dominican Republic, parts of South America (except Amazon region of Brazil): use chloroquine.
- Africa, Amazon region of Brazil, south-east Asia (except Thai–Cambodian border region): use mefloquine, doxycycline or Malarone.
- West Pacific, New Guinea: use mefloquine or doxycycline.
- Thai–Cambodian border region: use doxycycline or Malarone.

- Turkey, Egypt, Mauritius (rural, seasonal only): use chloroquine or proguanil.

(Malarone is an alternative to mefloquine or doxycycline in all areas, for those who can afford it!)

During pregnancy it is vital for the expectant mother to take antimalarials or, preferably, to avoid entering a malarious area. The hazards of getting malaria, particularly *P. falciparum* malaria, during pregnancy are great. The remote hazard of adverse effects on the baby of the antimalarial drugs is far outweighed by the advantages. Chloroquine plus proguanil as outlined above should be used. Maloprim and other pyrimethamine-containing drugs, mefloquine, doxycyline and Malarone, should be avoided during pregnancy.

It is wise to start weekly mefloquine 3 weeks before leaving for the malarious area in case side-effects develop and you have to switch to another drug. All antimalarial drugs except Malarone must be continued for 4 weeks after return.

Remember that no antimalarial drug is perfect. Much depends on whether it is taken regularly. If you are ill at all after your return you should consult your doctor and *mention the possibility of malaria.* If there is *any doubt* you should be referred to an infectious disease unit for exclusion of malaria. If you have been taking an antimalarial it may be difficult to find the parasites and yet you may be quite ill.

Standby treatment for malaria in high-risk areas

If you are going to a remote malarious area you would be wise to take a supply of quinine, 600mg to be taken 8 hourly for 7 days if you get a fever. Mefloquine, two tablets (each of 250mg) repeated after 8 hours (1,000mg total for an adult, 20mg/kg for children), is an alternative unless that is the drug you have been taking for prophylaxis. Fansidar and Malarone *are* also useful standby treatments. A new combination drug, artemether plus lumefantrine (Riamet or Co-artemether) will also be suitable for standby treatment.

Prevention of the "benign" malarias (*P. vivax*, *ovale* and *malariae*)

Weekly chloroquine or mefloquine will usually prevent *P. vivax*, *ovale* and *malariae* malarias. However, *P. vivax* and *P. ovale* can establish themselves in the liver despite chloroquine prophylaxis and may re-emerge to cause relapsing infections months or years later. Primaquine, 15mg a day for 2 weeks, will usually eradicate the liver cycle and should be given to travellers who have spent more than a few months in areas where these species are endemic. In parts of Indonesia, particularly Irian Jaya, and in Papua New Guinea, Thailand, the Philippines and the Solomon Islands, *P. vivax* malaria may not be eradicated by the usual 2-week course of primaquine. In these cases a 4-week course of primaquine should be given after the person returns home.

In New Guinea and adjacent areas of Indonesia (for example, Lombok), *P. vivax* malaria has become resistant to chloroquine. A double dose of chloroquine or the standard dose of mefloquine followed by a 4-week course of primaquine can be used to treat such resistant infections. Advice on malarial prophylaxis can be obtained from the following tropical medicine units.

Malaria Reference Laboratory
Tel. +44 20 7636 3924
Tel (24 hr): +44 9065 508908
Website: www.lshtm.ac.uk/centres/malaria

Hospital for Tropical Diseases
Tel. +44 20 7387 9300/4411
Healthline: +44 9061 337733
Fax: +44 20 7388 7645
Website: www.thehtd.org

London School of Tropical Medicine
Tel. +44 20 7636 8636
Website: www.lshtm.ac.uk

Liverpool School of Tropical Medicine
Tel. +44 151 708 9393
Fax: +44 151 708 8733
Website: www.liv.ac.uk/lstm/lstm.html

Oxford University Centre for Tropical Medicine
Tel. +44 1865 220968
Fax: +44 1865 220984

OTHER TROPICAL DISEASES

Bilharzia (schistosomiasis)

This fluke infection occurs in Africa, the Middle East, eastern South America, China and south-east Asia (Figure 19.3). Infection is acquired through contact with fresh water from lakes and sluggish rivers, usually by bathing or washing with water taken from these sources. Infected humans contaminate the lake by defecating or urinating into it and infect, in turn, the intermediate snail hosts. Snails release tiny cercariae into the water which burrow through the skin of bathers. The earliest symptom of possible infection is "swimmer's itch", experienced soon after contact with infected

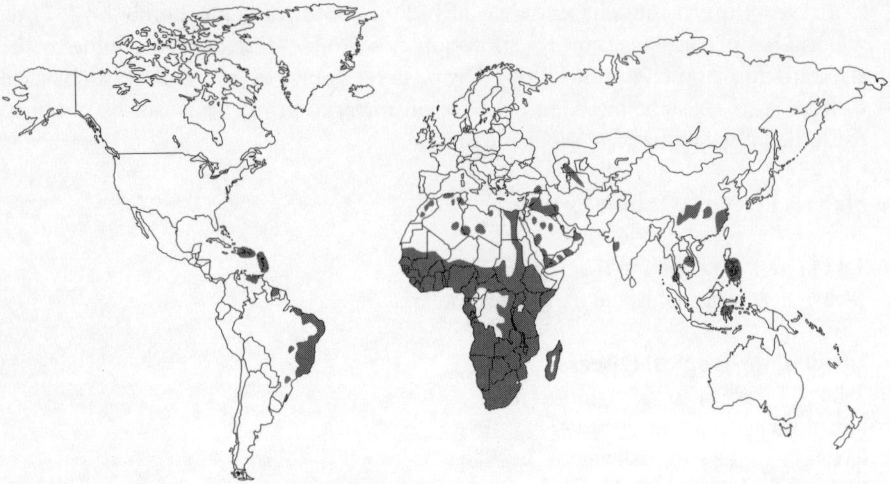

Figure 19.3 *Bilharzia (schistosomiasis)*

water. Some people develop an acute feverish illness associated with an urticarial rash and blood eosinophilia a few weeks after infection. Later symptoms include passage of cloudy or frankly bloodstained urine or dysentery and, rarely, ascending paralysis and loss of sensation in the lower limbs.

Travellers usually get worried about bilharzia when they get back from their trip and remember bathing in forbidden lakes or hear that another member of the party has been diagnosed as having schistosomiasis. Diagnosis is confirmed by finding ova in stool, urine or rectal biopsies, or by a blood test. Treatment is fairly simple with one to two doses of praziquantel (Biltricide).

Prevent bilharzia by not bathing in sluggish fresh water sources in endemic areas. Local advice may be misleading. Lake Malawi, officially declared free of bilharzia, has been the source of many imported cases of bilharzia in the UK over the last few years.

Dengue fever ("break bone" fever)

Mosquitoes such as *Aedes aegypti and A. albopictus* transmit dengue viruses from human to human in almost every part of the tropics, notably in south-east Asia and the Caribbean, and increasingly in urban areas (Figure 19.4). In most foreign travellers, dengue causes an acute fever associated with headache, backache and pains in the muscles and joints ("break bone" fever). The most obvious reddish blotchy rash often appears after a temporary lull in the fever. Petechial haemorrhages may be found in the skin and conjunctivae. The blood count usually shows leucopenia with relative lymphocytosis and thrombocytopenia. The diagnosis can be confirmed by testing two blood samples, one taken immediately and the other 2 weeks after the acute illness.

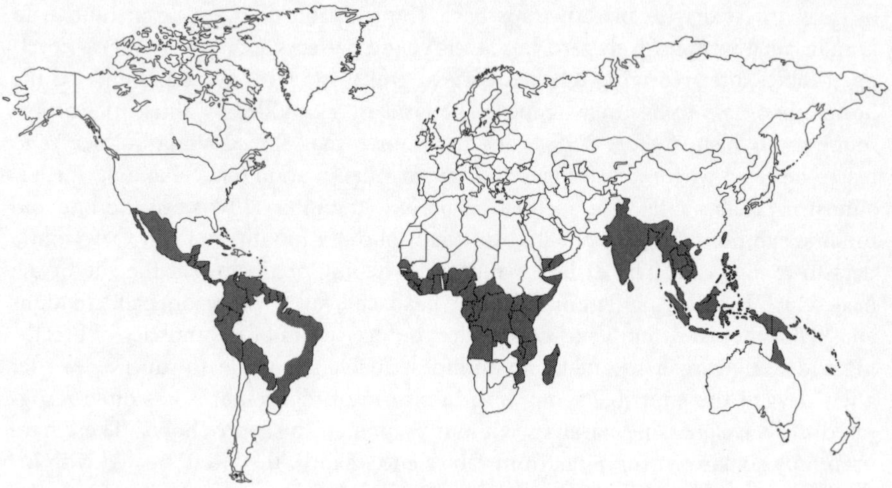

Figure 19.4 *Dengue fever ("break bone" fever)*

Severe, life-threatening forms of dengue (dengue haemorrhagic fever and dengue shock syndrome) occur almost exclusively in children who have been brought up in endemic areas and are suffering their second dengue infection.

Treatment of dengue fever is symptomatic (bed rest, control of fever and paracetamol).

Prevention is by wearing sensible clothing (see above) during the daytime biting period and applying DEET-containing repellents to exposed skin surfaces.

Rabies

Rabies or hydrophobia (literally fear of water) is a virus disease of mammals that is usually transmitted to humans by a dog bite. Although dogs are the most important source of human rabies worldwide, some countries have other vector species, such as cats, wolves, foxes, jackals, skunks, mongooses, racoons, vampire bats (Caribbean and Latin America only), flying foxes and insectivorous bats. Rabies occurs in almost every country (see Figure 2.5, page 15); the fortunate exceptions include Antarctica, Scandinavian countries (except Greenland and Svalbard), Malaysia, New Guinea, New Zealand, Japan, the UK and some smaller islands. It is especially common in parts of Latin America, the Indian subcontinent, Vietnam, Thailand and the Philippines. The disease probably causes at least 60,000 human deaths each year.

The rabies virus can enter the body in a number of ways. Virus in an animal's saliva can penetrate skin that has been broken by a bite or graze, and can invade unbroken mucous membranes, such as those covering the eye and lining the mouth and nose. Very rarely, the virus has been inhaled, for example, from the atmosphere of caves infested with insectivorous bats. Transmission of rabies from human to human must be excessively rare, but at least eight patients are known to have developed rabies after receiving infected corneal grafts. After the virus has entered the body, one of two things may happen. The virus may be killed by antiseptics or immune mechanisms before it does any harm, or it may spread along the nerves to reach the brain where it multiplies and causes inflammation (encephalitis), which is almost invariably fatal. The incubation period (the interval between the bite and the first symptoms of encephalitis) is usually about 2 months but can vary from 4 days to many years. The earliest symptom is itching or tingling at the site of the healed bite. Later the patient may develop headache, fever, confusion, hallucinations and hydrophobia. Attempts to drink water induce spasm of the muscles of breathing and swallowing associated with an indescribable terror. Death supervenes after a few days of these terrible symptoms. In a form of rabies that is less often recognised there is spreading paralysis without excitement or hydrophobia. There have been only six known survivors from rabies encephalitis: they were treated with intensive care.

Prevention

Details of pre-exposure immunisation are given in Chapter 2 (see Table 2.1, page 10).

Stroking stray dogs and apparently tame wild animals, keeping carnivores as pets and other unnecessary contact with mammals should be avoided in areas where rabies is endemic. Irrespective of the risk of rabies, mammal (including human) bites and scratches and licks on mucous membranes or broken skin should be cleaned immediately.

First, scrub with soap and water under a running tap if possible, or else immerse in water, for at least 5 minutes. The best virucidal agents are 40–70% alcohol (gin and whisky contain more than 40% alcohol) and povidone–iodine. Mammal bites are frequently contaminated by a variety of micro-organisms other than rabies virus, so a doctor or the expedition nurse should be consulted. Immediate thorough cleaning of the wound is of the utmost importance in preventing infection.

Second, rabies should be considered if it is known to occur in the area. The decision whether or not to give post-exposure vaccination and rabies immune serum is made by a doctor. Ideally, it is based on examination of the biting animal, but usually this is not possible. The species of animal, its behaviour, the circumstances of the bite and, in the case of a domestic animal, when it was last vaccinated are useful pieces of information. The decision must be made as soon as possible by a doctor working in the area where the bite occurrs. On no account should it be delayed until patients return to their own country. *If in doubt, vaccinate.* Modern vaccines such as HDCV, PVRV, PCEC and PDEV are potent and safe. They require fewer injections than the older type of nervous tissue vaccine which was given on at least 21 consecutive days under the skin of the abdomen. The old Semple vaccine deserved its reputation for being dangerous; the tissue culture vaccines are safe. Timely cleaning of the bite wound combined with vaccination and use of immune serum has proved very effective in preventing rabies. If a suspected rabid animal later bites someone who has received pre-exposure immunisation, immunity must be boosted with two injections of vaccine on days 0 and 7.

If the bitten person has not previously been immunised, a full course of post-exposure vaccination is required. The conventional course, using modern vaccines (detailed above), involves intramuscular injections of one whole vial (0.5ml or 1ml of reconstituted vaccine) intramuscularly on days 0, 3, 7, 14 and 30. These individuals should also receive a dose of rabies immune globulin. Half is infiltrated around the bite wound and the rest given intramuscularly into the front of the thigh. The dose of equine rabies immune globulin is 40 units/kg body weight; the dose of human rabies immune globulin is 20 units/kg body weight.

If rapid induction of active immunity is required and there is a shortage of vaccine, modern vaccines can be used effectively and economically by employing an alternative *multiple* site intradermal regime. On day 0, one ampoule of vaccine is divided between eight different sites (both deltoids, both thighs, both sides of the umbilicus and above both shoulder blades at the back). At each site 0.1ml (in the case of 1ml ampoules of vaccine) or 0.05ml (in the case of 0.5ml ampoules of vaccine) is injected intradermally (so that it raises a small *peau d'orange* papule). On day 7, four intradermal injections are given (both deltoids and both thighs) and single intradermal injections are given on days 30 and 90.

It is essential to take rabies seriously and minimise the risk of infection by avoiding potentially rabid animals. If bitten by a suspected rabid animal and no suitable vaccine is available, the individual should be repatriated without delay so as to start post-exposure prophylaxis as soon as possible.

For dog bite/rabies queries contact:

Public Health Laboratory Health Centre
Virus Reference Laboratory
Tel. +44 20 8200 4400 ext. 3204

River blindness (onchocerciasis)

In parts of east, west, central and southern Africa, Mexico and Central America and north-eastern South America (Figure 19.5), pernicious little black flies (for example, *Simulium damnosum*) transmit this infection from human to human in the vicinity of fast-flowing rivers and streams. The adult filarial worms live in subcutaneous nodules, especially around the waist. They produce enormous numbers of microfilariae which cause irritation and changes in the pigmentation and texture of the skin and damage the eyes, eventually causing river blindness. Foreign travellers have contracted onchocerciasis after only brief stops in the transmission zone.

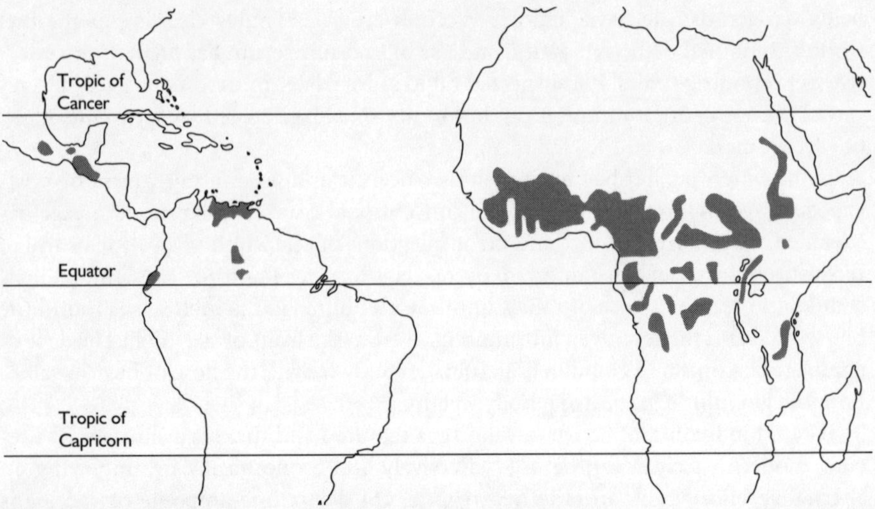

Figure 19.5 *River blindness (onchocerciasis) (D. Warrell)*

Diagnosis is supported by finding blood eosinophilia and is confirmed by microscopical detection of wriggling microfilariae in skin snips taken in affected areas. There is also a blood test of moderate specificity.

Treatment with ivermectin is effective, but may cause a temporary but damaging exacerbation of lesions in the eye and skin and should therefore be supervised in a hospital.

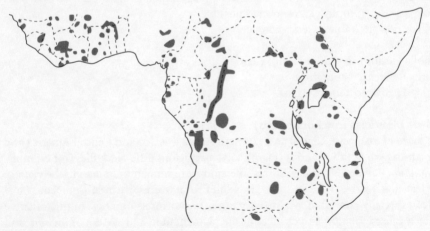

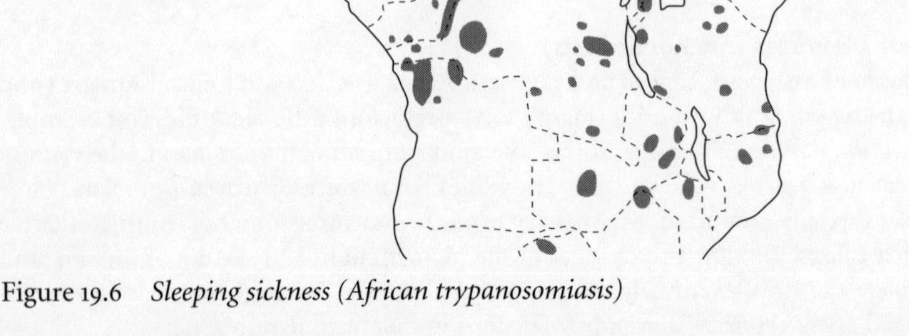

Figure 19.6 *Sleeping sickness (African trypanosomiasis)*

Prevent infection by wearing light-coloured clothing (long sleeves and long trousers) and applying DEET-containing repellents to exposed areas of skin.

Sleeping sickness (African trypanosomiasis)

Tsetse flies (*Glossina*) transmit trypanosomes (*Trypanosoma brucei gambiense*) between humans and *T. b. rhodesiense* between humans and animal reservoir hosts in a number of smallish areas scattered throughout West, Central, East and southern Africa (Figure 19.6). A small ulcer with a scab may appear at the site of the infected tsetse fly bite and, within the next few days, intermittent fever begins associated with headache, loss of appetite and enlargement of lymph glands, especially in the posterior triangle of the neck. Eventually, there is invasion of the central nervous system and patients become apathetic, sleepy and eventually comatose.

The diagnosis is confirmed by finding motile trypanosomes in lymph node aspirates, blood or cerebrospinal fluid. Treatment is difficult, especially after invasion of the central nervous system. Foreign travellers, especially to the game parks of eastern and southern Africa, have been infected and there is currently a massive resurgence of sleeping sickness in central/east Africa.

20 VENOMOUS AND POISONOUS ANIMALS

David Warrell

ATTACKS BY LARGE ANIMALS

Large animals, wild and domestic, should be treated with respect; they may not be as tame as they appear. Lions, leopards, hyenas, domestic dogs, jackals, wolves, elephants, rhinos, hippopotamuses, buffaloes, domestic cattle, domestic and wild pigs, ostriches and even rams have been responsible for occasional human deaths. In recent months, two campers in Kenya have been seized by the head and severely mauled by hyenas while sleeping in the open. Sharks kill about 50 people each year. Crocodiles (Figure 20.1) claim many human lives but in Africa hippopotamuses are thought to kill even more people. Recently in Kenya a man swimming to retrieve a duck he had shot was killed by a hippopotamus. It is extremely foolhardy for

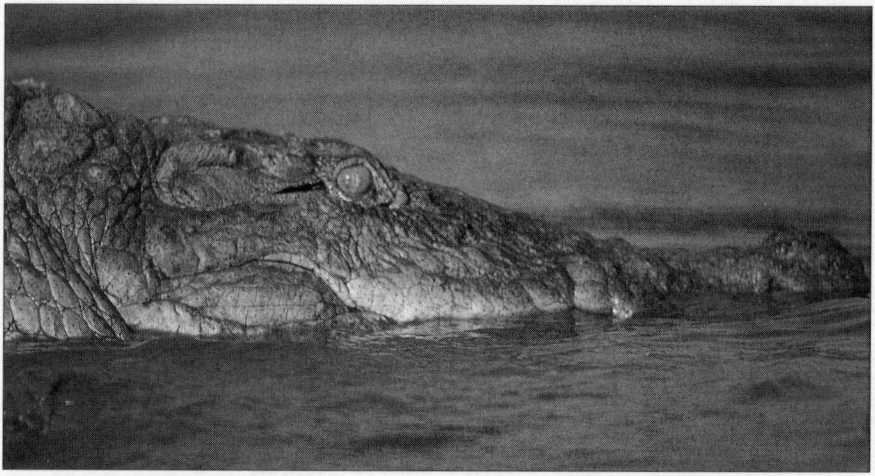

Figure 20.1 *The Nile crocodile* Crocodilus niloticus – *a threat to human lives (D. A. Warrell)*

travellers to bathe in rivers regarded as dangerous by the local inhabitants. A Peace Corps worker in Ethiopia did this in 1967 and was promptly killed and eaten by the resident crocodile. More recently, two British girls were killed by crocodiles in Tanzania and Kenya.

VENOMOUS ANIMALS

Travellers in tropical countries usually have an exaggerated fear of snakes, scorpions and other venomous animals. Most parts of the world, especially the tropical regions, harbour animals with potentially lethal venoms, but local farmers and children, rather than travellers, suffer. Thus snake bite is a major cause of death among some tribes of the Ecuadorian, Venezuelan and Brazilian jungles, and among the inhabitants of some parts of India, Burma, Nigeria and Sri Lanka; and many children die of scorpion stings in parts of Mexico and north Africa. Yet the author knows of no recent case of a European traveller being killed by a venomous bite or sting.

Before travelling to a tropical country it is worth finding out about local venomous species and trying to discover if there is a national centre for antivenom production, supply and treatment. The use of antivenom (also called antivenin, antivenene or anti-snake-bite serum) requires medical training. If an expedition is going to an extremely remote and snake-infested area it might be wise to collect some antivenom from the regional centre and to ensure that there is someone in the party who has been trained to use it safely. Otherwise, rely on local medical services but enquire about them in advance. Before buying antivenoms manufactured in Europe, seek expert advice about their effectiveness against the venoms of the species that are important causes of bites or stings in the area of your expedition.

Snake bite

Prevention

Snakes never attack humans without provocation and so the risk of snake bite can be reduced as follows. Avoid snakes and snake charmers. Do not disturb, corner or attack snakes and never handle them, even if they are said to be harmless or appear to be dead. Even a severed head can bite. If you corner a snake by mistake, keep absolutely still until it has slithered away (this demands enormous *sang froid*), because snakes strike only at moving objects. Never walk in undergrowth or deep sand without boots, socks and long trousers; and at night always carry a light. Never collect firewood or dislodge logs and boulders with your bare hands and never put your hand or push sticks into burrows or holes. Avoid climbing trees or rocks that are covered with dense foliage, and do not put your hands on sunbaked ledges you cannot see when climbing. Never swim in rivers matted with vegetation or in muddy estuaries where there are likely to be sea snakes. If you have to sleep on the ground, use a tent with sewn-in ground sheet, or tuck the mosquito net under your sleeping bag.

Otherwise use a hammock or raised camp bed. The danger is rolling over in your sleep and trapping a snake that has been attracted to the campsite by its natural prey, such as a small rodent.

Treatment of snake bite

First aid treatment of snake bite should be applied by the victim or other people who are on the spot.

TABLE 20.1 TREATMENT OF SNAKE BITE

1. Reassure the bitten patient
2. Cover the bite with a clean dressing but do not interfere with it in any way
3. Immobilise the bitten limb and encourage the patient to remain as still as possible
4. Treat pain with paracetamol or codeine tablets (not aspirin!)
5. Transport patient immediately to hospital but minimise the amount of movement
6. DO NOT attempt to catch or kill the snake
7. Avoid all traditional and "quack" remedies

First, reassure the patient, who may be terrified by the thought of sudden death. The grounds for reassurance are that only a small minority of snake species are dangerously venomous to humans and even the most notorious species, such as cobras, often bite without injecting enough venom to be harmful. The risk and rapidity of death from snake bite has been greatly exaggerated. Lethal doses of venom usually take hours (cobras, mambas, sea snakes and so on) or days (vipers, rattlesnakes and other pit vipers, and so on) to kill a human, not seconds or minutes as is commonly believed. *Correct treatment is very effective.*

Second, cover the site of the bite with a clean dressing.

Third, immobilise the bitten limb with a splint or sling and arrange immediate transport to a hospital, a dispensary or to the expedition medical officer. The patient must keep as still as possible and avoid exercising any part of the body, especially the bitten limb.

Do not attempt to catch or kill the snake, but if it has been killed already take it with you; it is useful clinical evidence. *However, it must not be handled with bare hands even if it appears to be dead.*

Avoid traditional remedies (incisions, suction, tourniquets, electric shock, snake stone and so on) which do more harm than good. For example:

- Do not apply a tourniquet (ligature or tight band). However, if the snake is one whose venom contains a dangerous neurotoxin (for example, cobra, krait, mamba, sea snake, Australian tiger snake, taipan, etc.) use the pressure-immobilisation (P-I) method. Bind the whole of the bitten limb as tightly as you would a sprained ankle, starting around the fingers or toes, using a long stretchy crepe bandage (10cm wide, 4.5m long) and incorporating a splint (Figure 20.2). This method should not be used after bites by snakes whose venoms cause a lot of local swelling and gangrene (for example, most vipers and some cobras).

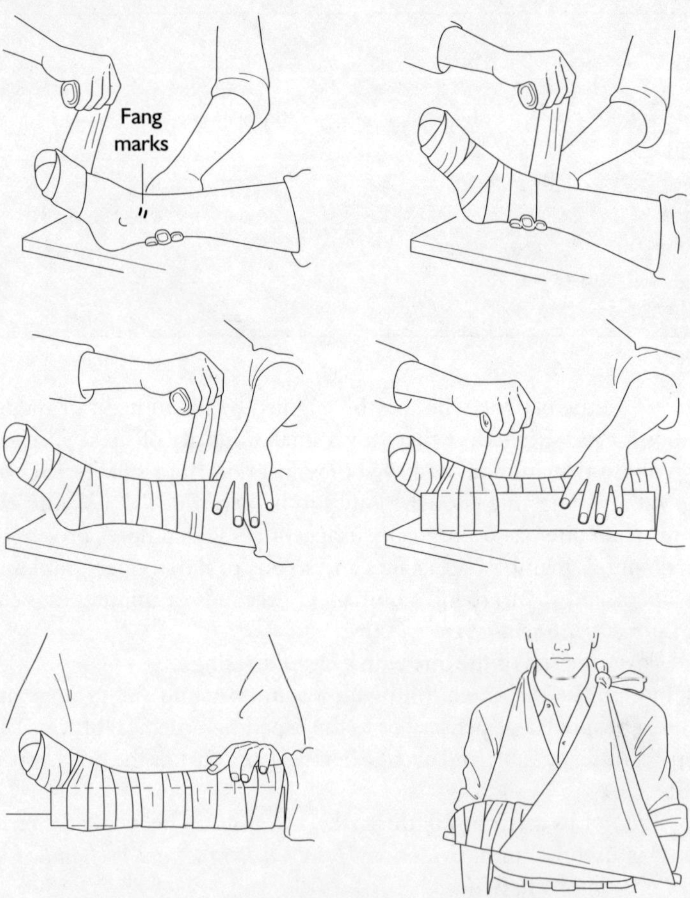

Figure 20.2 *Compression/immobilisation method for the treatment of snake bite on the leg or arm (Courtesy of Australian Venom Research Unit, University of Melbourne)*

- Do not suck at the wound with your mouth or a vacuum extractor apparatus, cut it with a razor blade, introduce potassium permanganate crystals, apply ice or electric shocks, or interfere in any other way.
- Do not give aspirin, which may cause bleeding.
- Do not give antivenom which can be dangerous and should be administered only by a doctor, nurse or dispenser who has emergency drugs (adrenaline/epinephrine, antihistamine and corticosteroid) to deal with antivenom reactions should they occur. If you have your own supply of antivenom take it with you to hospital where the doctor or other trained staff can administer it.

Advice for the expedition medical officer

Absence of local swelling 4 hours after a bite by a viper, rattlesnake or other pit viper suggests that no venom was injected and that no further treatment is necessary. However, bites by some snakes with neurotoxic venoms (mambas, kraits, cobras and so on) may not cause any local swelling, but may lead to serious systemic effects.

Indications for antivenom treatment

1. Bleeding from gums, nose, gastrointestinal tract or any other site distant from the bite itself, which started spontaneously after the bite, and persistent bleeding from wounds (such as venepuncture sites).
2. Failure of the patient's blood to clot if placed in a new, clean, dry, glass tube and left undisturbed for 20 minutes.
3. Signs of nervous system involvement such as drooping eyelids, difficulty in swallowing and breathing, pain, stiffness and paralysis of skeletal muscles, and extreme drowsiness or unconsciousness.
4. Passage of dark red, brown or black urine (haemoglobinuria or myoglobinuria).
5. Signs of heart involvement such as low or falling blood pressure, unusually slow pulse rate or irregular rhythm.
6. Swelling of more than half the bitten limb, swelling after bites on the fingers and toes, or swelling after bites by snakes whose venom is known to cause gangrene (for example, most vipers and rattlesnakes, some cobras).

Note: antivenom should never be given unless at least one of these six signs is definitely present.

Slight local swelling alone is not an indication for antivenom. Never give antivenom unless you have adrenaline (epinephrine) available to treat severe reactions to the antivenom. The adult dose of adrenaline is 0.5ml of a 1 in 1,000 solution (1mg/ml) given intramuscularly.

Choice of appropriate antivenom

Before giving antivenom make sure that its range of specificity includes the snake that has bitten your patient. Some knowledge of Latin scientific names is useful, for example: *Naja*, cobra; *Dendroaspis*, mamba; *Bungarus*, krait; *Micrurus*, coral snake; *Bitis*, African puff adder and relatives; *Echis*, saw-scaled *or* carpet viper; *Bothrops*, fer de lance; *Trimeresurus*, green pit vipers; *Crotalus*, rattlesnake. It may have been possible to identify the biting snake or its venom may have produced a diagnostic clinical sign, such as incoagulable blood caused by the saw-scaled viper in the northern third of Africa. Otherwise, a polyspecific antivenom with activity against the principal venomous species of the region is used.

Caution: do not give antivenom that is opaque. The change from a clear to cloudy solution indicates loss of activity and increased danger of reactions. Expiry dates can be ignored provided that the solution is crystal clear. Manufacturers' instructions included in packs of antivenom may be misleading.

How to give antivenom

For maximum effect, antivenom should be given directly into a vein, by slow intravenous injection (2ml per minute) or slow intravenous infusion of antivenom diluted approximately 50:50 in sterile isotonic saline. The initial dose depends on the type of antivenom, species of snake involved and severity of symptoms, but a typical starting dose is four to five 10ml ampoules. This is repeated after a few hours if a life-threatening condition such as bleeding or weakness of the breathing muscles is not cured, or if the blood is again incoagulable after 6 hours. The patient should be watched for signs of an antivenom reaction, namely fever, itching, rash, vomiting, breathlessness and wheezing, increase in pulse rate and fall in blood pressure. If this happens, give a 0.5ml injection of 1 in 1,000 adrenaline solution intramuscularly; this can be repeated after 10 minutes if it is not effective. Reactions are likely to be severe in those who suffer from asthma, eczema and other allergic disorders.

Only in an extreme emergency should medically unqualified people give antivenom; for example, when the victim is many hours away from medical care, has signs of severe envenoming (see above) and seems to be getting worse. Deep intramuscular injections at multiple sites into the front and side of the thighs (*not the buttocks*) can then be used. The sites should be massaged to increase absorption of antivenom and firm pressure then applied to injection sites to prevent bleeding (Figure 20.3).

Treatment of complications

1. Massive external bleeding or leakage of blood and tissue fluid into a swollen limb may leave the patient with an inadequate circulating volume so that the

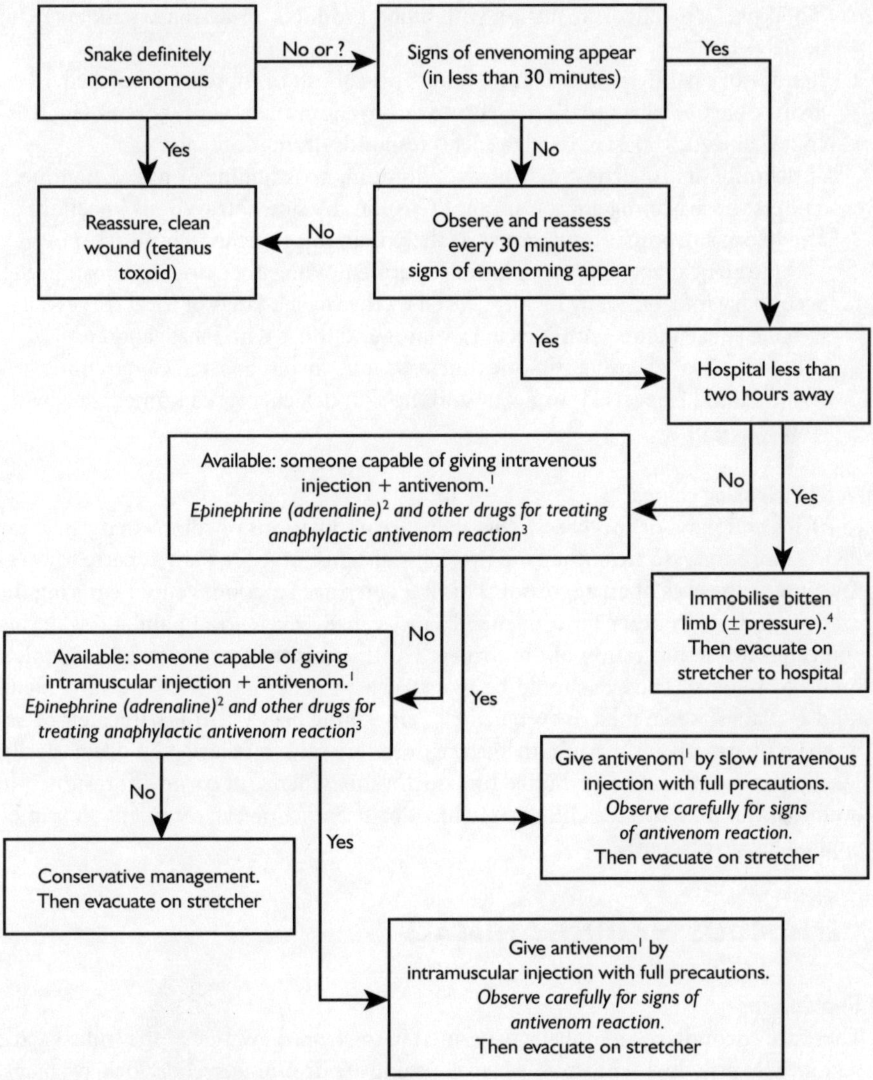

Notes:

1 "antivenom" means appropriate specific antivenom for the species of snake involved

2 "epinephrine (adrenaline)" means 0.1% (1:1000) adrenaline for intramuscular injection (adult dose 0.3–0.5ml)

3 "other drugs for treating anaphylactic antivenom reaction" means anthistamine and hydrocortisone for intravenous injection

4 "immobilise bitten limb (±pressure)" means immobilisation of the bitten limb with a splint or sling. "Pressure" means use of the pressure immobilisation method (Figure 20.2) using a long crepe bandage. This should only be used in the case of neurotoxic elapid snakes, *not* for viper bites

Figure 20.3 *Management of snake bite in remote locations*

blood pressure falls. Transfusion with blood products or plasma expanders may be needed.

2. Respiratory paralysis may require mouth-to-mouth or more sophisticated forms of artificial ventilation. Neurotoxic envenoming by some species (such as cobras and Australasian death adders) responds dramatically to anticholinesterase drugs such as edrophonium, neostigmine or physostigmine. The test dose is 10mg edrophonium (Tensilon) by slow intravenous injection after 0.6mg atropine (*adult doses*). If there is an improvement in muscle power within the next 20 minutes, continue treatment with subcutaneous neostigmine.
3. Secondary infection may be introduced by the snake's fangs or local surgery at the bite site. Patients with infected wounds and those with local gangrene should be treated with antibiotics and a tetanus toxoid booster. Gangrenous tissue should be excised surgically and the skin defect covered immediately with split skin grafts.

Note on spitting cobras

In Africa and parts of south-east Asia there are populations of cobras that can spray their venom forward from the fang tips for a distance of more than a metre towards the glint of the eyes of an aggressor. This is a defensive reaction. Venom entering the eyes or landing on other mucous membranes causes severe local pain and watering and can result in ulceration of the cornea. Treatment is the same as for any chemical injury to the eye. The eye should be irrigated with generous volumes of any bland fluid available (water, milk or even urine). Pain-killing drugs such as paracetamol can be given by mouth and 1% adrenaline eye drops are said to relieve pain dramatically. Ideally, the eye should be examined by a doctor for evidence of corneal abrasion. If in doubt, antibiotics such as chloramphenicol or tetracycline eye ointment should be applied for several days.

VENOMOUS MARINE ANIMALS

Sea snakes

These are encountered mainly by fishermen in the tropical waters of the Indo-Pacific region. The principal symptoms of envenoming are drooping eyelids, lockjaw, pains, stiffness, tenderness and paralysis of skeletal muscles, passing of dark (Coca-Cola-coloured) urine (myoglobinuria) and cardiac complications related to hyperkalaemia. Treatment is as described above.

Venomous fish

Many species of marine and freshwater fish have venomous spines on their gills, fins or tail. Stings occur when the fish are handled by fishermen or are trodden on or touched by bathers. Some species attack swimmers and scuba divers around coral reefs. There is immediate excruciating pain and swelling at the site of the sting. Severe systemic effects may follow. These include vomiting, diarrhoea, sweating, irregular heart beat, fall in blood pressure, spasm or paralysis of muscles including respiratory muscles, and fits.

Treatment

Forewarned is forearmed. If your expedition has an extensive programme, say on coral reefs, try to get maximum information about dangerous species locally. The venomous spine of stingrays, which is often barbed, should be removed. Local symptoms are rapidly relieved by immersing the stung limb in hot but not scalding water. Test the temperature with your elbow. If you have a thermometer, the temperature should not exceed 45°C. Alternatively, 1% lignocaine (lidocaine) or some other local anaesthetic can be injected, for example, as a ring block in the case of stung digits. Specific antivenom for some of the most dangerous species (such as stone fish, genus *Synanceja*) is available in some parts of the world. Patients may require mouth-to-mouth respiration and external cardiac massage. Atropine (0.6mg by subcutaneous injection for adults) should be given if there is a very slow pulse rate and low blood pressure.

Stingrays

The stingray attacks only when frightened and usually only when trodden upon. If it is known that there are stingrays about, it is wise to shuffle your feet or prod the ocean floor with a stick to make your presence known. Spines may be large enough to cause serious mechanical injury and are often left embedded in the wound together with the covering membrane. These foreign bodies are bound to cause infection if they are not removed. The stingray produces a heat-labile venom so immersion of the stung part in hot but not scolding water (not more than 45°C) will destroy the toxin and relieve the pain. *(Warning: there are stingrays in muddy tributaries of the Amazon. They sting people who step on them while fording rivers, usually in the dry season.)*

Jellyfish, Portuguese man o'war and other cnidarians (coelenterates)

Contact with the tentacles produces lines of very painful blisters. The venom of some species, such as the notorious box jellyfish (*Chironex, Chiropsalmus*) of tropical waters, can cause severe systemic effects, including cardiorespiratory arrest.

Treatment

Adherent fragments of tentacles must be removed (but *not* with your fingers) before more of their venomous nematocysts can discharge. Vinegar or dilute acetic acid effectively inactivates the nematocyst of box jellyfish, but many of the remedies that have been recommended in the past, such as methylated spirits, other alcohols and sunburn lotions, will stimulate massive discharge of nematocysts embedded in the patient. Antivenom is available in some of the worst-affected areas such as northern Australia. Severe cases may require mouth-to-mouth respiration and cardiac massage.

Sea urchins

The venomous spines and grapples of some sea urchins may become deeply embedded in the skin, usually of the sole of the foot when the animal has been trodden upon. Soften the skin with salicylic acid ointment and then pare down the epidermis to a depth at which the spines can be removed with forceps. Ordinary sea urchin prickles are absorbed quite rapidly provided they are broken into small pieces in the skin. Only if they have penetrated into a joint or if there is evidence of infection is surgical removal necessary.

Molluscs: octopuses and cone shells

Several species of small blue-ringed octopuses of the Indo-Australasian region can cause fatal envenoming by biting. There are many species of beautiful cone shells in tropical waters. These sting by harpooning and implanting a venom-charged arrowhead. Beware of handling these attractive animals. Deaths have occurred but no antivenoms are available.

Poisoning from ingestion of fish and shellfish

Extensive feelings of pins and needles, paralysis, itching, diarrhoea, vomiting and shock can follow a few minutes or hours after eating various molluscs and fish. A large number of species in many parts of the world can cause these symptoms at various seasons of the year. Famous examples are pufferfish, red snapper, barracuda, tuna and mackerel. Treatment attempts to eliminate the toxic materials from the gut by promoting vomiting and diarrhoea with emetics and purges. Symptoms of "scrombroid" (e.g. tuna) poisoning respond to antihistamine drugs and bronchodilators, but, in severe cases of paralytic poisoning, assisted ventilation will be required until paralysis of the breathing muscles has worn off. Prevent these poisonings by taking local advice. "Red tides" may warn of shellfish poisoning. Avoid eating very large reef fish (ciguatera poisoning), any parts of the fish other than the flesh (muscle) and some notorious species (such as Moray eels – ciguatera poisoning – and puffer fish – tetrodotoxic poisoning).

VENOMOUS ARTHROPODS

Stings by bees, wasps and hornets (*Hymenoptera*)

In normal people many stings, probably hundreds, would be required to introduce enough venom to kill. A man in Zimbabwe survived more than 2,000 stings. But a small number of people have acquired hypersensitivity and could be killed by a single sting. Systemic symptoms suggest hypersensitivity: generalised tingling with rashes (urticaria, weals, nettle rash or hives), swelling of the lips, tongue and throat, flushing, dizziness, collapse, wheezing, loss of control of bowels and bladder, and unconsciousness within minutes of the sting.

Prevention and treatment

It is possible to confirm hypersensitivity by blood or skin tests and to desensitise the patient using purified venom, but this takes time. People who know or suspect that they are hypersensitive should be taught how to give themselves a subcutaneous injection of 0.3ml or 0.5ml of 1 in 1,000 or 0.1% adrenaline (adult dose) and should carry this with them on the expedition (EpiPen, Anapen or Min-I-Jet self-injectable adrenaline kits with a ¼-inch long 25-gauge needle). They should wear a MedicAlert tag in case they are found unconscious (MedicAlert Foundation International, 12 Bridge Wharf, 156 Caledonian Road, London N1 9UU, tel. +44 20 7833 3034).

In tropical countries, especially Africa and Mexico, Central and South America, rock climbers and other travellers have occasionally been attacked by large swarms of angry bees, and some fatal falls have resulted. Some of these accidents could have been prevented if local advice had been sought. Thundery weather is known to upset bees. In the face of an attack, the best-tried methods of evasion seem to be to run very fast or to immerse yourself in water. The climber should appreciate that a fall is probably the greatest danger. After securing him- or herself he or she will have to rely on protection afforded by anorak, rucksack or tent. In South America about 100 people die each year after being attacked by furious swarms of Africanised honey bees. The principal effects of multiple stings in the non-hypersensitive subject are haemolysis, rhabdomyolysis (breakdown of skeletal muscle), bronchospasm, pneumonitis and kidney failure. No antivenom is readily available.

Stings by ants, beetles, moths and caterpillars

These insects, in particular the brightly coloured, hairy caterpillars, can cause severe problems: local pain, inflammation, nettle rash, blistering and arthritis on contact and, in Venezuela and Brazil, systemic bleeding and incoagulable blood.

Spider bites

Dangerous spiders occur mainly in the Americas, southern Africa, the Mediterranean region and Australia. The most notorious genera are *Latrodectus* (black/brown widow spiders), *Phoneutria* (Latin American armed or banana spiders, Figure 20.4), *Atrax* (Sydney funnel web spider) and *Loxosceles* (brown recluse spiders). Venoms of *Latrodectus, Phoneutria* and *Atrax* affect the nerves, muscles and heart, producing cramping pains, muscle spasms, weakness, sweating, salivation, gooseflesh, fever,

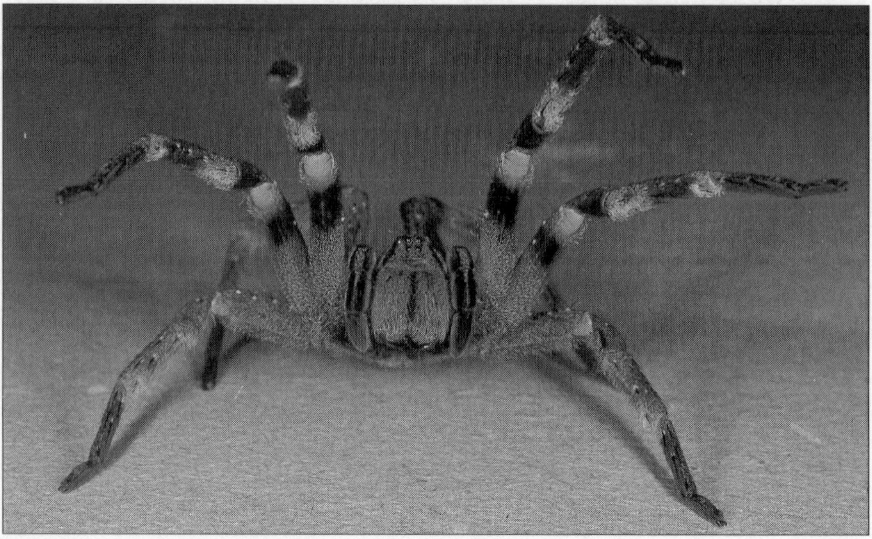

Figure 20.4 *Brazilian "armed" spider* Phoneutria nigriventer *in threatening posture (D. A. Warrell)*

nausea, vomiting, alterations in pulse rate and blood pressure, and convulsions. Loxosceles bites cause severe local necrosis, a generalised red rash, fever, dark urine (haemoglobinuria), blood clotting disturbances and kidney failure. Deaths are unusual except among children. Bites usually occur when the victim brushes against a spider that has crept into clothes or bedding. Antivenoms are manufactured in countries such as South Africa, Australia and Brazil, where spider bite is an important medical problem.

Scorpion stings

Dangerous scorpions (Figure 20.5) occur particularly in north and south Africa, the Middle East, the United States, Mexico, South America and India. The fatal cases are usually children. Most stings are not life threatening but cause excruciating local pain with little swelling. Symptoms reflect initial release of acetylcholine neurotransmitter (causing vomiting, abdominal pain, bradycardia, sweating, salivation and so on) followed by release of catecholamines (causing hypertension, tachycardia, pulmonary oedema, ECG abnormalities). The severe local pain is treated by injecting local anaesthetic at the site of the sting, e.g. 1–2% lignocaine (lidocaine), but a powerful analgesic such as tramadol injections may be required. Severe systemic symptoms should be treated with appropriate pharmacological agents (such as vasodilator drugs) and antivenom. Atropine, beta-blockers and digoxin are not generally recommended.

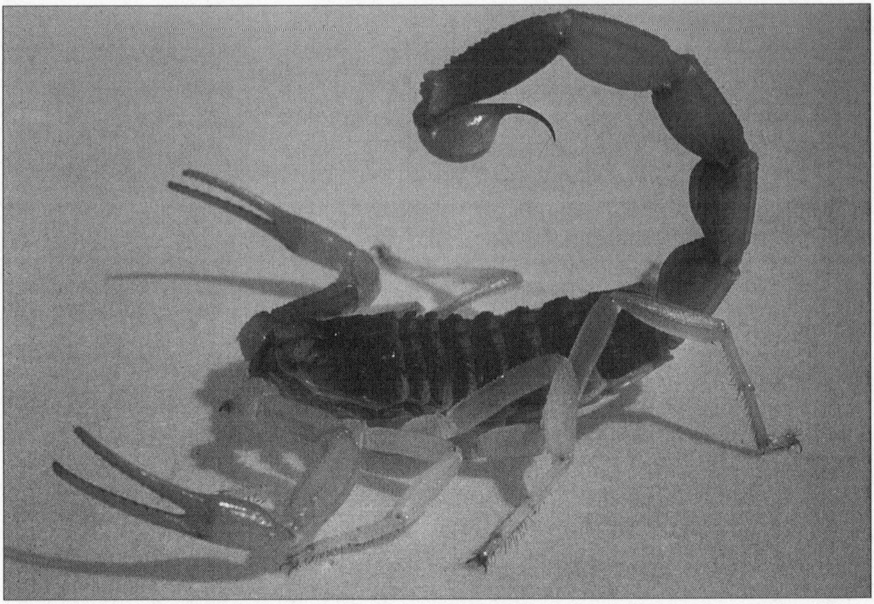

Figure 20.5 *Dangerous scorpion* Leiurus quinquestriatus *of north Africa and the Middle East*

Prevention is better than cure

When establishing a base camp in a scorpion-infested area, first dig out the scorpions. Their oval-shaped entry holes are usually easily recognisable. A thin twig should be used to guide the digging as the tunnel often changes direction. Always suspect there may be a scorpion under cases, logs and so on. *Always* shake your boots and shoes out before putting them on. *Always* look where you put your bare feet. The RGS Kora 1983 expedition dug out 180 scorpions in the base campsite. The exoskeleton of scorpions fluoresces in ultraviolet light, so use a UV lamp to search your chosen campsite.

OTHER VENOMOUS INVERTEBRATES

Bites by some tropical centipedes can be dangerous as well as painful (e.g. in the Seychelles), and some millipedes can squirt irritating defensive secretions. There is no specific treatment for either of these menaces. Many species of ticks can inject a paralysing toxin while they suck your blood. If a member of your party becomes progressively weak, it is important to search for the tick in hairy areas or inside the ears and to detach it as soon as possible. The symptoms should then subside.

Invasive arthropods

Various tropical arthropods have larvae which invade human tissue or are merely blood sucking.

Congo floor maggot (*Auchmeronyia luteola*)

The larvae live in the floors of huts. They attack humans who sleep on the ground and suck their blood, causing local swelling and itching. Fumigate the hut and treat the bites symptomatically, making sure that no secondary infection is introduced (wipe the skin with tincture of iodine, give systemic antimicrobials if there are signs of infection).

Tumbu fly, putsi fly, ver du cayor (*Cordylobia anthropophaga*)

This fly is common in sub-Saharan Africa. It lays its eggs on damp clothes laid out to dry and, if they are not ironed, the eggs will hatch and burrow into your skin. Do not spread your clothing on the ground to dry. A small boil develops with something moving in the middle; this is the posterior segment with the respiratory spiracles. There is a sensation of movement in these lesions.

Treatment

Cover with paraffin (Vaseline) and grasp the maggot, which will stick out its "head" to get air, or do a proper surgical excision.

Ver macaque, human botfly, Berne, El Torsalo, beefworm (*Dermatobia hominis*)

This fly is widely distributed in Central and South America from Mexico to Argentina and Chile. It lays its eggs on other insects. They hitchhike to the human skin and penetrate quickly. To begin with the maggot is bottle shaped and, although paraffin may cause the creature breathing difficulties, in the early stages you are likely to pull off the "neck" (actually the posterior segment with the spiracles) if you attempt to extract it. Wait until it is further developed, and you may succeed as with the tumbu fly. Otherwise make a cross incision to pull the maggot out, taking care not to cut it. An alternative is to cover the lesion with candle wax. The maggot will burrow its way into the candle wax, and you have got it.

Creeping eruptions (larva migrans)

The track made under the skin is caused by the larvae of animal nematodes, such as *Ancylostoma braziliense, Uncinaria stenocephala* and *Ancylostoma caninum*, the hookworms of cats and dogs. The larva moves day by day. The best treatment is thiabendazole applied topically in paraffin ointment.

Jigger fleas (*Tunga penetrans*)
After fertilisation the female of this little flea jumps (feebly) and burrows alongside the nailfold or into the skin of the groin, loses her legs and produces eggs each night. These must be curetted out and iodine applied. Jiggers and other unpleasant creatures can be avoided if you do not walk around barefoot.

Source of antivenom in the UK
Aventis Pasteur MSD Ltd

Tel.	+44 1628 785291
Fax:	+44 1628 411412
Website:	www.aventis-pasteur-msd.com

Advice on venomous bites and stings
National Poisons Centre

Tel.	+44 870 600 6266
Website:	www.doh.gov.uk/npis.htm

Centre for Tropical Medicine, University of Oxford

Tel.	+44 1865 220968
Fax:	+44 1865 220984

21 PSYCHOLOGICAL PROBLEMS ON EXPEDITIONS

Michael Phelan

"God knows it is just about as much as I can stand at times, and there is absolutely no escape. I have never had my temper so tried as it is everyday now," wrote Edward Wilson, a Polar explorer, in 1902. You do not have to spend the winter in the Antarctic to share some of the frustrations and annoyances that Wilson was describing to his wife. Expeditions are stressful and cause psychological difficulties for those involved. When organising or joining an expedition ensure that you are aware of the potential psychological disorders as well as the many physical conditions described elsewhere in this book. This chapter outlines steps to take at the planning stage to reduce psychological problems, and describes more common difficulties that can occur and the best way to manage them.

PLANNING STAGES

Start planning for an expedition at least a year before the anticipated departure date. Having decided the main aims and objectives, select a clearly defined leader. Ideally, he or she will have had experience of leading similar expeditions. Enthusiasm, maturity and hard work will, however, go a long way to compensate for lack of experience, but a clear understanding of leadership responsibilities is vital. There are different styles of leadership. Successful leaders understand their own strengths and weaknesses, and do not try to emulate someone else. Lack of confidence frequently results in excessive authoritarianism and subsequent resentment from team members. Confident leaders are able to accept that they are not always right and listen to the views of others, but at the same time make decisions, even if unpopular, when required. Any expedition leader should read a wide range of books about expeditions to develop a sense of the strains that will be imposed on him or her. It is also helpful to study a short paperback on management skills, which can provide useful hints on issues such as time management and delegation. Leaders of any expedition, however small, must appreciate that their lives will be dominated for months, and that their preoccupation will be a trial for people close to them.

Selecting the right team

This is likely to be one of the most vital factors in the eventual success of any expedition. The leader must be closely involved in selection. A formal interview process with the involvement of the leader helps to establish his or her authority from the outset. There are no hard and fast rules for picking the right team and instinct should not be ignored; it is often right. However, some principles should be borne in mind.

- **Background**. Past behaviour predicts future behaviour. Give more weight to what people have done than to what they say they are going to do. Find out about previous expedition experience, and any other relevant experience. Follow up references, and when possible speak to referees, as they may mention things that they have not felt comfortable to put down in writing.
- **Motivation**. Enthusiasm is a vital characteristic in any potential candidate. Look out for people who appear to be enthusiastic about life in general, not just about the proposed expedition. Discuss in detail with people why they want to go on your expedition, and what they are expecting. Ask them what they anticipate finding difficult about the trip, and also what they will do if they do not get selected. Many candidates may have negative reasons for escaping from their normal life, such as leaving a boring job or getting over a bereavement. Such reasons are not an absolute contraindication for selection, but they need to be discussed frankly.
- **Personality**. If there are such things as normal people, they do not go on expeditions. Equally, the perfect expedition person does not exist, and the happiest expeditions are those with a real mixture of characters on them. However, try to select people who have an open and friendly manner, and who are sensitive to others. Self-reliance is another vital characteristic, along with an ability to admit to failings and weaknesses with a smile. The psychological profile of the expedition members needs to be assessed, not so much by a qualified psychologist but by the expedition leader and co-organisers, with common sense and an understanding of human nature. A good psychological balance is what is needed.
- **Mental health**. Lastly, it is essential to ask about any mental health problems. If in any doubt do not hesitate to obtain a medical report from their GP (this will require written consent). Expeditions are not suitable for people convalescing from any mental illness.

Having made your final selection make sure that the group at the very least spends a weekend together before the expedition. This will begin the team building that is vital if the group is to work well together.

Personnel selection is only one aspect of the overall planning, albeit an important one. Attention to detail is needed in all other areas. Conflict and resentment will be reduced by ensuring that everyone has adequate equipment, and good-quality food is always a great boost to morale. However, the best-made plans may have to be changed at the last moment, and a degree of flexibility must be kept to cope with the unexpected.

OUT IN THE OPEN

Psychological problems that occur on expeditions can broadly be considered as those that affect the group as a whole and those that primarily affect individual members. These are described separately, but in reality there will always be some overlap.

Group dynamics

Humans are social animals, and are instinctively drawn to form groups with others. This behaviour is accentuated by the isolation and alien environment of most expeditions. As groups of people become more familiar with each other, individual members develop social roles within the group, such as being the joker who lifts morale, or the spokesperson who says what others are thinking. At the same time strong friendships are formed and members develop an intense sense of belonging to the group. This process is helped by joint decision-making and responsibility, as well as symbolic aspects such as expedition T-shirts.

Although being a member of a group is largely a positive experience it does have disadvantages. Intrusion into privacy and personal space can be overbearing, and there can be pressure to behave in a way that makes people feel uncomfortable. Scapegoating is a common phenomenon among any group of people. It can become a serious problem if not dealt with quickly. The leader needs to recognise when it is happening, and step in early to reinstate the excluded member. This can be done effectively by changing the person's role or giving him or her an essential task in order to increase the group's respect and sense of need.

A couple may have a particular problem in a group setting. The bond between them may be resented by other members and result in scapegoating of the couple. Alternatively, one of the couple may get on well with the rest of the group but leave the partner feeling rejected and isolated. The author's experience of couples on expeditions is limited to three male-dominated expeditions; however, on each occasion the woman was left isolated while her male partner integrated with the rest of the group. Anyone selecting a couple for an expedition must be ready for such problems, and the couple themselves need to understand the inevitable stress on their relationship.

Most expeditions have periods of general low morale, and these will be testing times for the leader. If such periods persist without obvious reason one member may be responsible for transmitting their own unhappiness to the entire group. Having one person going around saying "I'm really fed up with this aren't you?" can have a devastating effect on a previously happy expedition. The leader needs to detect if this is happening and try to help the person concerned.

An important role for any leader is to facilitate communication among the team. A formal structure should be in place for information to be shared and complaints to be aired early. This may be in the form of a daily meeting, or may involve maintaining regular radio contact on a more dispersed expedition. It is also important that all the members of the expedition have the opportunity to talk to the leader privately. Good leaders appreciate the importance of listening, and realise that being seen to understand the problems of others is often the only action that is required.

Individual disorders

Psychological and psychiatric disorders are far more common than generally recognised. It is estimated that one in six people will suffer from a formal mental illness at some stage in their lives, and many others will go through periods of great stress, to the extent that they have difficulty coping with their responsiblities. Although people with a family history of mental illness are more likely to be effected, no one is immune. Early adulthood is often when mental illness first becomes apparent, and it can be triggered by some exceptional stress, such as an expedition. If someone has a previous history of any mental disorder, it is essential that an expert opinion is sought, and advice taken, before departure.

Panic attacks

These may occur spontaneously, but are often precipitated by a feared situation. Attacks are characterised by extreme panic, to the extent that people may describe a feeling of impending death.

The panic is accompanied by physical symptoms such as:

- Chest pain
- Blurred vision
- Dizziness
- Tingling of the fingers and toes
- Feelings of extreme breathlessness accompanied by hyperventilation.

Bystanders who have not seen an attack before will be alarmed, and this only makes the sufferer worse. The correct immediate treatment for a panic attack is calm reassurance, and to get the person to breathe in and out of a paper or plastic bag held over their nose and mouth (if a plastic bag is used it must never be put over the head). In the longer term panic attacks usually become less frequent and less severe. If they persist an expert opinion should be sought, and medication and/or specific psychological therapies will be prescribed.

Depression

Everyone becomes miserable from time to time, and this is quite normal on an expedition. Occasionally, someone may develop a depressive illness, which is quantitatively different. It may follow an infective illness or some other clear trigger, such as bad news from home, but the cause may not be immediately obvious to others, or indeed to the person concerned. As well as a depressed mood and a lack of energy, other characteristic features include:

- Poor sleep, especially early morning wakening
- Loss of appetite
- Mood worse in the morning
- Poor concentration
- Frequent tearful episodes
- Preoccupation with worries and a sense of guilt
- Thoughts of suicide or self-harm.

If all or some of these features are present then the matter must be taken seriously. There is often an understandable reluctance to ask about suicidal thoughts, but embarrassment must be put aside, and the subject broached with anyone who is depressed (around 1% of all deaths are due to suicide, and the proportion is far greater in young people). If they are feeling suicidal they will be reassured by having the opportunity to discuss their thoughts. They may well get better, but if their condition deteriorates, or it is felt that they are a suicide risk, they should be evacuated home.

Acute confusional and psychotic states

In contrast to panic attacks and depression, which are common, acute confusional states, psychoses are rare. Characteristic features include:

- Bizarre and inexplicable behaviour
- Preoccupation with strange and frequently persecutory beliefs
- Hallucinations, either visual or auditory
- Disorientation in time, place and person
- Fluctuations in the level of consciousness.

On an expedition malaria and heat stroke are two of the most likely conditions to cause a confusional or psychotic state. Drugs may also be responsible. Clearly, no member of the expedition should take recreational drugs, and it is important that people do not take local drugs, herbal or otherwise. Occasionally prescribed drugs may also cause a confusional state. For instance, there are some reports of the antimalarial drug mefloquine (Lariam) causing temporary mood disturbances and confusion (this is rare and should *not* stop you taking vital prophylaxis against malaria). The onset of schizophrenia is another possible cause, but far less likely.

Confusional states may follow head injuries. The onset may be delayed by some days. This is a major emergency, and the sufferer must be evacuated immediately.

Psychiatric medication

Psychiatric drugs should not be a routine part of expedition medical kits, and should never be used by someone who is not medically qualified. However, on expeditions where immediate evacuation is not possible a doctor, experienced in their use, may consider including the following:

- Antidepressants (for example, fluoxetine 20mg), which, although effective in relieving the symptoms of depression in approximately 65% of cases, takes at least 2 weeks to work.
- Anxiloytics/hypnotics (for example, diazepam 5mg). There may be an occasional role for such drugs in the treatment of acute anxiety or severe stress reactions, but they are addictive and their use should be limited to a few days.
- Antipsychotics (for example, chlorpromazine 50mg) may help to settle someone in an acute confusional state, but there is a risk that their use will mask a dangerous deterioration in the patient, and extra-pyramidal side-effects may require the concurrent use of anticholinergic drugs (for example, procyclidine 5mg).

Returning home

If there has been a major disaster or near disaster on an expedition this must be given attention on returning home. During the last decade there has been an increasing recognition of the severe psychological sequelae for many people involved in accidents or near-death experiences. The term post-traumatic stress disorder describes the common symptoms of intrusive thoughts and flashbacks to the traumatic experience, nightmares, disturbed sleep and avoidance of specific situations or places which can follow any traumatic experience. If others have been killed or severely injured, survivors may feel guilty that they escaped, even if they were not responsible for what happened. If untreated these symptoms can persist for years, and result in significant disability and distress. Expert help should therefore be obtained.

Most expeditions pass without disaster. Hugh Robert Mill, once the RGS librarian, described "the fine tradition of British explorers [in] passing over ... little squabbles and jealousies", and there is no doubt that minor disagreements and personality clashes will soon be forgotten once everyone is back home. However, after the initial excitement of returning, it is common to miss the camaraderie of the expedition; a feeling of anticlimax is an inevitable consequence of a successful trip. Far more attention is given to the process of team building at the beginning of an expedition than to team separation at the end. A responsible leader will recognise that this is a painful process, and pay attention to the sense of loss felt by the team. Practical steps can include circulating a list of contact details for expedition members to help people stay in touch with each other. An organised reunion a few months after coming home may help (as well as being a chance to chase people up for their contribution to the report). However, the best solution is to start planning the next expedition.

22 EXPEDITION DENTISTRY

David Geddes

PREPARING FOR A TRIP

High on Everest during 1994 a UK doctor, thoroughly prepared in all other respects for his summit bid, decided enough was enough – his continual toothache was overwhelming his chance of a lifetime. He descended through base camp, ran 26 miles to Namche Bazaar where he was able to be treated by one of the Sherpa dental therapists in the only effective remote dental facility in Nepal. Subsequently he was fortunate to progress through all the camps and stand on the summit of Everest. Pre-monsoon in 1999, Russian, Slovenian, American, Korean and Nepalese climbers with summit chances on Lhotse Shar, Everest, Nuptse and Pumori all presented for difficult emergency dental treatment at Namche Bazaar. All these climbers had dental conditions that could have been prevented had they considered treatment before leaving their home country.

Prevention is better than cure, and much better than a ruined trip
A dental exam, if possible including panoramic X-rays, should be carried out 3 months prior to departure. Treatment waiting lists and complex therapies may take a surprisingly long time to achieve

RISK AWARENESS

The remote traveller will find dentists few and far between and dental problems surprisingly frequent. If in desperation you feel compelled to seek treatment, you should be aware that where standards of cross-infection control are not assured, the risk of transfer of HIV and hepatitis or enteroviruses may be unacceptably high. The dental exam prior to departure is of the utmost importance. Almost all dental problems are predictable, especially when supported by comprehensive X-rays. It would be wise to accept professional advice that even mildly suspicious observations should be electively treated. A root treatment may occasionally take some months to settle.

Third molar (wisdom teeth) problems are relatively common in young adults. Waiting lists for surgical extraction under general anaesthetic can be excessively long in the UK (9–18 months). In remote areas, when personal hygiene has slipped for a week or two, bacterial infections of the gum structure around the part-erupted lower third molars can be debilitating. Treatment involves much more detailed oral hygiene after all meals, hot concentrated salt-water mouthwashing and broad-spectrum antibiotics capable of dealing with anaerobic bacteria.

As *dental pain* often results from a pressurised swelling in a constricted space normally full of nervous tissue, it can be controlled for weeks with a combination of antibiotics and suitable painkillers (non-steroidal anti-inflammatories, e.g. ibuprofen). This will preserve the option of seeking further treatment later.

The expedition medical officer will need to decide during the planning phase, pre-expedition, just what dental treatment is to be offered. There is a choice between using drugs only (prescription dentistry) and being prepared to attempt emergency extractions. The black arts of successful extraction technique and local anaesthetic placement take some decades to learn!

The expedition medical officer may be called upon to treat the following:

- Minor tooth and filling fractures
- Major tooth fractures from trauma
- Soft-tissue infections associated with wisdom teeth (third molars)
- Acute and transient dental pulpal pain in response to stimulation by hot, cold and sugary stimuli
- Chronic dental pulp pain which is often spontaneous and very protracted
- Mandibular and maxillary bone fractures
- Avulsed teeth.

Prior to leaving home, a decision should be made by the medical officer to offer treatment based on:

- Drugs only – be prepared for cross-border import of drugs
- Instrumentation – requires equipment, materials, training and costs
- Evacuation and referral – depends on local treatment availability, insurance and cost

In preparation the expedition medical officer should consider whether it would be possible to carry out some of the following skills to any advantage over the option of palliative treatment using pharmaceuticals.

- Do I have sufficient expertise to cope?

- Can I guarantee successful clinical outcomes?
- Does my knowledge allow a realistic differential diagnosis?
- Equipment – have I practised the manipulative surgical skills including working in a mirror image?
- Materials – have I practised their critical mixing and setting times?
- Will cross-infection control be adequate?
- Do I have the resources to treat postoperative problems?

In concluding risk awareness, the importance of travel, illness and evacuation insurance should be considered. It would be unusual for predictable dental problems to be covered. Health insurance generally does not cover dental problems adequately as first-world dental risks and costs are high. The replacement of a tooth lost when on expedition, by a bridge or implant, will be very costly and will not be covered by insurance, or state-funded dental schemes. Private dental capitation schemes will cover most costs and for that reason are particularly worth considering. While advising fellow travellers to examine the small print of any travel insurance, the "expedition dentists" should consult their indemnity insurers who will be capable of offering advice on medico-legal responsibilities concerning appropriate "duty of care".

> Expedition doctors would be well advised to consider dental treatment by prescription only, unless involved in a long expedition in extremely remote circumstances, such as polar regions.

DENTAL PROBLEMS AND THEIR TREATMENT

Lost fillings and broken teeth

- *Symptoms* – vary. Nil to transient reaction to hot, cold and sweet stimuli, sometimes leading to mild short-lasting toothache. Tongue getting "cut to ribbons".
- *Treatment* – press a small ball of temporary filling material into as dry a cavity as possible (to dry the cavity consider using cotton wool twisted on to the end of a match).
- *Requirements* – gloves, temporary filling material, mirror and flat-bladed plugger, cotton-wool rolls for saliva control.
- *Problems* – mixing filling material, working in mirror, saliva control, having to repeat the procedure.
- *Tip 1* – if it causes no symptoms leave alone.
- *Tip 2* – divers should beware hyperbaric pressure changes under damaged fillings. These should be thoroughly sealed with temporary filling material.

Chronic toothache

- *Symptoms* – continual tormenting toothache, soft-tissue swelling – which is often large – sleepless, distracted and irritable.
- *Treatment* – lance and drain any large swellings
  – antibiotics and non-steroidal anti-inflammatory drugs (NSAIDs), with initial high dosage
  – extraction if no adequate resolution of symptoms.
- *Requirements* – drugs, local anaesthetic, syringe, forceps, knowledge and practice of both local anaesthetic application and extraction technique.
- *Tip* – avoid extraction if possible.

Loose crowns and bridges

- *Symptoms* – obviously loose or avulsed crown or bridge.
- *Treatment* – clean and thoroughly dry both prosthesis and anchoring teeth. Practise reseating crown then re-cement using proprietary cement.
- *Requirements* – cotton wool for moisture control, cement.
- *Tip* – Supaglue is a cyano-acrylic. Do not use in the mouth in any circumstances.

Lower third molar and associated gum problems

- *Symptoms* – swelling at angle of mandible, trismus, earache.
- *Treatment 1* – antibiotics for anaerobic infection, NSAIDs, hot salt-water mouthwashes, rigorously improved oral hygiene and/or extraction.
- *Treatment 2* – The same treatment rationale applies to general gum problems, even if uncomfortable to apply and sustain.
- *Requirements* – drugs, knowledge of placement of inferior dental block, local anaesthetic, aspirating syringe, forceps and elevators, and how to use them.
- *Tip* – lower third molars are often impacted and among the most difficult of extractions without a surgical approach. Avoid extraction.

Traumatically damaged teeth

- *Examination* – approach is decided by the severity of the enamel and dentine fracture and whether pulpal blood is visible in the fracture area.
- *Symptoms* – acute reaction to hot, cold and sweet stimuli through fractured dentine tubules. Hypersensitive to touch, sometimes local anaesthetic not effective.
- *Treatment* – if no blood, attempt to seal and cover exposed dentine with

temporary filling (glass ionomer material). If pulpal blood present, attempt to seal with calcium hydroxide paste and glass ionomer temporary filling. Give broad-spectrum antibiotics and NSAIDs; extract if acute pulpal pain becomes uncontrollable.

- *Requirements* – drugs, calcium hydroxide lining, glass ionomer temporary filling, local anaesthetic, syringe, forceps.
- *Tip 1* – hot and cold hyper-reaction fades considerably in a few days.
- *Tip 2* – pulpal blood in a remote situation means almost inevitable nerve necrosis and eventual root treatment. Counsel patient of cost of tooth replacement before extraction. Implants and/or bridge work is very expensive and not covered by most insurance.

Avulsed teeth

- *Symptoms* – patient presents with whole tooth and root knocked out.
- *Treatment* – if kept in warm isotonic solution (saliva is best) the tooth can be replanted into the socket after the evacuation of any solid blood clot.
- *Requirements* – ability to splint into place. This will be almost impossible in remote locations. Splint using filaments of copper electrical wire.
- *Tip 1* – counsel on cost of prosthetic replacement but advise that success of replantation is beyond reasonable expectation, and unsplinted teeth have no hope.
- *Tip 2* – Supaglue is a cyano-acrylic. Do not use in the mouth in any circumstances.

Fractures to mandible and maxilla

- *Symptoms* of fractured mandible – inability to eat, independent movement of different groups of lower teeth, typically history of trauma to chin, not excessively painful.
- *Symptoms* of fractured maxilla – difficulty in eating, depressed or spongy zygomatic arch, not excessively painful.
- *Treatment* – prioritise and treat all wounds
  - consider extent of head injuries
  - protect airway
  - immobilise fracture by well-padded external vertical bandaging, if possible with upper and lower teeth in occlusion
  - pain relief, high-calorie soft-food diet
  - immediate accompanied evacuation to specialist care.

DENTAL EQUIPMENT AND DRUGS FOR REMOTE DENTISTY

Aim to keep the weight of your dental first aid kit to less than 1.5kg
Contact: The Dental Directory, 6 Perry Way, Witham, Essex CM8 3SX
Tel. +44 800 585586
Online purchasing: www.dental-directory.co.uk

TABLE 22.1 MINIMAL DENTAL EQUIPMENT
Sterile surgical gloves
Cotton-wool rolls
Sealed alcohol swabs
Sachets of instrument sterilisation solution
2 dental mirrors
1 sickle probe
1 pair locking tweezers
1 flat-bladed filling plugger
1 spatula to mix filling material/glazed paper pad
1 pair Spencer Wells fine suturing forceps
Black suture silk on fine semi-lunar needle
1 pair fine-curved surgical scissors
Disposable scalpels
Extraction forceps of your choice – 4 forceps would be the minimum
Aspirating local anaesthetic (LA) syringe, gauge 30 needles (3cm), LA cartridges

SUMMARY

1. Almost all routine dental problems can be prevented by a timely comprehensive dental inspection and elective treatment.
2. Dental pain will compromise and may ruin an expedition.
3. Expedition dental symptoms can be palliatively treated by antibiotics and non-steriodal anti-inflamatory drugs such as ibuprofen.
4. Hyperbaric pressure changes under damaged fillings will cause severe dental pain, whereas hypobaric changes at altitude will not (although prolonged exposure to extreme cold can cause pain).
5. A decision by the medical officer pre-expedition needs to be made as to whether to include extraction as a treatment option, bearing in mind the likelihood of oral trauma (rockfall, avalanche, bar-room brawls, etc!).
6. Most proprietary "emergency" dental kits are not worth having.
7. General travel/health insurance covers few dental situations.

8. Duty of care and responsibilities need to be discussed with your indemnity insurers.

TABLE 22.2 DENTAL PHARMACEUTICALS AND MATERIALS

Antibiotics
Metronidazole 200mg for anaerobic gum infections: one four times a day for 4 days
Augmentin 500mg for all dental swellings and pain: one three times a day for 5–7 days

Pain relief
Ibuprofen 400mg for all dental pain of routine origin (up to three times a day)

Mouthwashing
Sachets of hydrogen peroxide mouthwash, table salt

Temporary filling materials
Dycal – a two-liquid opaque calcium hydroxide lining to place under deep temporary fillings or over traumatically exposed live pulpal tissue
Cavit – a soft, easy-to-use, calming, temporary filling material
Glass ionomer filling material – a permanent filling material made up by mixing powder and water in a careful ratio. Normally contains fluoride. Can also be used in a thin preparation to re-cement crown

SECTION 3

MEDICAL PROBLEMS OF ENVIRONMENTAL EXTREMES

23 DESERT EXPEDITIONS

Sundeep Dhillon

Humans are well equipped to live in hot areas provided they are acclimatised to the environment. Yet many people fall victim to the effects of heat, not only in the tropics, but also while exercising in temperate latitudes. This chapter aims to provide a greater understanding of the mechanism, diagnosis, treatment and prevention of heat-related illnesses and other problems associated with deserts.

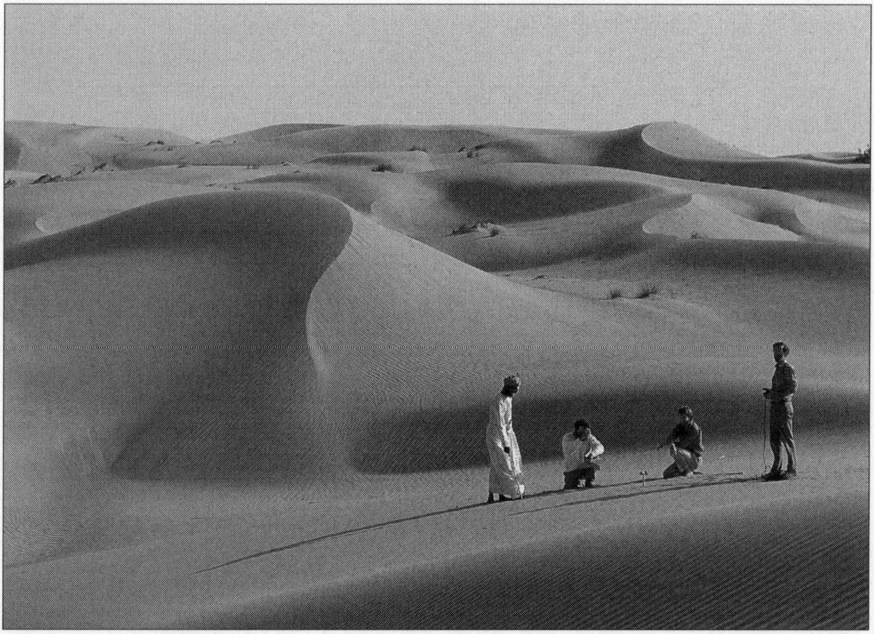

Figure 23.1 *Working with the Bedu in the Wahiba Sands, Sultanate of Oman (RGS/R. Turpin)*

Climate

Most people have a romantic view of deserts with huge undulating sand dunes as far as the eye can see, punctuated with lush oases. The reality is rather different. It is convenient to divide deserts into three types as identified by Maria Harding in *Weather to Travel*:

- Hot desert
  - High day-time temperatures dropping sharply at night
  - Little precipitation
  - No cool season
  - Sahara, Middle East, Australia
- Steppe
  - Semi-arid edges of hot deserts
  - Tropical grasslands
  - Rainy season
  - Sahel, central India
- Cold desert
  - Higher latitudes
  - Extremes of temperatures with severe winter season
  - Gobi desert in Mongolia, Antarctica.

Most deserts do, however, share some common features:

- High day-time temperatures
- Low night-time temperatures
- Minimal surface water
- Poor vegetation
- Cloudless sky
- Variable wind speed with dust/sand (and snow) storms
- Sparsely populated.

Preparation

Most desert expeditions are vehicle based. The most comprehensive resource for these expeditions is the *Vehicle-dependent Expedition Guide* by Tom Sheppard, available from the Expedition Advisory Centre at the RGS. It covers all aspects of planning, communications and equipment for vehicle expeditions. *Sahara Overland* by Scott is also excellent. It contains detailed information including GPS waypoints for a range of expeditions and has a linked website (www.sahara-overland.com) with up-to-date reports from travellers.

Medical planning for desert expeditions starts with a thorough pre-expedition questionnaire and health assessment including a dental check. Deserts are among the most remote and isolated regions in the world, and medical assistance may be non-existent. A simple delay of a re-supply vehicle or a navigation error may be potentially disastrous when water supplies are running low. The psychological effects of this challenging environment should not be underestimated, and planning must be meticulous and allow a large safety margin of time, water, fuel and food. As much advice as possible should be sought from previous expeditions. Local knowledge is invaluable and every opportunity should be taken to check details of proposed route and conditions prior to each leg of the journey. Maps are often scarce or unreliable, as most "roads" may simply be nomadic tracks, which vary from season to season. It is easy to overestimate the distance that can be covered either on foot or by vehicle.

Clothing, footwear and shelter

In deserts, *light, loose-fitting clothes* made of natural materials covering the body and a *hat*, scarf or *khaffieh* covering the head provide protection from the sun and allow air to circulate and so evaporate sweat. Shorts and T-shirts are also convenient and generally perfectly adequate, but it is important to use sun block on exposed skin. The colour of clothes is not of great importance. In direct sunlight white will reflect heat, black will absorb it. Logically, lighter-coloured clothes should be cooler; in practice loose clothing, whatever its colour, will be most comfortable. Sunglasses and goggles are essential eye protection for desert travel.

Footwear needs to be light, comfortable and tough. Shoes, trainers and boots all have disadvantages. Feet enclosed in footwear in hot climates become sweaty, smelly, soft, wrinkled and often infected with fungi. The disadvantage of bare feet or flip-flops is the lack of protection from the heat of the ground, from rocks or thorns or occasionally snakes and parasitic infections. The choice must depend on the conditions. For sand and gravel deserts go for walking sandals, trainers or desert boots; rock and volcanic larva may require heavier footwear. Whatever you choose, make sure you care for your feet. Treat blisters early and take every opportunity to allow your feet to air and dry.

It is possible to travel for months in desert, scrub and bush land without the need for shelter. A camp bed off the ground as protection against snakes, scorpions and spiders makes a perfect bed, but remember to shake out your shoes in the morning. A tent will protect you from flies and the unwanted attention of domestic dogs near human habitation. A tent and a decent campfire will provide a reasonable sense of security against hyena and lion for those dubious about the protection of fire alone. Where large animals and domestic dogs are present, keep food in a secure position away from you, preferably in a locked vehicle. If there is wind or a sandstorm, bivouac against a natural shelter such as rocks or stay in your vehicle. Beware of making camp in wadis or dry river courses; flash flooding from rain many miles away can be very rapid and, if not lethal, it will be inconvenient.

HEAT-RELATED ILLNESSES

Heat-related illnesses are preventable, yet are a potential life-threatening hazard for all expeditions. It is essential that all expedition members are aware of the risk factors, recognition and treatment of heat illness.

Heat-related illnesses cover a range of symptoms from lethargy and headache to death. They result from combinations of high environmental temperature/humidity, ineffective heat loss and increased bodily heat production, especially from exercise. They can occur at any temperature, but are most common in hot, humid environments. They are serious but preventable conditions which are underdiagnosed. Heat stroke carries a case fatality of between 17 and 70%.

Definitions

Traditionally, heat-related illness has been described using a variety of terms including heat syncope, heat cramps, heat stress, heat exhaustion and heatstroke. These terms are misleading as they are not necessarily caused by an increase in core temperature. In this chapter the term "heat-related illness" refers to any debilitating condition resulting from an increase in core temperature.

Incidence

Heat stroke is responsible for around 240 deaths per year in the United States. In the UK there are over 200 cases of heat stroke every year. Both of these figures are probably underestimates. Among military populations in a hot, humid climate (Singapore), the incidence may be as high as 3.5 cases per 1,000 soldiers.

Prevention

- Identify individuals at risk
- Monitor environmental heat stress
- Adjust the daily aims of the expedition accordingly
- Educate expedition members about heat illness, its early recognition and treatment
- Provide adequate clean drinking water, shade and latrines
- Prepare a robust medical evacuation plan.

Acclimatisation

Effective acclimatisation takes about 2 weeks. To acclimatise expeditioners should exercise for a *minimum* of 60 minutes a day in the heat. Light clothing (e.g. T-shirt and shorts) should be worn to encourage evaporative heat loss. Ideally individuals should undertake light-to-moderate exercise for 2–3 hours daily. Those who are less fit should adopt work/rest cycles to make up the required acclimatisation time (e.g. 45 minutes of exercise followed by 15 minutes of rest in the shade and fluid replacement). They should be supervised at all times. The body increases the amount of

TABLE 23.1 RISK FACTORS FOR HEAT-RELATED ILLNESS

Environmental
- High temperature
- High humidity
- Poor shade

Constitutional
- Extremes of age
- Reduced physical fitness
- Women are less heat tolerant than men
- Obesity
- Previous heat intolerance

Behavioural
- Lack of acclimatisation
- High physical workload
- Excessive/inappropriate clothing
- Inadequate water intake
- Dehydration (e.g. from flying, diarrhoea, alcohol)
- Recreational drug use (e.g. "ecstasy")

Medical
- Any intercurrent illness (e.g. chest infection, diarrhoea)
- Any chronic disease (e.g. diabetes, heart disease)
- Heat rash (prickly heat) and other skin diseases
- Inappropriate diuresis or other renal diseases
- Medication (e.g. beta-blockers, diuretics, antidepressants, antihistamines)

sweat produced (but it is more dilute), which increases evaporative cooling and keeps the core temperature down. As a result, an acclimatised person has a higher fluid requirement than a non-acclimatised person and may require up to 1.5 litres of water an hour.

The intensity of exercise should be gradually increased each day, working up to an appropriate physical training schedule adapted for the environment. Physical training should be conducted in the morning or evening, when it is cooler. Air-conditioned vehicles and hotel rooms should be avoided.

Some degree of acclimatisation can be obtained in temperate climates prior to departure. Hot baths twice a day, and wearing more clothing than normal when exercising, are both effective. Physical fitness is also crucial. Any strenuous physical activity raises the core temperature, but this needs to be done regularly in order to have a protective effect. Any change of environment with significant additional heat stress will require an additional period of acclimatisation.

The benefits of acclimatisation are lost over 20–40 days after returning to a temperate climate.

Assessment of heat risk

There are four environmental characteristics that influence heat stress:

- Air temperature
- Solar (or radiant heat) load
- Absolute humidity
- Wind speed.

Measuring these factors is difficult. A wet bulb globe thermometer (WBGT) measures the first three, but is expensive. Further details are available on the RGS website. The following method is designed for use in the field with no equipment.

- Each individual should work out their maximum heart rate (220 minus age) (e.g. a 40-year-old will have a maximum heart rate of 220 minus 40 = 180 beats/minute).
- The group should all work to the lowest figure obtained.
- The group should undertake the proposed activity for one work period (e.g. 30 minutes) under close supervision.
- Immediately after this initial work period all should recheck their heart rates. If anyone's heart rate exceeds 75% of the age-adjusted maximum (e.g. 180 × 0.75 = 135 beats/minute) the next working period should be reduced by one third (e.g. to 20 minutes with 40 minutes' rest).
- The group should rest in the shade and rehydrate for the remainder of the hour.
- Repeat the process until the 75% age-adjusted maximum has not been exceeded.

Fluids

Maintain an adequate fluid intake. Fluid must be drunk before, during and after exercise. Thirst is a poor guide to fluid requirement, as 2–3% dehydration significantly impairs exercise tolerance but does not initiate thirst. If individuals drink only enough to satisfy their thirst they will be dehydrated. To avoid dehydration it is essential that all expeditioners are encouraged to drink water despite not feeling thirsty. Individuals may not drink enough in certain situations, e.g. before going to sleep (to avoid having to wake up and dress to urinate) or before long journeys. Expedition leaders should therefore be aware of these factors and allow plenty of breaks during any activity along with an adequate number of suitable latrines. An inability to be able to spit is another indicator of dehydration.

Acclimatisation results in larger quantities of more dilute sweat being produced, so fluid requirements increase during the first 2 weeks of exposure.

The colour, volume and frequency of urine give the best guide to the adequacy of hydration. Dark yellow urine is a sure indicator that the individual is dehydrated, as is the desire to urinate less than twice a day. Changes in body weight offer a less useful guide, as weight loss is common, and caused not only by dehydration, but also by increased workload, gastrointestinal upset and decreased appetite due to heat and unfamiliar food.

Thirsty = dehydrated, dehydrated ***does not*** *= thirsty*

In hot environments, water losses can reach 15 litres per day per person. Complete replacement requires realistic estimates of potable water requirements, an adequate water logistic system, and individuals who understand and act on their water requirement.

Electrolytes

Sports drink manufacturers have heavily promoted their products as the ideal way to replace the water and salt lost in sweat. The principle that both water and salt should be replaced is correct, but for this to be effective the drink must contain a sodium concentration of at least 50mmol/l. Most sports drinks have a sodium concentration of 10–25mmol/l. The oral rehydration solution (ORS) recommended by the World Health Organization has a sodium content of 60–90mmol/l, but this is unpalatable in the quantities required. Whilst lifesaving for diarrhoeal illnesses, its use cannot be advocated for healthy people in the heat.

Some people have advocated salt tablets, but these irritate the stomach and provide an unknown amount and concentration of sodium as they are consumed with a variable amount of water. They are best avoided. In a study comparing the effectiveness of solid food and water with a commercial sports drink in fluid replacement, the former was more effective in restoring whole body water balance as the food contained more solutes than the sports drink.

Over-drinking

Whilst it is impossible to rely on thirst to drink enough water to avoid dehydration, it is equally important not to drink too much water as this can dilute the sodium content of the blood to such a level that fits, unconsciousness and death may occur. As a general guide if drinking causes distension of the stomach and feelings of nausea, then there is a possibility of over-drinking. The urine should be checked for colour and, if it is clear, the amount of water drunk should be reduced. It is not usual for young, healthy adults to get up more than once a night to urinate.

TABLE 23.2 **A COMPARISON OF RECTAL, TYMPANIC AND ORAL METHODS OF MEASURING CORE TEMPERATURE**

	Rectal	*Tympanic*	*Oral*
Pros	Most accepted and validated method for measuring core temperature	• Easy to measure • Increasingly used by GPs and hospitals • Fast and accurate in experienced users • Easy to monitor changes in temperature	• Easy to measure • Known by most people
Cons	• Expedition personnel, especially teenagers, may be reluctant to use • Rectal lag	• Operator dependent • Correct placement required in order to get an accurate temperature	• Unreliable – requires a conscious co-operative patient who has not recently drunk any cold or hot fluids • Thermometer must be placed under the tongue • Casualty should not breathe through mouth

In conclusion plenty of water should be made freely available to expedition members. Water drinking discipline should be imposed during and after work periods, and food should be provided during rest periods. Table salt should be available, but salt tablets are not necessary. Soups are an excellent source of both fluid and electrolytes. Sports drinks should be used only by athletes competing in the heat who are familiar with the products, and ORS reserved for those with diarrhoea.

Note: the above guidelines apply to hot, dry environments such as deserts. The potential for evaporative heat loss is much reduced by hot, wet environments (e.g. jungles), resulting in a larger increase in body temperature for a given intensity of work. In jungles acclimatisation sessions should be conducted at a lower intensity than for hot, dry environments with mandatory rest/work cycles. The importance of maintaining and restoring fluid balance applies equally for hot, wet environments.

Measurement of core temperature

Traditionally the gold standard for measuring core temperature has been measurement of rectal temperature. However, there is poor correlation between the rectal temperature and the severity of symptoms, and the critical core temperature remains unknown (fatalities have been reported with rectal temperatures of 39.5°C and survivors with temperatures of 47°C). There is a well-documented lag between the measurement of core temperature and the rectal temperature. It is important that medical personnel are aware of the limitations of the measurement of core temperature. Two other methods are available. Their pros and cons are summarised below. Rectal temperatures remain the accepted gold standard, but tympanic (ear drum) temperatures may be acceptable in experienced hands.

RECOGNITION OF HEAT ILLNESSES

Anyone suffering the following symptoms in a hot (and/or humid) environment, or during increased physical activity in a temperate environment, should be treated as a victim of heat illness until proven otherwise:

- Weakness
- Lethargy
- Headache
- Dizziness
- Confusion
- Nausea
- Vomiting
- Muscle cramps
- Fatigue
- Hysteria
- Anxiety
- Impaired judgement
- Hyperventilation/tachypnoea
- Diarrhoea
- Staggering
- Collapse
- Convulsions
- Loss of consciousness

MANAGEMENT OF HEAT ILLNESSES

The 7 Rs:

1. Recognise signs and symptoms – if in doubt treat as heat injury.
2. Rest casualty in shade – get rest of group under cover and drinking water.
3. Remove all clothing – strip to underwear.
4. Resuscitate – maintain airway.
5. Reduce temperature ASAP – evaporative cooling and intravenous fluids.
6. Rehydrate – oral or intravenous fluids.
7. Rush to hospital – consider evacuation.

The most important thing to remember is to remove the casualty from the source of heat and place him or her in the shade. Remember that the ground can be a continued source of heat and the ideal position is on a stretcher or bed, which allows circulation of air. A hammock is ideal for encouraging heat loss. It is not necessary, or indeed desirable, to use ice-cold water. This causes constriction of the surface blood vessels and a reduction in blood flow to the skin. The skin therefore appears cool, while the warm blood circulates beneath, rising in temperature from metabolic processes.

The patient should be sprayed or splashed with water and fanned to encourage evaporative cooling. A wet sheet may be used instead. The administration of a cold intravenous solution of less than 1 litre of saline within an hour has been shown to result in significant reduction in core temperature and an improvement in the clinical condition of the patient.

Heat-injured casualties who have not been cooled and are shivering are seriously ill. Their temperature has risen so quickly that they have lost the ability to control their temperature and will complain of feeling cold. They will not feel hot or thirsty. They will be pale with cold skin. They will want to be wrapped in warm clothing, which only increases their core temperature, as does shivering. This is not normal and they must have their core temperature measured to exclude heat illness or a febrile illness such as malaria.

With cooling, the return to a normal temperature is often associated with shivering. It is important to continue to monitor the core temperature, as an individual's thermoregulatory capacity has been damaged. These individuals are at continued risk of both hyperthermia and hypothermia.

Stop the activity for all participants

Measure core temperature, pulse rate, blood pressure and conscious level (see Chapter 12). While a fall in systolic blood pressure is a poor indicator of early volume depletion, its presence reliably indicates that the patient is seriously ill and is a sign of impending cardiorespiratory collapse. Aspirin and/or paracetamol is of no value in heat illness and treatment should not be given. Glucose should be given orally or intravenously as casualties are often hypoglycaemic.

If conscious

- Lay the casualty down in the shade.
- Raise their feet.
- Strip them to their underwear.
- Spray their whole body with water.
- Fan their skin vigorously to aid evaporation.
- Give them water to drink.

If unconscious

- Place them in the recovery position (risk of vomiting).
- Protect their airway.
- Give them intravenous fluids (isotonic saline).
- Cool them by spraying the body with water and fanning the skin.
- Evacuate as an emergency.

MINOR HEAT ILLNESSES

Sunburn

Sunburn reduces the thermoregulatory capacity of skin and also affects central thermoregulation. Sunburn should be prevented by the use of adequate sun protection. When it does occur, affected individuals should be kept from significant heat strain until the burn has healed.

Heat syncope

Fainting on standing in the heat is thought to occur due to blood pooling in the legs and increased blood flow to the skin. Upon standing the blood supply to the brain is temporarily interrupted, causing loss of consciousness. Although most cases of heat syncope are harmless, the potential for heat illness should be considered, especially following physical work in the heat, or after the acclimatisation period.

Heat oedema

Mild swelling of the limbs may be experienced during the first few days of exposure to heat, during which time the plasma volume increases to allow for the increased blood flow to the skin.

Heat cramps

The precise mechanism behind heat cramps is unknown. Heat cramps may occur in salt-depleted individuals recovering after a period of work in the heat, but also with any unaccustomed exercise, even in cool conditions, e.g. swimming. Salt supplementation has been found to reduce the incidence of heat cramps. Cramp is painful and can recur but does not have any long-term effects. If the individual is otherwise well, there is no association with heat illness. Treatment is supportive with salt supplementation to food for a few days. Intravenous fluids are rarely required.

Miliaria rubra

Miliaria rubra is an inflammatory skin eruption, which appears in actively sweating skin in humid conditions. In dry climates, miliaria may be seen on skin covered by clothing. Each lesion represents a blocked sweat gland, which cannot function efficiently, and therefore the risk of heat illness is increased in proportion to the amount of skin surface involved. Sleeplessness due to itching and secondary infection of occluded glands may further affect thermoregulation. Miliaria is treated by cooling and drying affected skin, avoidance of sweating, controlling infection and relieving itching. Sweat gland function recovers with replacement of the damaged skin, which takes 7–10 days.

Eyes

Eyes are prone to damage from sand and direct sunlight. A sand-filled eye can be cleared by bathing the open eye in clean water. The eye may have an abrasion or retained foreign body, which should be dealt with as described in Chapter 13. Several pairs of sunglasses and goggles are needed to prevent sand getting in during storms. Sunglasses should be worn at all times during the day, even when overcast.

Throat

Dry air, sand and insects make breathing difficult, and the development of a dry persistent cough likely. A loose cloth (muslin) over the nose and mouth can prevent foreign bodies entering and prevent some loss of moisture.

SUMMARY

Heat-related illnesses can present a real threat to any expedition, but with proper preparation and management all are preventable. It is essential that all expedition members are aware of the risk factors, recognition and treatment of heat illness. Expedition organisers need to take account of the lengthy time required to acclimatise properly, and construct a suitable, flexible itinerary and programme of physical work. Unusually energetic individuals may need to be restrained from excessive physical effort. The medical plan should include a medical briefing to all personnel, adequate work/rest cycles with suitable hydration, provision for taking the core temperature and administering intravenous fluids, and a pre-arranged casualty evacuation plan which can be relied upon 24 hours a day.

24 TROPICAL FOREST EXPEDITIONS

Paul Richards

"Jungle" to many people evokes an image of an unbearably hot suburb of hell where unfortunate travellers suffer endless torment from clouds of disease-carrying bugs, while the trees, dripping with poisonous snakes, serve only as cover for vicious animals waiting to pounce.

The truth, of course, is that tropical rainforests are home to many indigenous peoples and are hospitable once one knows how to live in them. Certainly, they can afford equal or greater comfort than many other expedition destinations though, as with all environments, such comfort is greatly facilitated by good planning and appropriate equipment. Many of the health problems encountered in the tropical environment such as infectious diseases or animal bites and stings are covered in Chapter 20. The purpose of this chapter, therefore, is to give an overview of expeditions in a tropical rainforest and draw attention to a selection of specific points.

The environment

Tropical rainforests cover a dwindling 6% of the Earth's land mass and are defined by their location (between the Tropic of Cancer 23° 27' N and Tropic of Capricorn 23° 27' S) and by their high rainfall, which can be several metres a year. They are thus hot and humid, often with little breeze or respite, though upland forests may chill enough through the night to require a blanket or lightweight sleeping bag. Some forest floors may be under water for much of the year.

Preparation

Much of the success of any expedition relies heavily on the pre-departure preparation. The team should be selected not only for the appropriate combination of skills to complete whatever task the expedition is undertaking, but also for the ability to live with one another for prolonged periods in sometimes trying circumstances. Previous successful expedition participation is a good predictor. Expeditions are often physically challenging but fitness can be improved by training and sometimes a bright sense of humour can be a more desirable asset!

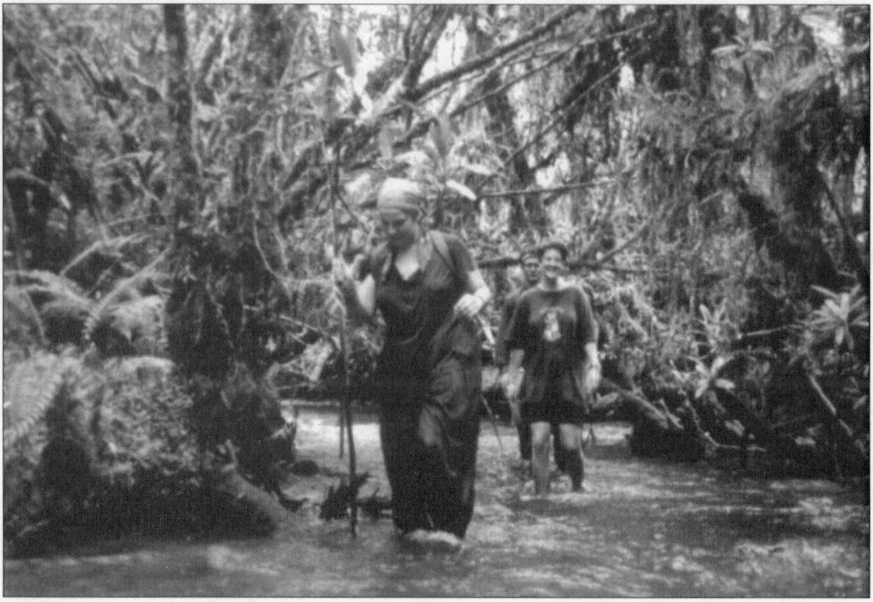

Figure 24.1 *Wading through a jungle river – Irian Jaya (P. Richards)*

The command structure is best decided at the outset with roles and areas of responsibility such as food, medical kits, science data and so on defined and, importantly, agreed by all members to avoid potential conflict in the field. Team bonding and a sense of ownership are helped enormously by shared preparation and realistic "trial runs" before the expedition departs.

Ensure that the team receives appropriate immunisations and advice on hygiene and bite avoidance. All members should know first aid and navigation. Organise jungle training for those new to the environment and training in any special techniques that projects may require. Other chapters in this book are useful sources of advice on pre-expedition preparation.

Water and food

Obtaining water is not usually a problem in tropical forests, although the quality can be variable. In savannah or scrubland water may be scarce. Consider from where you will obtain water and how you will purify, store and carry it. If operating from a base camp then boiling is the most effective sterilisation even for water containing particulate matter, but on the trail removal of sediment by coarse filter (e.g. Millbank bag) and sterilisation with iodine enable regular filling of water bottles. Each member should carry at least 2 litres of personal water. Commercial water purifiers rapidly become clogged unless sediment is first removed by prior filtration. In some parts of the world water may be contaminated by heavy metals, for example mercury from the gold-mining process in the Amazon basin.

Friendly villages may be able to supply smaller groups with (sometimes unfamiliar) food but large expeditions should be provisioned in case requirements exceed supply. In uninhabited areas sometimes several days' worth of food may need to be carried. Living off the land by trapping, shooting and foraging is ambitious and unlikely to be viable except for the most experienced of jungle travellers. Fresh food deteriorates rapidly and must be stored out of reach of ants and other wildlife. Tins have long shelf life and are relatively immune to predation. Packet or dehydrated food requiring little preparation is useful and is lighter to carry. Food must be cooked hygienically (see Chapter 10) and raw food is best avoided to minimise gastrointestinal illness.

Acclimatisation

Humans may once have been "tropical animals" but for many this is definitely past tense. Those transported abruptly by aircraft from temperate climes are likely to suffer from fatigue, lethargy, poor sleep and reduced exercise tolerance. They should maintain hydration and exercise little in the first few days and this limit on activity should be considered when formulating the expedition itinerary. Acclimatisation is assisted by slower transit overland or on a boat but otherwise takes about 8–10 days (slightly longer in children). Not surprisingly, air conditioning delays acclimatisation and is best avoided. In preparation, careful exercise in a hot humid environment, as simulated by exercising in warm clothing indoors for an hour a day for at least a week preceding jungle exposure, will aid acclimatisation, although the benefit is lost within a week if not maintained. Care must be taken to maintain hydration and the exercise halted if any signs of heat stress develop.

Clothing and equipment

Nudity aids evaporation of perspiration, which in humans is the main method of cooling, but provides no protection from bites or scratches. This and the possibility of offending cultural taboos necessitate clothing for expeditioners. Women in particular need to be mindful of local dress codes in exposing bare legs or even arms. In some forests shorts may be suitable but in others insects and sharp or irritant plants make long trousers and long-sleeved shirts a must. Covering up is especially important in preventing insect bites, particularly from dusk to dawn when malaria-carrying mosquitoes are active. Clothing should be cotton, light, loose and airy. Tight clothing impairs air circulation and evaporation, and predisposes individuals to prickly heat. Pale colours attract fewer mosquitoes and are theoretically cooler.

Both clothing and skin tend to rot when continuously wet. Try to dry the skin at night if possible and reserve a dry set of clothes for camp. A wet set for day travel can be rinsed in camp to remove salt and drying attempted over the fire but can be worn damp next morning if necessary. A plastic bag large enough to line your rucksack and twisted, folded and taped at the neck will protect dry kit in tropical storms or if the rucksack falls in a stream.

A hat is useful to protect the head from rattan-barbed leaves hanging across trails, for comfort in rains, and for sun protection in open areas. An umbrella is carried by some for open trails or forest downpours but can snag if used when walking. It is, however, useful in camp; tied at the top of a 2-metre tree branch which has been stuck in the ground and denuded of leaves it will make an effective sheltered clothes stand.

Footwear is subject to opinion. Bare feet or sandals provide no protection from thorns, snakes and infections such as hookworm and larva migrans, which burrow through skin in contact with infected soil. Heavy rigid boots can be difficult on slippery logs but a good tread is important in mud. On firm open trails some prefer trainers though these provide no ankle support. In very wet or muddy conditions, rubber boots are simple and provide good protection. The author's preference is for light, quick-drying, cordura-type boots. A flap covering the laces to prevent snagging on foliage is a bonus. Needless to say, all footwear should be well broken-in; "Vietnam Jungle Boots" in particular seem to predispose to blisters. For camp, comfortable lightweight shoes such as trainers are useful but remember you may need to trek in your "spare" footwear.

A machete is essential for jungle survival and generally for making trails or camp. The tool should be respected and care taken to learn safe use. Some locally produced machetes can be of suspect quality, as illustrated when the author narrowly missed impalement by a fast-flying blade that buried itself 4 centimetres into a nearby tree after departing its handle. Its flat edge was being used by a novice to play baseball!! There is the potential for major injury if one slips when carrying a live blade so it should be sheathed when not in active use. Gloves are useful as hands can sustain many small cuts from sharp grass when cutting foliage.

Shelter

Sleeping on the ground is not recommended due to exposure to scorpions, snakes, ants and other wildlife. Options include constructing a raised platform, a tent (although these can be stiflingly hot and are heavy when wet) or a hammock. A tent with a sewn-in bucket-type groundsheet offers a barrier to ground wildlife and a groove cut into the ground around the tent will drain rainwater runoff. Hammocks are favoured by many, as they can be slung just about anywhere, are quick to erect, light and take advantage of every slight breeze. Hammocks should be slung fairly tight, as sleeping is difficult when sagged to a banana shape. A tarpaulin or poncho rain shelter can then be strung over the hammock and a permethrin-impregnated mosquito net suspended beneath it so that it covers the occupant without leaving gaps or touching the skin. The ground beneath the hammock, and for a few feet surrounding, should be cleared so that the occupant can step clearly on to earth. Leaf

Figure 24.2 *Sleeping off the ground (C. Caldicott)*

litter can hide all sorts of fauna and, although snakes will depart if they detect your approach, to surprise a resting snake by stepping on it from your hammock may provoke a defensive bite. Whatever form of shelter is chosen, a sleeping mat enhances comfort and a silk sleeping bag liner used alone may give sufficient warmth. Group areas such as communal dining can be protected by large tarpaulins.

MEDICAL PROBLEMS SPECIFIC TO TROPICAL EXPEDITIONS

Skin

Stop as soon as practical when you feel any "hot spots" and treat them before they become blisters. Damp and encased in shoes, feet become waterlogged, smelly and infected with fungi, so take every opportunity to air them and avoid sleeping in wet socks. Bacteria can gain entry through soggy broken skin giving secondary infections. Fungal infections are also common in the groin. Wash and dry the skin daily where possible and apply prophylactic antifungal powder to the feet and skin folds. Using a combination antifungal/weak steroid cream (hydrocortisone) economises on weight, speeds relief of inflammation and can double up as anti-irritant on non-infected bites.

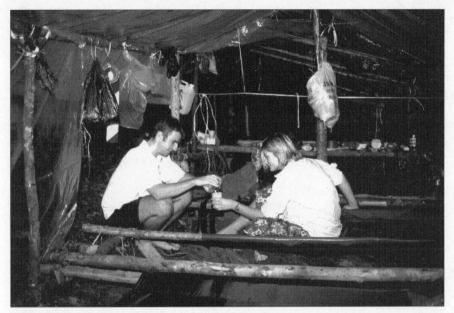

Wound infections

In this humid environment, even small scratches can quickly become infected. Minor infection may progress to spreading skin infection (cellulitis) requiring antibiotics, or abscesses, or, at worst, become a life-threatening generalised sepsis (septicaemia). It is prudent, therefore, to examine the skin, particularly legs and arms, each evening. Using carefully cleaned hands, wounds should be washed with soap and water as soon as possible, dried with clean gauze or similar, antiseptic applied and covered if open. Iodine tincture 2% for water sterilisation is an effective antiseptic but traditional cream stings less. Spray-on iodine (Savlon Dry) avoids the need to touch the cleaned wound. Healing is more likely if the wound is kept dry.

Prickly heat (miliaria rubra)

This is an intensely irritating prickly rash, which arises in skin waterlogged from continual perspiration. The sweat pores become blocked and inflamed giving a rash of tiny blisters on a background of red skin. Common sites are the waist, armpits, neck, upper back and chest, scalp and flexures. Treatment is to bathe in cool water, gently pat dry and apply talcum powder or calamine lotion.

Insects

Insects are often tiresome nuisances but their importance lies in the large range of diseases they can transmit (see Chapter 19). Malaria is probably the most significant disease in terms of numbers affected. Fortunately, the same methods of bite avoidance work for all. Some people hardly seem to respond to bites whilst others suffer intensely irritating reactions.

Topical or oral antihistamines or Eurax all help with itching, although there is a small risk of skin sensitisation with topical antihistamines. The breach of skin in-

TABLE 24.1 **INSECT AVOIDANCE**

Cover up	Long sleeves, trousers, hat. Especially dusk to dawn
Insect repellent	DEET, eucalyptus, citronella. Cover all exposed skin. Spray or liquid better than solid stick which may leave gaps
Mosquito net	Especially for sleeping. Avoid gaps; tape tears More effective if permethrin impregnated If touches skin, insects may reach skin through the net pores
In buildings	Net-screened windows/doors. Air conditioning 'Knock down' spray Mosquito coils/permethrin-impregnated heated pads

tegrity or subsequent scratching can produce secondary bacterial infection, which should be treated with antibiotics as above.

Dehydration and heat illness

These are covered in Chapter 23.

Symptoms and signs of dehydration

- Fatigue
- Confusion
- Thirst
- Rapid pulse
- Poor urine output
- Dry mouth and membranes
- Loss of skin turgor (feels "porridgey").

Maintaining hydration
Thirst is a poor indicator of hydration
Urine should be of good volume and mostly clear
Drink beyond the point when you stop feeling thirsty
(Concentrated urine = dark or tea colour = dehydration)

Gastroenteritis and hygiene

Personal and camp hygiene are particularly important in the tropical environment (see Chapter 10). Acceptable contact lens hygiene may not be practicable in an expedition setting due to the risk of eye infection. Antibiotic eye drops and back-up spectacles must be carried. Diarrhoea and vomiting can spread quickly through the expedition team and hands should be washed with antiseptic soap after use of the latrine and before handling or eating food. I take personal responsibility for cleaning and storing of my own spoon and mess kit and avoid sharing of personal water bottles. As daily fluid requirement is already high due to perspiration, added loss from gastroenteritis can quickly lead to dehydration, particularly where vomiting makes extra intake difficult.

Treatment to replace lost fluid and body salts should begin at the onset of the illness before dehydration becomes apparent. Losses should be minimised by ceasing exercise and remaining in the shade as much as possible. Glucose is rapidly absorbed across the bowel wall, taking water and sodium with it, and is more effective mixed with water in rehydrating than water alone. It is the basis for oral rehydration solution (ORS), which also contains important salts such as sodium and potassium. A

TABLE 24.2 ADDITIONAL SUPPLIES FOR TROPICAL RAINFOREST EXPEDITIONS (SEE CHAPTER 3 FOR DETAILED MEDICAL KIT)

Useful Items in a Jungle Formulary	*Examples/notes*
Dry iodine spray	Savlon Dry
Soap!	
Insect repellent	DEET
Suntan cream	Factor 15+, water resistant
Antihistamine	Loratdine or cetirizine
Antifungal dusting powder	
Antifungal cream	Clotrimazole with hydrocortisone
Antifungal vaginal cream/pessary	
Eurax cream	(Itchy bites)
Antibiotic for skin	Erythromycin
Antibiotic for gut	Ciprofloxacin, metronidazole
Standby malaria treatment	Seek contemporary advice
Loperamide	
Oral rehydration solution (ORS)	Diorylate
Antiemetic	Prochlorperazine (+ Buccastem)
Gauze	
Non-adherent dressings	Melolin
Blister kit	Compeed/Spenco/Comfeel

TABLE 24.3 OTHER USEFUL KIT

- Swiss Army penknife or Leatherman multi-tool
- Paracord
- Bungees
- Plastic bags (+ziplock)
- Duct tape (repairs!)
- Torch
- Candles
- Whistle
- Camera polarising filter
- Cigarette lighter
- Jay cloth (face flannel)
- Machete sharpening stone
- Learn basic knots

rough guide is 200–300ml with each bout of loose stool in addition to normal daily fluid requirement. If no commercial preparation is available, it can be made by:

Eight level teaspoons of sugar + two level teaspoons of salt in 1 litre of sterilised water

A surprising amount of fluid can be taken by frequent sipping; although some may vomit back, some will stay down. Severe dehydration may require rectal (controversial) or intravenous fluids and evacuation (see Chapter 18 for more details).

In contrast to in Britain, where gastroenteritis is usually viral, in this environment it is often bacterial. This is associated with acute onset, fever and general toxicity, and responds rapidly to antibiotics such as ciprofloxacin. Other useful drugs are loperamide, which slows the diarrhoea, and antiemetic drugs such as prochlorperazine to reduce vomiting. This is available as suppositories or special tablets which can be dissolved under the upper lip (Buccastem).

Psychological problems

Unfamiliar sounds, smells, fear of animals, disease, the intense darkness of night or the isolation of sleeping exposed in a hammock in a strange place may contribute to anxiety. The best tip is to be interested in the jungle around you, learn about the environment and listen to local guides. In other words, become informed. Fear arises from uncertainty and unfamiliarity and knowledge makes the forest accommodating rather than intimidating. Prolonged exposure to wet discomfort saps morale so regular return to a comfortable environment, which might be a well-constructed base camp, is important. "Social time" particularly for sharing of the evening meal and general relaxed chat, is important for team integrity and morale.

HAZARDS AND NUISANCES

Be aware of hazards when choosing a site for the night. Look up! Loose or rotting branches can, and frequently do, crash down. Seemingly attractive abandoned native shelters can harbour spiders, ants or rodents and the snakes that feed off them. Even when it is dry locally, rivers can rise quickly from rain upstream and drown the camp. Routine jungle travel may involve wading through water but care must be taken with fast-flowing or deep rivers. Learn and practise river-crossing techniques in advance but avoid the hazard itself where possible. Do not enter gorges without thought to escape routes.

Trauma may be associated with falls, sprains, use of knives, lacerations on foliage, road traffic accidents or expedition activities such as kayaking. A stout walking pole made from a small tree or branch is useful on steep or slippy ground. Log bridges are often several feet off the floor and fixing the eye on the far end rather than the feet aids balance.

Getting lost in rainforests is very easy. A few steps off a trail and the forest looks the same in every direction. Use local guides who know the area and ensure they

Fig. 24.3 *Log bridge (C. Caldicott)*

don't inadvertently leave behind their inevitably slower charges. On trails keep the persons ahead and behind in sight at all times. Navigation with map and compass can be difficult over any distance but global positioning systems (GPS), although accurate, may be unreliable. The forest canopy interferes with reception and capturing enough satellites for a fix may be slow or impossible. Wide clearings offer the best hope. Batteries do flatten and the humidity is unkind to electronics.

Leeches cause psychological distress out of all proportion to any physical harm. Aquatic leeches attack swimmers and will enter orifices like the nose, mouth, etc. Land leeches tend to attach on the lower limb but can climb rapidly. Socks, trousers

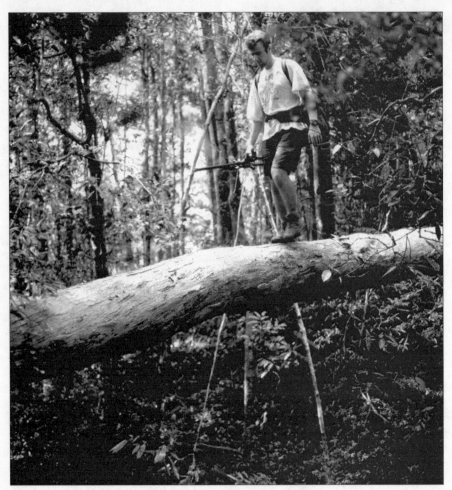

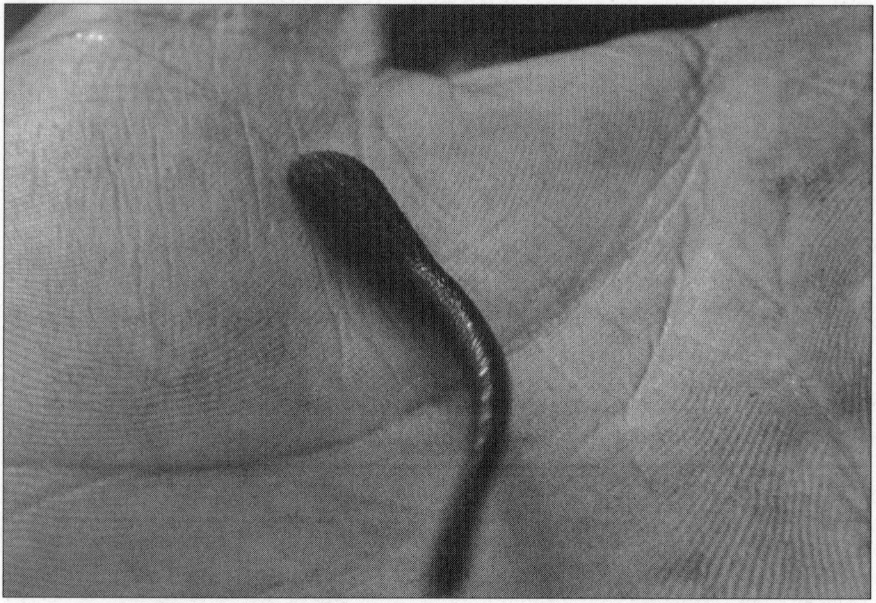

Fig. 24.4 *Leech on hand (P. Richards)*

and boots provide little protection but DEET offers some deterrence. A tickling sensation or sharpness as they bite may give them away but often the first indication is blood-stained clothing. As they inject an anticoagulant, bleeding persists but a single bite is more messy than serious. Before attachment, they can be flicked off but pulling them off after they have taken hold may leave mouth parts behind and predispose to infection. Of themselves, they are not thought to transmit infections. Application of iodine tincture, salt kept dry in a film canister, other chemical irritants or a lighted cigarette all persuade leeches to let go. Burning them off with a lighter is hazardous to both parties! Apply pressure if necessary to stop the bleeding and treat leech bites as wounds.

Snakes can be so well camouflaged and tend to detect the approach of heavy footfall so quickly that it is possible for non-natives rarely to see them. Humans are not prey but snakes may attack defensively if disturbed. Scorpions are easier to detect as they fluoresce under a portable ultraviolet light. Centipedes can give nasty bites. The following precautions will minimise the risk of snake and scorpion bites:

- Sleep off the forest floor.
- Open up and shake out sleeping bag before use.
- Shake out clothing before wearing.

- Check ground before sitting at the base of trees.
- Store boots inverted on sticks – prevents wildlife crawling in.
- Always routinely tap boots to jolt out any unwanted inhabitants.
- Don't put hands into holes.
- Don't poke holes with sticks.
- Don't straddle logs. Step on to them then away.
- Don't put hands blind into the depths of rucksacks.
- Avoid swimming in water containing matted foliage.
- Don't put hands on branches or ledges that can't be seen.
- Remember banks of rivers and streams are common snake haunts.
- Always use a torch and wear boots to visit latrines – snakes hunt at night.

TABLE 24.4 **EXAMPLES OF OTHER BIOHAZARDS FOUND IN TROPICAL RAINFORESTS (SEE CHAPTERS 19 AND 20)**

Arthropods	**Larger animals**
Ants	Bats, dogs (rabies), crocodiles,
Jiggers	
Chiggers	**Aquatic**
Myiasis	Stingray
Bees, wasps	Electric eels
Irritant moths, caterpillars, butterflies	Piranha
Plants	**Scorpions**
Spines or sharp plants	**Snakes**
Irritant foliage	**Spiders**
Hallucinogenic plants used by locals	**Poison-dart frogs**
Poisonous plants	**Centipedes**

SUMMARY

Tropical rainforests are wet and hot and everything thrives including disease. They can nevertheless be comfortable if attention is paid to personal and camp hygiene, construction of shelters and care of equipment. Hazards can be anticipated and mitigated. Venomous, stinging or biting animals can be avoided and minimising insect bites is essential. Be prepared for serious illnesses but realise that they are rare, the majority being minor. Most of all, enjoy the forest. Few environments reveal such abundance and richness of life, and to lie in a hammock, listening to the many sounds of the forest as dawn breaks through the morning-mist-shrouded trees, will long enchant the memory.

25 POLAR EXPEDITIONS

Chris Johnson

The polar traveller encounters meteorological extremes: strong winds can combine with low temperatures to create conditions similar to a blast-freezer but, in contrast, a cloudless summer's day may lead to heat exhaustion, sunburn or snow blindness. The first-time traveller will encounter many unfamiliar hazards. Good training and risk-management procedures can reduce the dangers of these hazards. The weather often makes travel difficult and electrical storms may disrupt radio communications. It can be difficult, dangerous and expensive to evacuate casualties.

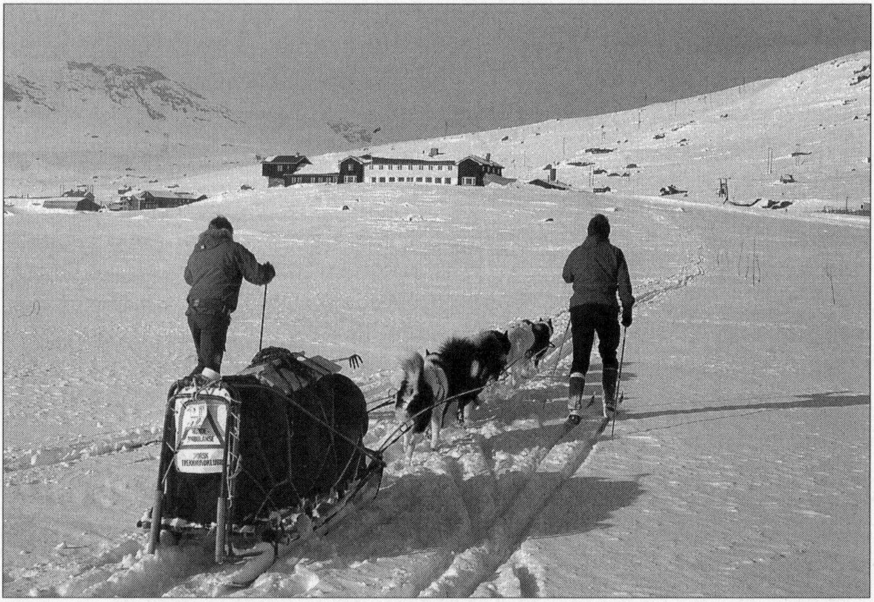

Figure 25.1 *A dog ambulance approaches Finse in Norway (C. Johnson)*

Independent groups should have sufficient medical equipment and expertise to care for casualties for several days. Tents, clothing and equipment must be capable of surviving extreme conditions.

TABLE 25.1 POLAR HAZARDS

• Low temperatures	• Sunburn
• High winds	• Snowblindness
• Whiteout	• Frostnip
• Avalanche	• Frostbite
• Crevasse	• Hypothermia
• Shifting sea-ice	• Wildlife (bears)
• Thin lake and river ice	• Contaminated water
• Dehydration	• Transport (ski/skidoo)

PREPARATION

All expedition members should be instructed in basic first aid, personal hygiene and the hazards of the area they are to visit before departure. The expedition medical officer (MO) should contact the emergency services, if they exist, in the area to be visited and find out how they can be contacted and how casualties could be evacuated. Satellite beacons (emergency position indicating beacons – EPIRBs) may be worth taking if there are sophisticated emergency services in the area. Avalanche transceivers are required if you plan to travel in mountainous areas. You must have adequate medical insurance and some countries demand that expeditions hold search-and-rescue insurance.

To reiterate previous chapters, all travellers should have medical and dental examinations well before the date of departure so that any necessary treatments can be completed. Conditions such as toothache or piles which are merely a nuisance at home can become a serious problem on an expedition. People with a stable medical condition such as well-controlled hypertension, diabetes or epilepsy can take part in expeditions, but the expedition leader and the MO should be aware of their condition as worsening of the disease could cause problems to everyone. Several separate sets of their usual drugs should be carried in case some are lost. People with unstable medical conditions, for example those prone to hypoglycaemic attacks, grand-mal epilepsy or inflammatory bowel disease, should not travel to remote areas unless comprehensive medical support will be available nearby. The condition may worsen under stress and the infirmity of one expedition member may threaten the lives of all. People with poor peripheral circulation in the cold (Raynaud's disease) are more likely to suffer from cold injuries in severe conditions.

Eyes

Anyone whose vision is so poor that they always need to wear glasses or contact lenses must plan to avoid the difficulties that might arise from loss or breakage: as a minimum, a spare pair should be taken. When the air temperature is below –20°C glasses invariably mist over. Metal-rimmed spectacle frames can become very cold and cause frostbite if they are in direct contact with the skin; opticians sell silicon sheaths to cover the side arms of the currently fashionable metal spectacles. Plastic-framed glasses or snow goggles are preferable. For the same reason, exposed metal studs and earrings should not be worn in extreme conditions.

Infectious diseases

These are uncommon in polar areas. However, some sledge dogs carry rabies and a course of rabies inoculations is advisable if the expedition is to work with these animals. Other immunisations may be needed for the journey to and from the expedition base. It is always sensible to ensure that you are covered against tetanus.

Medical supplies

Medical supplies must be compatible with the potential needs of the party. Drugs and dressings are both bulky and expensive, and over-enthusiastic ordering of medical supplies may deprive the team of funds better spent elsewhere. Some aqueous drugs crystallise and degrade in the cold; therefore powdered preparations and plastic containers should be selected whenever possible. Careful packing is essential to prevent breakages. Most medical supplies will be stored together, but a standby kit should be available in case the bulk of the supplies is lost in an accident. Suggestions for basic medical supplies are given in Chapter 3.

FIELD ARRANGEMENTS

At base camp the MO should be responsible for supervising the water supply and sanitary arrangements (see Chapter 10). Fresh water can usually be obtained by melting snow, and this is safe to drink unless it comes from an area frequented by animals or birds. Deer and beaver live near to many apparently pristine melt streams. They can contaminate the water with giardia spores which, if drunk, cause chronic diarrhoea and crampy abdominal pain. Beware of glacier outwash streams, which contain fine, highly abrasive rock dust in suspension (see B. Dawson, 1994); this is a powerful laxative. If in doubt, boil water or use a filtration and sterilising system. Bathing in cold climates is a masochistic pastime, but both people and clothes must be washed whenever possible as skin infections are common among sweaty, unwashed individuals.

Toilet facilities and rubbish dumps should be well demarcated and sited downwind and downstream of the campsite and water supply. In cold climates human waste and packaging materials break down very slowly and are your gift to future generations. As far as possible *all* waste should be removed from the area you visit. It may be hidden by a covering of snow during winter and spring, but it will be horribly visible at the end of the summer melt. There is now evidence that exposing excrement to direct sunlight results in less environmental pollution than hiding it away, as UV light sterilises harmful bacteria. Some North American National Parks are now recommending "smearing" rather than "digging" for small groups in very remote areas, but a properly designed field latrine is necessary whenever groups are bigger and stay longer.

Dehydration

Because polar air is very dry, sweat evaporates quickly and it is easy to underestimate the amount of fluid that is lost. Dehydration is a risk during the first days of an expedition, and everyone should be encouraged to drink enough to ensure that they produce plenty of urine even if they do not feel thirsty. A combination of malaise, headache and raised body temperature is common when parties first arrive in the cold, and this may be a mild form of heat exhaustion.

Food

Food is a much discussed topic on any expedition. It is necessary to balance variety with the need to obtain sufficient energy. While at base camp, or travelling using motorised transport, energy requirements will be similar to those of an outdoor worker in the UK (3,000cal/12,000kJ per day), but heavy outdoor work such as hauling sledges is an extremely energetic pastime requiring two or even three times this energy intake. In cold climates a greater proportion of the diet is likely to be made up of fatty foods. In the past polar expeditions have lived off the land, but nowadays many animal and bird species are protected and licences required before they are hunted. The internal organs of many polar animals contain toxic amounts of vitamin A and must be discarded; they are in any case not a gastronomic treat.

Fuel

As well as for heating food, fuel is required in polar areas to melt drinking water and dry clothing. It takes twice the energy to boil ice from –30°C as it does to boil water from 0°C. These additional energy demands must be considered when fuel needs are calculated.

Travel

Skidoos must be used with caution in areas where there are fences as garrotting injuries are a recognised risk. Tracked vehicles are usually noisy and should not be approached when moving. Expeditions should define safety procedures before entering avalanche and crevasse zones. Snow is an opportunity for recreation. Travellers on polar trips should enjoy themselves, but expeditions may need policies to limit the risks of leisure activities. A ski injury that would merely be a nuisance in a resort may threaten life in the wilderness.

MEDICAL PROBLEMS SPECIFIC TO POLAR REGIONS

Cold injury is a risk whenever it is cold and windy. The risk of frostbite is low when air temperature is above –10°C, but becomes significant whenever the air temperature falls below –25°C. Prevention of cold injury requires constant vigilance on the part of expedition members who should be paired off in the "buddy" system to check each other regularly for the telltale signs. Peripheral parts of the body such as fingers, toes and ears may become chilled causing frostnip or frostbite or, far more seriously, the victim may be unable to maintain his or her body temperature and become hypothermic.

Hypothermia

Hypothermia is a fall of the victim's core temperature to an extent that the ability to function normally is impaired. Normal core temperature is 36.5–37°C, and a fall below 35°C usually causes symptoms. Hypothermia is uncommon in a properly clothed, fit person, but may develop if someone is injured, or if clothing is inadequate

Wind speed		Ambient temperature (°C)							
mph	kph	–40	–30	–20	–10	–5	0	+5	+10
		Equivalent temperatures (°C) and danger of hypothermia for a fully clothed person							
		GREAT (exposed flesh may freeze)			INCREASING			SMALL	
46	74	–87	–71	–54	–38	–29	–21	–13	–4
35	56	–84	–68	–52	–36	–28	–20	–12	–3
23	38	–77	–62	–49	–31	–24	–16	–9	–1
12	20	–62	–49	–36	–23	–16	–10	–3	+2
6	10	–48	–37	–26	–15	–9	–3	+1	+7
0	0	–40	–30	–20	–10	–5	0	+5	+10

Figure 25.2 *Wind chill index*

or wet. It usually develops insidiously over several hours, although it can happen within minutes if someone falls into cold water. The symptoms are similar to drunkenness: poor co-ordination, falling over, confusion. They may shiver uncontrollably, but do not always do so. They may vehemently deny that anything is wrong and refuse help. Untreated, they will eventually become comatose and die. In the field diagnosis can be difficult, but anyone whose torso feels "as cold as marble" should be treated as a cold casualty.

TABLE 25.2 **FEATURES OF HYPOTHERMIA**

Body core temperature (°C)	*Associated symptoms*
37	Normal body temperature
36	
35	Judgement may be affected; poor decision-making Feels cold, looks cold, shivering
34	Change of personality, usually withdrawn – "switches off/doesn't care" Inappropriate behaviour – may shed clothing Stumbling, falling, confused
33	Consciousness clouded, incoherent Shivering stops
32	Serious risk of cardiac arrest Body cannot restore temperature without help Limbs stiffen
31	Unconscious
30	Pulse and breathing undetectable
29	
28	Pupils become fixed and dilated
27	
26	
25	
24	Few victims recover from this temperature
23	
22	
21	
20	
19	
18	Lowest recorded temperature of survival

Experts have disagreed about the best treatment for severe hypothermia and this has led to conflicting advice in textbooks. E. L. Lloyd gives an excellent review of these controversies in his 1996 article (see References and Further Reading). However, the controversies are irrelevant to most expeditions as they are unlikely to have the types of advanced resuscitation equipment that some mountain rescue groups now carry. The aim of treatment is to restore the body heat of the victim.

TABLE 25.3 **TREATMENT FOR HYPOTHERMIA**

- Seek shelter
- Remove damp outer clothing
- Wrap casualty in additional dry insulation such as a sleeping bag
- Lie down and insulate from the ground

If conscious:

- Restore body heat by providing warm drinks, warming the air with a stove and sharing the body heat of unaffected rescuers
- Chemical heat pads can be helpful if they are available, but ensure that they do not cause burns
- Do not give alcohol
- Ensure casualty rests and is kept under close supervision for at least 24 hours

If unconscious or body temperature is very low: evacuate urgently, if feasible

Rescuers must be careful not to put themselves at risk by giving up too much of their own clothing. Even after body temperature has been restored the casualty may remain confused.

Severe hypothermia is most likely to be encountered following a serious accident, for instance an avalanche. All cases of severe hypothermia should be evacuated urgently. In hospital, the policy is that all cold casualties should be re-warmed, but in the mountains a more pragmatic approach is needed, particularly if there are several casualties. The Scottish Mountain Safety Forum in 1997 produced guidelines to assist with decision-making (Table 25.4).

Frostnip

In contrast to hypothermia, which usually develops quite slowly, peripheral cold injury can develop within seconds. The earliest change is termed frostnip and is a numb, waxy white patch of skin most commonly seen on the earlobe or over the cheekbone. It is painless and its onset is usually unnoticed, although some

TABLE 25.4 **RECOMMENDATIONS FOR EVACUATION OF COLD INJURED**

	Criteria	*Action*
Definitely alive	Conscious	Insulate from heat loss Rewarm Monitor regularly Evacuate
Definitely alive	Unconscious Respiration and/or pulse present	Insulate from heat loss Rewarm only once in hospital Maintain airway Evacuate in recovery position
May be alive	No respiration No circulation (1 min) Clear airway No obvious fatal injury. Temperature below 32°C	Radio/phone for medical advice with evacuation plan Rewarm only once in hospital
Definitely dead	No respiration No circulation (1 min) Airway blocked Obvious fatal injury Temperature below 32°C	Evacuate as dead

experienced polar travellers may detect a sudden burning "ping" as it develops.

Treatment

Rewarm the body part by covering it with a gloved hand or blowing warm exhaled air over the skin. *Do not rub nipped skin.* No permanent injury is done if skin is nipped and quickly rewarmed, although redness and swelling may persist for a day or two. In some Scandinavian countries, ointments are sold that it is claimed have a protective effect against cold injury. The evidence is that they are not effective and indeed may increase the risk of injury.

Frostbite

Frostbite – freezing of the underlying tissue – is the progression of the superficial injury of frostnip if it is left untreated. A frostbitten part should be thawed only if the victim can rest for a prolonged period afterwards. Although it is desirable to protect a damaged limb, it is possible for the victim to walk to safety on a frostbitten foot, but once thawed the limb will be useless.

Treatment

- Rewarm the affected body part by putting it in clean water.
- Slowly warm the water to 40°C.
- Give strong painkillers as this process can be very painful.
- Protect body part from pressure and do not allow to refreeze.
- Cover raw areas with sterile dressings and change regularly.
- Take the tops off white blisters, but *not* blood blisters (see Auerbach, 1995).
- Give penicillin and painkillers (e.g. ibuprofen) regularly.
- Evacuate as soon as possible.

After circulation has been restored, the affected part will look red, blistered and severely swollen. Once treatment has begun, the damaged part must be protected against all forms of pressure and must not be allowed to refreeze. Severe frostbite takes months to heal, and the patient should be evacuated to a hospital used to dealing with the problem. Most doctors have seen dry gangrene associated with poor circulation; this causes death of the digit or limb from the inside. Frostbite injuries look similar, but are less serious as they are generally associated with superficial damage while the core of the limb is healthy. Unless infection develops, amputation should be undertaken only when a line of demarcation between healthy and dead tissue has become obvious. Improved scanning techniques and anti-prostaglandin drugs are improving the outlook for hospitalised patients with serious frostbite injuries.

Sunburn

Solar energy is intense in polar areas with strong reflection off the snow, and the radiation may exceed that in equatorial regions. High latitude (owing to thinning of the ozone layer) and altitude increase the risk of sunburn and a high factor sun cream should be applied liberally. Sunburn is particularly uncomfortable when rays reflected upwards off the snow burn the eyelids and underside of the chin and nostrils. Lips are particularly vulnerable to chapping and a suitable protective cream should be used.

Snowblindness

This is the term given to sunburn of the surfaces of the eye. The sensation is similar to having sand ground into the eyes. It can be extremely debilitating, being painful but more importantly causing a significant reduction in vision. In mild cases, the eye surface will heal in a few hours; however, in severe cases, where the eyelids may swell up and close, the patient may be incapacitated for several days and should rest in a darkened room or tent.

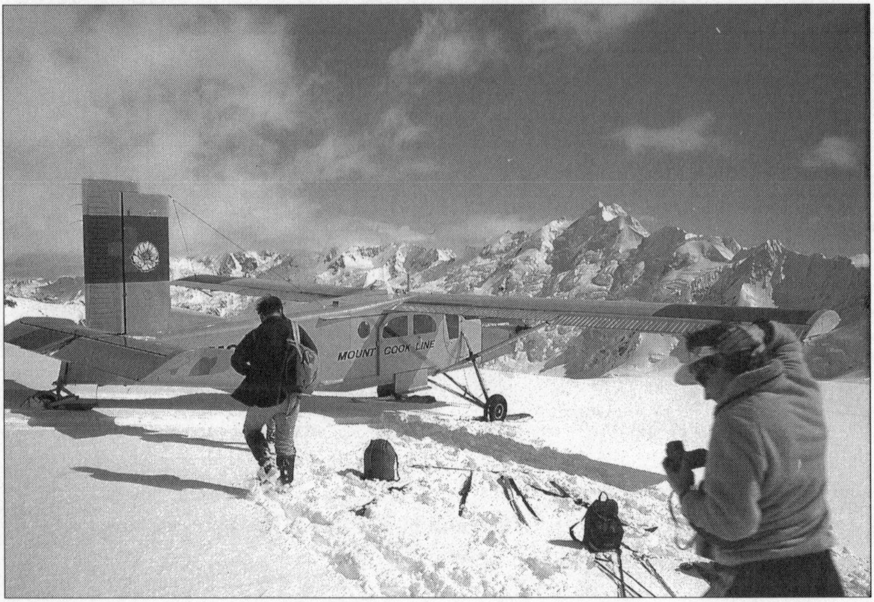

Figure 25.3 *Party arriving on Tasman Glacier in New Zealand (C. Johnson)*

Treatment

- Rest in a darkened room or tent.
- One dose of local anaesthetic eyedrops (e.g. amethocaine) relieves the initial discomfort, but further painkilling tablets will be required.
- Eyedrops that prevent spasm of the ciliary muscles of the pupil (e.g. tropicamide) can help, but repeated use of local anaesthetic drugs is no longer recommended.
- Chloramphenicol ointment can be used to soothe the eye, applied four times a day.

Ultraviolet light can penetrate cloud and snowblindness may develop even on overcast days. Expedition personnel should wear goggles or dark glasses with side protectors whenever they are working in bright conditions. If sunglasses are lost or damaged, an eye covering fashioned by making a couple of small horizontal slits in a sheet of card will provide an effective emergency alternative. Some experienced polar travellers have found that they are almost immune to snowblindness, but their apparent resistance should not entice newcomers to discard their eye protection.

Other hazards

Other polar hazards include the risk of suffocation or *carbon monoxide poisoning* in snowed-in tents and snow-holes. Ventilation holes must be checked regularly to ensure that crystals of water vapour do not block them. Some polar expeditions climb high enough for *mountain sickness* to be a problem (this topic is covered in Chapter 26). Although *wildlife* in the southern hemisphere is usually friendly, the same cannot be said of grizzly and polar bears which may take an unwanted interest in your presence; seek local advice and, if recommended, take a firearm.

Medical personnel attached to government polar research groups have studied many aspects of medicine and physiology, but the results of their investigations may be difficult to obtain as they are published in specialist professional journals. It is difficult to conduct field research in extreme conditions, but there remain opportunities for an enthusiastic MO to undertake a small research project. *Man in the Antarctic* (see References and Further Reading) is a good place to start reading about polar medical research.

The major hazard of the polar environment lies in its unfamiliarity. Once the hazards have been realised and guarded against, the cleanliness, beauty and remoteness of the polar wilderness provide inexhaustible pleasure for those fortunate enough to venture into it.

Evidence base

This article was based upon information from major textbooks on the subject including those by Auerbach (1995) and Lloyd (1986), updated following a search of Medline articles for 1990–2000 using the keywords "accidental hypothermia" and "frostbite".

26 HIGH-ALTITUDE AND MOUNTAINEERING EXPEDITIONS

Charles Clarke

A number of related medical conditions develop when people travel to altitudes above 3,000m (10,500ft). There is a wide variation in both the speed of onset and severity of symptoms and also the height at which they develop. The problems are caused by lack of oxygen.

In Nepal, the country with most high-altitude visitors (probably over 50,000 per year), the mortality rate of trekkers is believed to be around seven per year, with a quarter of the deaths due to altitude-related illness. In other words, several people on holiday die each year from potentially treatable conditions. On high-altitude climbing expeditions to peaks over 7,000m death rates are much higher, at around 4%. It is difficult to ascertain the importance of altitude illness compared with accident. In practical terms, for the expedition organiser or doctor, on a trip to heights over 5,000m, illness due to lack of oxygen demands recognition, chiefly because it is an unpleasant hindrance, but also, rarely, because it is a cause of fatalities.

MEDICAL PROBLEMS SPECIFIC TO HIGH ALTITUDE

Acute mountain sickness

Most people feel unwell if they drive, fly or travel by train from sea level to 3,000–3,500m. Headache, fatigue, undue breathlessness on exertion, the sensation of the heart beating forcibly, loss of appetite, nausea, vomiting, dizziness, difficulty sleeping and irregular breathing during sleep are the common complaints. Shivering and feeling the cold are also common. These are symptoms of acute mountain sickness (AMS), which usually develop during the first 36 hours at altitude and not immediately on arrival. The symptoms pass after several days.

Well over 50% of travellers develop some form of AMS at 3,500m, but almost all do so if they ascend rapidly to 5,000m (16,400ft). On a personal level I feel unpleasantly exhausted and headachy for several days every time I fly to Lhasa, which is at 3,620m – this is the usual situation for most people.

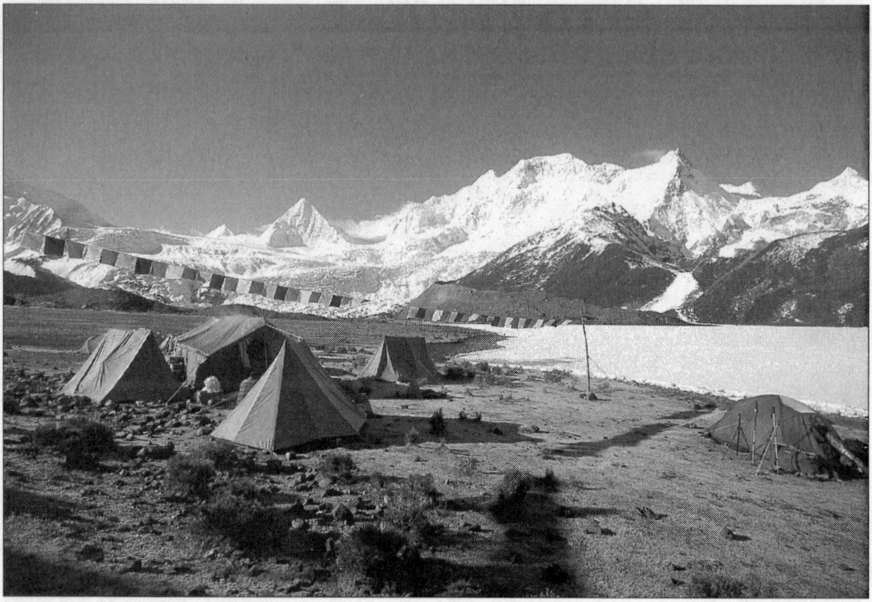

Figure 26.1 *Sepu Kangri, 4,700m, eastern Tibet, May 1997. Serious altitude sickness is a problem at these altitudes, despite the gentle terrain of base camp (C. Bonington, Chris Bonington Picture Library)*

Acclimatisation and ascent profiles

Acclimatisation, i.e. feeling well again, takes place over several days. Once travellers are acclimatised in this way, further gradual height gain can take place although symptoms may recur. Acclimatisation to, say, 4,000m, allows the body to adapt to this altitude, but not higher until further acclimatisation has taken place.

The question "How high, how fast?" has no absolute answer because of individual variation, but it is reasonable for healthy people of any age to travel rapidly to 3,500m. One often has to fly to this sort of altitude (Lhasa, for example, is 3,620m). Many people will develop AMS after arrival. It is unwise to travel much above 3,500m immediately from sea level. Accepted guidelines for Himalayan trekking groups (rarely adhered to in practice) are 300m of height gain per day above 3,000m with a rest day every third day. This profile seems tiresomely slow for many but it is well worth advocating – many altitude-related incidents occur in large groups where the slow acclimatiser is swept along by fitter members. By endorsing this profile would-be trekkers can encourage their trekking agent/team leader to adopt a safe schedule before departure – and make a journey at high altitude more enjoyable.

Above 4,000m the speed of further height gain should continue to be gradual and it is advisable to spend a week above 4,000m before sleeping above 5,000m.

The highest altitude where humans live permanently is about 5,500m (18,000ft), but on mountaineering expeditions or treks, residence for several weeks around 6,000m (20,000ft) is quite possible. At these altitudes people who are acclimatised should feel entirely well, being limited only by breathlessness on exertion. It is often impossible (for example on the Tibetan plateau) to keep to this counsel of perfection.

Prediction and prevention of AMS

There is unfortunately no way of predicting who will be seriously troubled by AMS and who will escape it. It is tempting to suppose that being physically fit and avoiding smoking would help in prevention, but unfortunately this is not so. Strenuous exercise at altitude, whether or not the subject is fit, makes AMS worse. Undue exertion and carrying heavy loads should therefore be avoided until acclimatised.

Patients with heart or lung disease or high blood pressure should seek specialist advice before travelling above 3,500m. Occasionally an individual develops AMS on every occasion they go to altitude.

Prevention of AMS

- Graded ascent (see above)
- Consider acetazolamide (Diamox) 125mg (half a 250mg tablet) twice a day.

Graded ascent is the best preventer of AMS. However, there has been much research on acetazolamide (Diamox), a drug used to reduce fluid retention (it makes you urinate) and in the treatment of glaucoma. Diamox also stimulates respiration – and this is probably why it is helpful. There is no doubt that Diamox is genuinely useful in the prevention of AMS if taken for several days before ascent. If Diamox is being used, half of one 250mg tablet should be given twice daily for 3 days before 3,500–5,000 metres is reached.

Travellers who take Diamox should be aware of its unwanted effects (all drugs have their dangers). Diamox makes some people feel nauseated and generally unwell and quite commonly causes tingling of the fingers. These cease when the drug is stopped. More unusual reported side-effects include flushing, rashes, thirst, drowsiness or excitement. People who are allergic to sulphonamide antibiotics are likely to develop allergic reactions to Diamox (e.g. rashes).

I do not recommend the drug routinely, and do not take it myself. If someone wants to take Diamox (e.g. because of previous problems) I suggest a trial of Diamox at sea level (i.e. before leaving home) for 2 days, so that its effects are known to the individual.

Treatment of AMS

It is important to emphasise that AMS, although unpleasant, is usually a self-limiting condition without serious sequelae. Principles of treatment include:

- Rest days, relaxation, descent? Do not go higher!
- Simple analgesia for headache: aspirin, paracetamol
- Consider dexamethasone 4mg every 4 hours (three doses)
- Consider hyperbaric chamber (portable pressure bag).

Portable pressure bags (hyperbaric chambers) are of some value in buying time while plans for descent are under way. They are, however, bulky (the size of a small rubber dinghy).

I use no drugs unless really necessary because symptoms usually resolve; the only real cure is to become acclimatised to the lack of oxygen. It is most important not to go higher if symptoms develop and to consider losing altitude if recovery does not take place within several days – and certainly if symptoms worsen.

Pulmonary and cerebral oedema: severe forms of AMS

In less than 2% of travellers AMS occurs in several serious forms at 4,000–5,000m and occasionally lower.

High-altitude pulmonary oedema

This is a condition in which fluid accumulates in the lung causing severe illness (which may come on in minutes). It is characterised by breathlessness and sometimes frothy sputum (phlegm). Early pulmonary oedema should be suspected if a member of a party is unduly short of breath (certainly at rest) or if they have a persistent dry cough or apparent chest infection causing breathlessness. Pulmonary oedema may be preceded by AMS.

Prevention of high-altitude pulmonary oedema

- Ascend slowly, avoiding heavy loads.
- Do not climb with a chest infection, a bad cold or flu-like symptoms.

Treatment of high-altitude pulmonary oedema

Patients with pulmonary oedema are dangerously ill and should be evacuated to a lower altitude as an emergency. Frequently, a descent of only 500m (1,500ft) is sufficient to improve the situation dramatically. Principles of treatment include:

- Sitting the patient upright.
- DESCENT, evacuation, oxygen (treat the problem seriously).

- Nifedipine (Adalat). Take a 10mg tablet under the tongue and then a 20mg slow-release tablet four times daily.
- Hyperbaric chambers (portable pressure bags). These require the patient to lie flat and are difficult to use in this setting.

Cerebral oedema

Cerebral oedema is another severe form of altitude-related illness. It is usually preceded by AMS. It is due to fluid collecting within the brain. Patients become headachy, irrational, drowsy and confused over a period of hours, and their walking becomes unsteady. Double vision may occur. The condition is a serious one and evacuation to lower altitudes is mandatory. Principles of treatment include:

- DESCENT, evacuation, oxygen
- Dexamethasone 8mg by mouth, followed by 4mg every 4 hours for 24 hours
- Hyperbaric chamber (portable pressure bag).

In both pulmonary and cerebral oedema medical advice is desirable, although it may not be available. Those who are suspected of having pulmonary or cerebral oedema should be evacuated to lower altitude promptly. This frequently causes difficulties for the party as a whole. Patients should certainly not go high again until they have been seen by a doctor. Complete recovery is usual in both conditions if patients have been treated early and appropriately.

Treatment of severe altitude sickness, type unknown

- DESCENT, evacuation, oxygen
- Dexamethasone as above
- Nifedipine as above
- Hyperbaric chamber.

Peripheral oedema and retinal haemorrhages

Fluid retention causing swelling of an arm, a leg or the face is sometimes noticed on waking or after a long march. This is peripheral oedema. It usually subsides over several days and does not herald pulmonary or cerebral oedema.

Haemorrhages into the retina (minute blood blisters in the back of the eye) are known to occur quite commonly around 5,000m but rarely cause any problems, being unnoticed by the subject and visible only to a trained observer with specialist equipment (an ophthalmoscope). Very occasionally these tiny haemorrhages interfere with vision (causing a "hole" in the vision); descent is advised and complete recovery is usual.

Other problems

Cold and frostbite and their prevention and treatment are dealt with in Chapter 25.

Prevention of sunburn is essential. Although many proprietary creams and blocks are available, RoC Crème Ecran Total Protection Extreme (SPF 25) and Uvistat are particularly recommended. Simply covering exposed parts with silk or cotton masks is equally effective.

Snowblindness is a severe conjunctivitis (inflammation of the white of the eye) and keratitis (inflammation of the cornea) caused by exposure to UV light reflected off snow. This can happen in a matter of hours. Spare sunglasses should always be carried, and if these are not available a simple mask of cardboard or material with a thin slit to peer through can be used. Snowblindness is recognised by intensely red, painful eyes (see Chapter 25 for details on treatment). Recovery is usual within several days.

Patients who have had treatment for short-sightedness using laser or radial keratotomy should seek specialist ophthalmic advice before climbing to high altitude, as some recent studies have reported a change in refractive power at high altitude that may be visually disabling.

Summary

AMS is a common and minor, although debilitating, problem of high altitude. Rarely it leads to two potentially fatal conditions – pulmonary and cerebral oedema – both of which are medical emergencies.

In giving advice about travel to high altitudes it must be stressed that the simple adage of travelling slowly and descending if you are ill – advice known for generations in all high-altitude countries – cannot be bettered.

SUPPLIES FOR HIGH-ALTITUDE EXPEDITIONS

Medication

1. Acetazolamide (Diamox) 125mg by mouth twice daily for 5 days.
2. Dexamethasone 4mg tablets. Take 8mg at once and 4mg every 4 hours for up to 2 days.
3. Nifedipine (Adalat) 10mg under the tongue at once and 20mg slow-release tablets every 6 hours for 2 days.
4. Oxygen by mask, if available.
5. Portable hyperbaric chamber.

Pressure bags

Portable hyperbaric pressure chambers, which are bags inflated by a foot pump, can be life-saving and can buy time. The patient is placed in a sleeping bag and then in the chamber which is finally zipped up. A simulated descent of 500m or more can be

Figure 26.2 *Testing a portable pressure chamber at high altitude – Sepu Kangri Base Camp, 4,700m, eastern Tibet (C. Bonington, Chris Bonington Picture Library)*

achieved in less than 15 minutes. Any expedition to altitudes of over 5,000m should consider carrying a pressure bag. They weigh less than 10kg.

Pressure bag suppliers

GAMOW Bag
Hyperbaric Technologies Inc.
PO Box 69, Amsterdam
NY 12010, USA
Tel. +1 800 382 2491, fax +1 800 842 1031

CERTEC Bag
CERTEC
Sourcieux-les-Mines
69210 France
Tel. +33 74 70 39 82

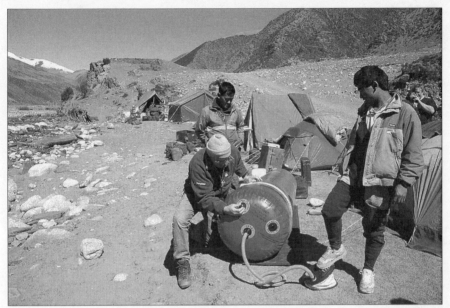

Portable Altitude Chamber
CE Bartlett Pty Ltd
PO Box 49, Wendouree
VIC 3355, Australia
Tel. +61 3 5339 3103, fax +61 3 5338 1241

Each of these systems is reliable. The Portable Altitude Chamber is the cheapest at present. Offers are sometimes made by the manufacturers, and it may be possible to borrow or hire equipment in Kathmandu (try Himalayan Rescue Association, PO Box 4044, Thamel, Kathmandu) and other centres.

UIAA Mountain Medicine Centre via the British Mountaineering Council

The MMC produce eleven useful Information Sheets for climbers and trekkers:

1. Mountain Sickness, Oedemas and Travel to High Altitude
2. Climbing at Extreme Altitudes above 7,000m
3. Diamox, Decadron and Nifedipine at High Altitudes
4. Portable Compression Chamber in Acute Mountain Sickness
5. First Aid Kits
6. Sunscreens and Altitude
7. International Transport of Drugs and Oxygen from Britain
8. Oxygen Systems Available for Use at High Altitudes
9. Causes of Death at Extreme Altitude
10. Frostbite – Practical Suggestions
11. The Oral Contraceptive Pill and High Altitudes

These are available from:
British Mountaineering Council (BMC)
177–179 Burton Road
West Didsbury
Manchester M20 2BB
Tel. +44 161 445 4747, fax +44 161 445 4500
Email: info@thebmc.co.uk

27 UNDERWATER EXPEDITIONS

Andrew Pitkin

The increasing use of diving as a means of exploration in the underwater environment has resulted in a substantial rise in the popularity of underwater expeditions. Many such projects have additional scientific or ecological objectives and may involve large numbers of participants over many months or years. It is therefore unsurprising that most expeditions desire or require medical support.

Diving is an equipment-centred activity and, because of this, diving expeditions usually remain within closer reach of "civilisation" than many others. A notable feature of diving-related expeditions is that the variety of illnesses caused uniquely by hyperbaric exposure requires a recompression chamber for definitive treatment; this is not an item easily carried in a medical kit.

Fitness to dive

Participants in a diving expedition may have diving qualifications from any of a number of training organisations, which have varying requirements for fitness to dive. In the UK the medical examination for commercial divers is much more comprehensive than for sports divers, reflecting the occupational nature of the risk. In recent years the UK's Health and Safety Executive (HSE) has adopted a pragmatic risk assessment approach to diving regulations and fitness to dive; the standards required for a North Sea saturation diver are not necessarily those required of an underwater cameraman filming marine life in a tropical aquarium, although both may be employed as divers. A similar approach should be adopted for expedition divers with the obvious proviso that diving, for any form of reward, brings such diving within the jurisdiction of the HSE or analogous industrial health organisation. Some general standards apply, which may be modified according to the diving activity; these are shown in Table 27.1.

TABLE 27.1 **GENERAL CONTRAINDICATIONS TO DIVING**

Category	*Condition*	*Notes*
Absolute	Epilepsy	
	Cardiac disease	Ischaemic or arrhythmogenic
	Obstructive airway disease	COPD, emphysema, asthma
	Pregnancy	
	Middle-ear disease	
	Insulin-dependent diabetes mellitus	In the context of an expedition
Relative	Obesity	e.g. BMI > 35kg/m^2
	Lack of physical fitness	e.g. $\dot{V}O_{2\,max}$ < 40ml/kg per min or equivalent
	Psychiatric disease	Requiring medication (e.g. antidepressants)
	Previous penetrating chest wound/ lung injury	Unless cleared by a diving physician
Temporary	Acute upper respiratory tract infection	Until resolved
	Tympanic membrane (TM) barotrauma	TM perforation 4 weeks, otherwise 5–10 days

Expert and impartial advice about fitness to dive, whether for recreational, expeditionary, commercial or military diving, can be obtained from the Institute of Naval Medicine, Alverstone, Gosport, Hants PO12 2DL.

Diving activities and techniques

Most expeditionary diving has used conventional sport diving techniques (open-circuit scuba). As sport diving evolves to use more advanced procedures, such as Nitrox, helium-based mixed gas and rebreathers, expedition organisers increasingly seek to apply these techniques (often collectively called "technical diving") for exploration purposes; indeed, many aspects of technical diving were developed by explorers for specific projects. The decompression advantages of Nitrox, the deep diving capabilities of Trimix/Heliox and the logistical benefits of rebreathers mean that expeditions are likely to use one or more of these techniques. Expedition medical officers should be familiar with at least the principles, if not the details, of their use.

Nitrox

Nitrox strictly means any gas mixture containing air and oxygen, but in practice is used for air enriched with oxygen (i.e. > 21% oxygen). The lower partial pressure of nitrogen and higher partial pressure of oxygen reduces decompression requirements compared with air. Alternatively Nitrox can be used with air decompression tables or computers for an additional safety margin. The depth at which a Nitrox mix can be used is limited by the maximum safe partial pressure of oxygen that can be breathed with an acceptably low risk of central nervous system (CNS) oxygen toxicity (see below). For simple diving, mixtures of 25–35% oxygen are usually used, but higher percentages up to 100% oxygen may be used during decompression to speed up elimination of inert gas (nitrogen or helium).

Helium (Trimix and Heliox)

At depths beyond 30 metres, divers may become impaired by nitrogen narcosis. This becomes a substantial problem at depths greater than 50 metres and has led to the use of helium and oxygen mixtures (Heliox) and Trimix (a mixture of helium, nitrogen and oxygen) by sports divers wishing to dive deeper. Prevention of CNS oxygen toxicity means that the gas breathed on the bottom is low in oxygen and therefore is inefficient for decompression purposes; divers therefore typically breathe one or more different mixtures, often Nitrox, for decompression. This necessitates carrying additional cylinders on the dive unless they can be placed at a reliable retrieval point (e.g. a cave entrance). The breathing of a decompression gas at depth can cause acute oxygen toxicity with possibly lethal consequences (such as an underwater convulsion).

Rebreathers

Traditional open-circuit scuba is inefficient, as all the gas breathed is wasted into the water despite having had very little of its oxygen used. The concept of recycling the gases via a reservoir ('counterlung') is as old as diving but until recently such units were available only for use by military divers. Rebreathers employ a canister of soda lime to remove waste carbon dioxide; additional oxygen is added to the breathing loop either at a constant rate (semi-closed circuit) or by a computer-controlled valve only as it is needed to maintain a constant partial pressure of oxygen (closed circuit).

Rebreathers have a number of advantages, the most important of which is their low gas usage; unlike open-circuit scuba this is largely independent of depth. It is quite possible to build a compact closed-circuit rebreather with an underwater duration of 24 hours *at any depth.* This enormous logistical advantage over open-circuit systems, an advantage that increases with greater depths, means rebreather use on advanced diving expeditions will inevitably become more common in the future. Other benefits are that the inhaled gas is already warmed and humidified, minimising respiratory heat loss, and the lack of bubbles – necessary for covert military operations, but also useful for underwater photographers and videographers.

The main disadvantage of rebreathers, apart from their expense, is that dangerous malfunctions can occur without the diver being aware of the problem (e.g. too low or high a partial pressure of oxygen) and which may cause diver loss of consciousness under water; without a full-face mask drowning is likely. Such risks are minimised in

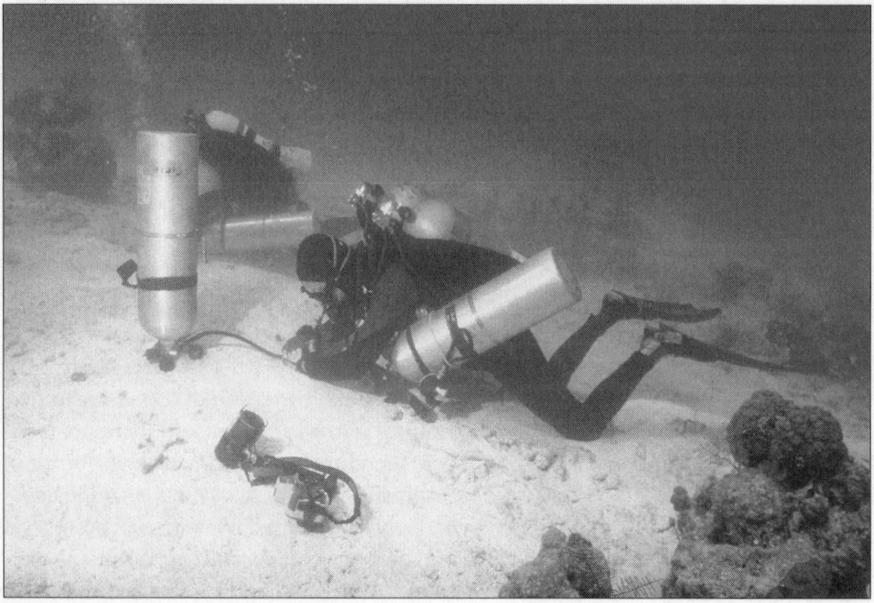

Figure 27.1 *Decompression after a deep mixed-gas dive (A. Pitkin)*

the military setting by rigorous training and very high maintenance standards; most non-military users of rebreathers do not have the same level of training or technical support.

Overhead environments (cave, wreck and ice diving)

Most recreational dive training is based upon the premise that a diver who has a major problem can ascend directly to the surface. Inside a cave or wreck this is clearly impossible and therefore any problem that occurs must be solved under water. This requires training and additional equipment which is based on the principle of redundancy: any vital piece of equipment is backed up by an alternative so that a single failure under water will not pose an immediate threat to the diver's well-being. In cave diving, where caves may be penetrated under water for distances of several miles or more, elaborate and formalised techniques and equipment configurations have been evolved to minimise the chance of a problem becoming fatal. These include the "thirds rule" (using only one third of available gas for cave ingress, leaving a third for exit and a third for emergency use), maintaining a continuous guideline to the surface and having at least two back-up lights. Wreck penetration often uses these procedures but poses somewhat different hazards of entanglement and silting. Ice diving requires similar techniques but poses additional problems from the effects of cold on equipment and humans. Decompression diving tends to be the norm in all types of

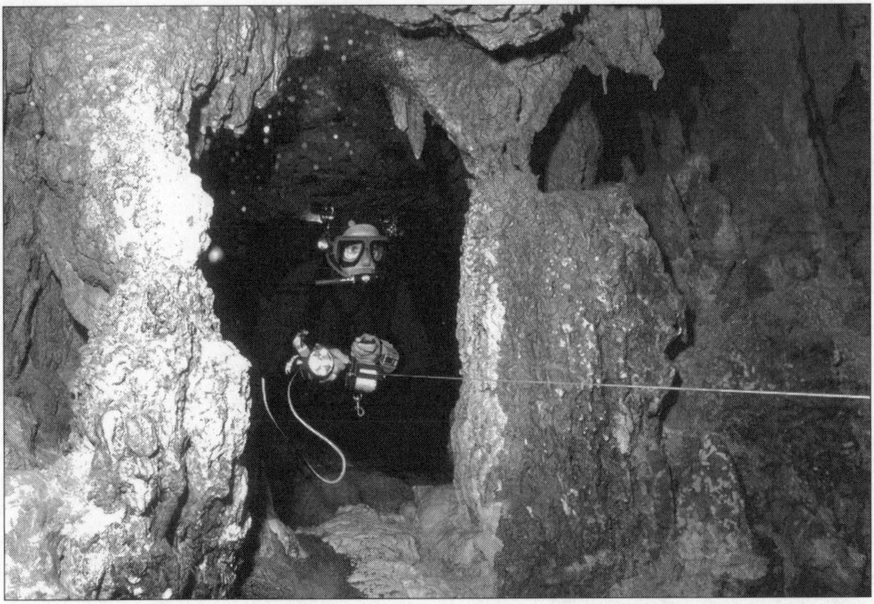

Figure 27.2 *Cenote Carwash, a popular cave diving site in Mexico (A. Pitkin)*

overhead environment diving, and open-water dives with a significant decompression obligation may be regarded as having a "virtual" decompression ceiling, necessitating a similar approach to dive planning and equipment configuration.

MEDICAL PROBLEMS SPECIFIC TO DIVING EXPEDITIONS

Participants in diving expeditions are exposed to general hazards related to being in or near the water (e.g. hypothermia, near-drowning) as well as those related exclusively to diving. These arise either as a result of exposure to increased ambient pressure under water or to the use of one of the many forms of underwater breathing systems available.

General hazards

Hypothermia and near-drowning are dealt with in Chapters 25 and 29 respectively. Divers are vulnerable to trauma, particularly while at the surface and boarding a boat, especially in heavy seas. A small but persistent number of fatalities occur from propeller injuries to divers from surface craft. Hazards posed by dangerous marine life are covered in Chapter 20.

Decompression illness (DCI)

This term covers clinical syndromes caused by intravascular or extravascular gas bubbles generated during ascent from depth. Breathing compressed gas at depth results in nitrogen (or helium) being dissolved in blood and body tissues at a rate determined by partial pressure gradient (i.e. depth), temperature and molecular weight (Graham's law). The time spent at depth obviously directly affects the amount absorbed. In addition delivery of gas to body tissues is affected by perfusion, so that lipid-rich and well-perfused tissues such as brain and spinal cord may have relatively large amounts of inert gas dissolved in them. When the diver ascends the gas in the tissues becomes 'supersaturated' and gaseous bubbles are formed, which may cause clinical effects in a range between none and physiological dysfunction severe enough to result in death, and which is usually referred to as decompression sickness (DCS). Traditionally DCS has been divided into type 1 (mild) and type 2 (severe) forms, a classification still used in the United States but falling into disuse in Europe where a descriptive classification is now favoured (Table 27.2).

TABLE 27.2 DESCRIPTIVE CLASSIFICATION OF DECOMPRESSION ILLNESS

Manifestations	Neurological pain Limb pain Girdle pain Pulmonary Cutaneous Lymphatic Constitutional	*Evolution*	Progressive Relapsing Static Spontaneously improving Resolved
Inert gas load	Depth/time profile Decompression obligation Gas mixture(s) used	*Evidence of barotrauma*	Lung Sinus Ear Dental

A different mechanism of injury is expansion of gas in the diver's lungs during a rapid ascent, which enters the pulmonary veins and is carried through the left side of the heart to the brain causing cerebral arterial gas embolism (AGE). In practice a distinction between this and the effects of dissolved inert gas (DCS) is very difficult and now both entities are commonly encompassed within the term decompression illness. This can be usefully divided into neurological (75%) and

TABLE 27.3 COMMON CLINICAL SYNDROMES SEEN IN DECOMPRESSION ILLNESS

Clinical scenario	*Cause*	*Management*
Rapid ascent to surface • Loss of consciousness or seizure (may be within 10 min of surfacing) • Weakness of half the body (one arm and leg: hemiparesis) • Confusion/cognitive impairment	DCI (cerebral arterial gas embolism)	• Resuscitation: ABC • Give oxygen • Lie flat • Immediate recompression
Rapid ascent to surface • Breathlessness • Chest pain	Pneumothorax	• Give oxygen • Vent chest with intravenous cannula (or chest drain) • See Chapter 14
Rapid ascent/omitted decompression • Back pain • Weakness/numbness of legs • Loss of bladder control	Neurological DCI (spinal cord)	• Give oxygen • Give fluids • Urgent recompression
After any dive • Tingling/numbness of fingers (both sides, often asymmetrical) • Weakness, altered reflexes • Inco-ordination	Neurological DCI	• Give oxygen • Give fluids • Recompression as soon as possible
After any dive • Dull pain in/near the shoulder or elbow, often improved slightly by movement • Weakness/numbness of same arm or hand (easily overlooked)	Limb pain DCI	• Give oxygen • Give fluids • Recompression as soon as possible
Possible difficulty equalising ears • Vertigo, unsteadiness • Severe nausea and vomiting • Nystagmus (jerking movement of eyes)	Inner-ear DCI or barotrauma	• Give oxygen • Give intravenous fluids • Recompression as soon as possible
After multiple or deep/long dives • Extreme fatigue, sleepiness • Malaise, shivers • Nausea, anorexia	Constitutional DCI	• Give oxygen • Give fluids • Consider recompression

non-neurological DCI (25%). The former can cause permanent disability and should be treated aggressively with recompression therapy, even if this is delayed. The latter will resolve eventually without specific treatment although recompression will usually result in more rapid recovery. About a quarter of cases of neurological DCI will be left with a permanent neurological deficit even after treatment.

Symptoms and signs of decompression illness are extremely variable and may be bizarre; unexplained symptoms occurring after diving should be assumed to be due to decompression illness until proven otherwise. Sensory symptoms (tingling, numbness, particularly of the hands) are seen in 60% of cases; motor symptoms (weakness, inco-ordination) are present in 30% of cases and imply more severe disease. There are a number of common patterns of decompression illness which are shown in Table 27.3. *It is important to remember that the* sine qua non *of DCI is that it occurs during or after a decompression* (which may be a previous dive); symptoms appearing during the descent or bottom phases of a dive need an alternative explanation. A relatively common (15%) but easily overlooked feature of DCI is that of disordered thought or personality change, which may result in a diver inappropriately refusing treatment or evacuation.

First aid treatment of decompression illness is simple, but relies on recognising that there is a problem. The diver may be unable to self-diagnose the problem due to cognitive impairment. Concealment and denial are common because of the 'stigma' attached to DCI by many divers.

First aid treatment of DCI

1. Resuscitation: ABC.
2. Administer 100% oxygen. This is most efficiently done with a demand regulator; constant-flow systems rarely deliver close to 100%, even when they incorporate a reservoir bag.
3. Keep the diver lying flat. This is most important for cerebral gas embolism, but is also useful in other forms of DCI.
4. Give fluids, oral if possible, otherwise intravenously. Immersion in water, cold and increased hydrostatic pressure all contribute to dehydration after every dive. Bubbles in the bloodstream cause blood vessels to become 'leaky' allowing further fluid loss from the blood into the tissues. If the diver is alert and able to speak give fluids orally; if there is any doubt about the airway nothing should be given by mouth.
5. Keep the diver comfortably cool, but not to the point of shivering. Most diving casualties have a degree of hypothermia, but in tropical regions conditions on the surface can get extremely hot; the diver should be kept as cool as is practicable.
6. Seek expert advice and consider evacuation to recompression facility.

Further treatment of a casualty with decompression illness depends on the nature of the problem and the logistics of transfer to a recompression chamber. It is essential to consider the possibility of urgent evacuation during the planning phase of a diving expedition, as few are fortunate enough to have a recompression chamber on site. Whether an individual casualty needs urgent recompression treatment can be a difficult decision; expert advice can and should be obtained 24 hours a day from the Royal Navy's Duty Diving Medical Officer at the Institute of Naval Medicine. *Any diver with neurological symptoms should be recompressed to minimise the chance of permanent neurological damage*; this applies even if symptoms have disappeared while breathing 100% oxygen. It is very common for symptoms to reappear hours or even days later and vital time for transport to a chamber may have been lost. The effectiveness of oxygen as a first aid measure does not mean that hyperbaric treatment is not necessary; this phenomenon of the "oxygen ostrich" has been responsible for poor eventual outcome in a number of DCI cases.

Expedition organisers may raise the possibility of using a portable monoplace chamber (such as the Hyperlite) for treatment of DCI in the field. The main problem with these is that they do not allow access to the patient during treatment and this will be of greatest concern inpatients with severe DCI who should be treated as quickly as possible. This is the "portable paradox": cases that most need to be treated immediately are least suitable for treatment in monoplace chambers that can be used on site. Most experienced diving physicians would therefore advise continuing resuscitation with oxygen and fluids while awaiting evacuation to a multiplace chamber.

Similar considerations apply to in-water recompression. There may be situations where the potential benefit outweighs the risks but the hazards are not trivial and should be considered very carefully. The casualty is exposed to hypothermia, further dehydration and oxygen toxicity; additional symptoms can evolve which may not be noticed under water or which may be life threatening (e.g. loss of consciousness). In-water recompression has on occasion been used successfully in remote locations for divers with stable DCI, but the technique remains controversial.

Other treatments that may be of use in decompression illness include non-steroidal anti-inflammatory drugs (NSAIDs) such as ibuprofen or diclofenac. These can be very useful as an adjunctive treatment for limb pain DCI but, like aspirin, they should be avoided in neurological DCI where the antiplatelet effects could promote secondary haemorrhage in the spinal cord. Another drug that appears to have been useful in occasional cases of neurological DCI is lignocaine (lidocaine), given intravenously in the same doses used for ventricular arrhythmias. None of these experimental treatments should interfere with the proven ones, which are oxygen and fluids.

Nitrogen narcosis

At high partial pressures under water nitrogen has effects similar to anaesthetic

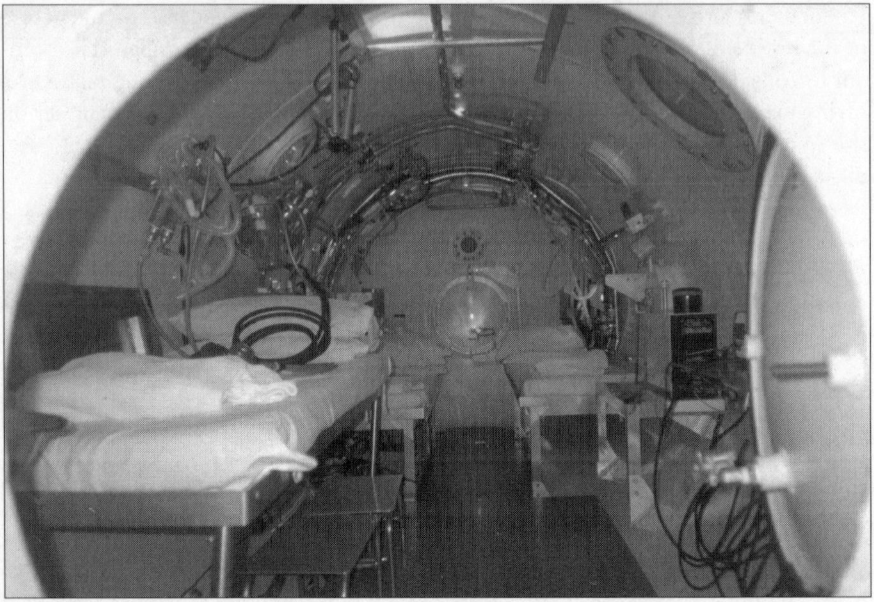

Figure 27.3 *A modern multiplace hyperbaric chamber (A. Pitkin)*

agents, causing a variety of symptoms including tunnel vision, euphoria, apprehension, tinnitus, inability to carry out complex tasks, loss of co-ordination, drowsiness and eventually loss of consciousness. Hypercapnia (excessive CO_2) and exertion increase the effects, which can vary considerably between divers and dive sites (worse in cold, dark, poor-visibility conditions). As the symptoms invariably resolve rapidly on ascent the main problem is the impairment of the diver's performance, which may lead to other problems such as DCI or near-drowning.

Hypercapnia (carbon dioxide poisoning)

Carbon dioxide (CO_2) is the main waste product of the body's use of oxygen, and is removed by breathing out of the lungs. A sensitive control mechanism exists to regulate breathing directly from the partial pressure of CO_2 in the blood, which is thus kept remarkably constant, even during extreme exertion. The diver can also learn to override the 'urge to breathe' (as in free diving). A diver who is exerting hard and trying to eke out a limited supply of air through poor-quality breathing apparatus is at risk of hypercapnia. Rebreather divers whose absorbent is exhausted (more quickly in cold conditions) and cave divers breathing from exhausted air spaces in flooded caves can be exposed directly to high levels of carbon dioxide. The symptoms include headache, flushing, palpitations, drowsiness, and potentiation of both oxygen toxicity and nitrogen narcosis. It is often said that hypercapnia causes breathlessness: this is *rare* in the diving scenario where the sensation of breathlessness appears to be inhibited by high partial pressures of oxygen. Under water the diver should stop exerting and abort the dive if symptoms do not resolve rapidly. At the surface symptoms will quickly disappear once the diver is breathing fresh air or oxygen.

Oxygen toxicity

Oxygen can have toxic effects at the partial pressures encountered in diving, but oxygen toxicity rarely occurs using air. This is because the threshold for acute oxygen toxicity (about 1.6 atmospheres absolute, ATA) occurs at 66 metres, where nitrogen narcosis is likely to be a much more serious problem. Use of Nitrox mixtures means that this partial pressure may be reached at much shallower depths. The risk is increased by time of exposure, immersion in water, exertion and extremes of temperature. It is decreased by air breaks and avoidance of hypercapnia and heavy exertion. Acute oxygen toxicity mainly affects the central nervous system, causing visual disturbances, hearing disturbances, muscle twitching (especially in the face and diaphragm), nausea and convulsions; these may occur without any prior warning and have often been fatal when they have occurred under water. Rebreather divers may be at risk from malfunctions, inappropriate choice of gas mixture (semi-closed circuit) or rapid descents (closed circuit).

If a diver has any symptoms that suggest oxygen toxicity, he or she should stop any exertion and either ascend or change to a gas mixture with a lower oxygen content. For closed-circuit rebreathers this may entail flushing the loop with diluent. Rescue of a diver suffering a convulsion under water is rarely ultimately successful unless the diver is using a full-face mask. The initial 30 seconds of a convulsion typically comprises a tonic phase where the diver is rigid and has a closed glottis; decompression to the surface during this phase should be avoided as it is likely to cause arterial gas embolism. During the clonic phase (rhythmic jerking movements) the diver can be surfaced and resuscitated. It should then be assumed that the diver has suffered arterial gas embolism and should be recompressed as a matter of urgency; in the meantime oxygen administered at the surface is unlikely to cause further problems.

Pulmonary oxygen toxicity, whilst occasionally seen during hyperbaric oxygen treatment of a diving casualty, is not a problem in self-contained diving.

Hypoxia

There are few situations where a diver is exposed to hypoxia, but like oxygen toxicity it can cause sudden loss of consciousness under water without warning. Deep divers use mixtures with oxygen fractions of less than 12% at great depths which if breathed at the surface could cause hypoxia. Almost any mixture used in self-contained diving will be safe to breathe at depths of 10 metres or more. Of more concern are rebreather divers whose variable oxygen consumption (by exertion) must be matched by oxygen added to the loop at a steady flow rate in semi-closed systems and according to directly measured loop partial pressure in closed-circuit systems. Hypoxia is notorious for its insidious effects on mental function; lack of insight is characteristic. Other features are euphoria, loss of fine motor control and unconsciousness. These are likely to occur when the inspired partial pressure of oxygen is less than 0.1ATA. Like oxygen toxicity loss of consciousness under water due to hypoxia may easily be fatal. Treatment once on the surface is with oxygen, or air if oxygen is unavailable.

Barotrauma

The volume of an enclosed gas-filled space varies inversely with pressure (Boyle's law). If air-containing spaces within the body are not equalised with the pressurised breathing gas on descent they will be compressed ('squeezed'). In practice this causes problems only with normally rigid cavities such as the middle ear and facial sinuses, although abnormal air spaces such as under dental fillings can also be very painful.

Middle-ear barotrauma affects the tympanic membrane and is extremely common. Even mild eustachian tube dysfunction may lead to painful stretching of the tympanic membrane and if the diver continues to descend it will perforate. Characteristically this results in a sudden disappearance in the pain and sometimes a salty taste in the throat (blood or salt water). Cold water entering the middle ear may cause temporary vertigo. On examination the tympanic membrane will appear reddened and usually the perforation can be seen. A fluid level, sometimes haemorrhagic, is often present behind the tympanic membrane. Simple non-perforating barotrauma heals within a few days, but a diver with a perforation should not dive again for at least 4 weeks.

Inner-ear barotrauma causes similar but more severe symptoms. High pressures in the skull from overenthusiastic Valsalva manouevres can rupture the round window of the cochlea (the organ of hearing), resulting in leakage of perilymph and damage to the cochlea and vestibular apparatus (organ of balance). Vertigo is severe and usually associated with a hearing loss; these symptoms continuing after a dive are a sinister sign and expert advice should be sought. Occasionally the inner ear is directly affected by decompression illness and distinguishing this from inner-ear barotrauma can be impossible. One other cause of transient vertigo that can occur during ascent is due to the eustachian tubes venting air at different rates (alternobaric vertigo). It always disappears within minutes.

Pulmonary barotrauma (affecting the lungs) is the most serious form and can be fatal. If gas in the lungs is not able to vent freely during ascent it can escape through the delicate lung tissue: into the pleural cavity, causing a pneumothorax (chest pain, breathlessness); into the mediastinum, causing pneumomediastinum (central chest pain, voice change, neck swelling); and, most seriously, into the bloodstream, causing gas embolism to the brain and sometimes the coronary arteries that supply the heart with blood. Typically the diver has made a rapid ascent and is unconscious on surfacing or loses consciousness shortly thereafter. Convulsions are common. Less severe embolism causes stroke-like symptoms with one-sided weakness (hemiparesis) and speech/language difficulties. Treatment is discussed above along with other forms of decompression illness.

Carbon monoxide poisoning

Carbon monoxide poisoning is now rare since most divers are aware of the problem of compressor air intakes being close to or downwind of an exhaust. The symptoms appear at depth and can be bizarre. Jacques Cousteau's account of his near-fatal dive in the Fontaine de Vaucluse in *The Silent World* is characteristic of the disorientation, loss of sense of time, inco-ordination, headache and vomiting that carbon monoxide poisoning causes. The 'cherry-red' coloration described by some authors is almost never seen. Treatment is with 100% oxygen and persisting symptoms are an indication for hyperbaric oxygen treatment.

Expert advice

Diving diseases are complex and can be difficult to manage even by experts with long experience in the field. Expedition medical officers are urged to make use of the excellent service provided by Royal Navy diving physicians at the Institute of Naval Medicine in Alverstoke, Hampshire. At least one Royal Navy diving physician is available 24 hours a day, 365 days a year, for advice on management of a diving accident anywhere in the world. Contact them on:

+44 7831 151 523

Less urgent enquiries (for example on fitness to dive) can also be made through the above number or by letter to:

Senior Medical Officer (Diving Medicine)
Institute of Naval Medicine
Alverstoke
Gosport
Hants PO12 2DL

ADDITIONAL MEDICAL SUPPLIES FOR DIVING EXPEDITIONS

Base camp medical kit

Additional items to those listed in Chapter 3:

Oxygen with mask and tubing
0.9% saline 500ml × 4

Intravenous fluid infusion sets
Intravenous cannulae 18g × 4 (e.g. Venflon)
Inflatable splints
Plaster of Paris bandage
Velband
Chest drains, tubing and Heimlich valves
Urinary catheter and drainage bag
Laryngoscope and batteries
Endotracheal tubes
Airways
Artery forceps
Suction catheter and apparatus
Syringes 10ml, 20ml and 50ml
Nasogastric tube
Aneroid sphygmomanometer and BP cuff
50% dextrose injection
Ventolin inhaler and spacer device
Diazepam injection
Ketamine injection

Dive site/mobile camp medical kit

Additional items to those listed in Chapter 3, Table 3.3:

Auroscope
Stethoscope
Sleek adhesive tape (two rolls)
Sutures:
  0/0 black silk on hand needle
  3/0 Dexon
  5/0 nylon
Syringes 2ml and 5ml
Injection needles and cannulac (assorted)
Sofratulle – dressing for a wide range of infected lesions
Fusidic acid cream 30g – topical antibacterial cream for skin infections
Miconazole cream 30g – topical antifungal cream for feet infections
Betnovate cream 30g
Neutrogena hand cream
Antacid tablets
Cinnarizine tablets 15mg – anti-sea sickness medication
Buccastem 3mg – anti-sea sickness medication
Glyceryl trinitrate spray

Lip salve
Calamine cream
Space blanket

Emergency injections box
Adrenaline (epinephrine) 1 in 1,000 solution
Atropine 600mcg/ml
Dexamethasone 4mg/ml, 20mg/ml
Benzylpenicillin 600mg vial
Hydrocortisone 100mg/2ml vial
Metoclopramide 5mg/ml
Chlorpheniramine 10mg/ml

28 CAVING EXPEDITIONS

Andrew Pitkin

Caving activities share some medical hazards with other activities (climbing and diving in particular), but in addition a few are unique to the subterranean environment. Caves are restricted spaces formed by flowing water which present dangers from flooding, restricted air exchange, and unusual flora and fauna. Sections of the deepest caves may be among the most remote places on earth. Intercurrent illness therefore can be, and has been, fatal among cave explorers. Most medical problems are predictable; as data collected by the British Cave Rescue Council (Table 28.1) show, hypothermia and injuries from falls represent the majority of emergencies requiring evacuation from caves in the UK.

TABLE 28.1 EMERGENCIES REQUIRING CAVE RESCUE IN THE UNITED KINGDOM 1989–98

Emergency	*Number*	*(%)*
Upper limb injuries	22	(12)
Pelvis and lower limb injuries	38	(21)
Head injuries	13	(7)
Chest injuries	7	(4)
Spinal injuries	19	(11)
Multiple major trauma	9	(5)
Exhaustion and hypothermia	45	(25)
Medical conditions	13	(7)
Drowning	11	(6)

Supplied by the British Cave Rescue Council.

MEDICAL PROBLEMS NOT SPECIFIC TO CAVING EXPEDITIONS

Near-drowning

Cave systems are formed by flowing water and sudden ("flash") flooding is a major hazard to cavers. The medical officer (MO) may have to deal with cases of near-drowning while being trapped in part of the cave system waiting for the water levels to recede. Cave diving is used increasingly to pass sumps (passages completely filled with water) into more distant passages; equipment failure during a cave dive may also require the MO to deal with near-drowning.

The exact sequence of events that occurs in drowning in humans has not been fully worked out. Breath holding occurs on initial submersion. Its duration will vary according to the victim's age, physical condition, exertion, water temperature, etc. Submersion in very cold water can cause a reflex involuntary gasp with immediate water inhalation. If this does not happen, the rising carbon dioxide in the blood will at some point force the victim to breathe in; water in the larynx may cause laryngospasm (reflex closure of the vocal cords) and prevent water entering the lungs. Water in the mouth and pharynx is often swallowed and subsequently inhaled along with stomach contents. Eventually the falling level of oxygen in the blood overrides the "protective" laryngospasm and water enters the lungs. In about 10% of cases laryngospasm persists until respiratory arrest occurs and no water enters the lungs ("dry drowning").

Symptoms and signs of near-drowning

- Difficulty breathing
- Retrosternal chest pain
- Cyanosis
- Coughing frothy bloodstained sputum
- Cardiorespiratory arrest in severe cases
- Convulsions and impaired conscious level maybe to the point of coma.

Hypothermia may complicate matters, but has been associated with survival following prolonged immersion (rarely up to 60 minutes).

In the cave environment the ability to care for a survivor of near-drowning is extremely limited. Follow the guidelines in Chapter 29, page 328. In addition provide resuscitation with basic life support as needed, paying particular attention to the airway, and arrange immediate evacuation to the surface.

Hypothermia

Hypothermia is the commonest single problem requiring rescue from caves in the UK, accounting for a quarter of the callouts for cave rescue organisations (see Table

28.1). Cavers are not exposed to high winds like climbers, but may be unable to avoid immersion in cold water during a caving trip. Conductive heat loss from bare skin immersed in water is approximately 25 times that in air and most textiles lose almost all their thermal insulting properties when wet. Even wetsuits permit considerable evaporative heat loss when removed from water. Heat production must balance heat loss to prevent hypothermia; heat production can be increased by shivering or purposeful activity (ideally to get to a warmer environment), such as climbing a pitch or lifting equipment. Forced inactivity such as waiting to ascend a pitch leaves the wet caver vulnerable to hypothermia. There is marked individual variation in susceptibility to hypothermia and some evidence that resistance to cold can be increased by repeated exposure.

TABLE 28.2 **FEATURES OF HYPOTHERMIA**

Core temperature (°C)	*Manifestation*
37–35 "Mild"	Feeling cold, pale skin, shivering, "goose bumps", disinterest in group activities, impairment of precise hand movements
35–32 "Moderate"	Uncontrollable shivering, generalised inco-ordination, mental slowing, lack of co-operation, memory impairment
< 32 "Severe"	Cessation of shivering, confusion, strong desire to sleep, incoherent speech, visual disturbances, urinary incontinence, coma. Slow, possibly irregular pulse, low blood pressure, slow shallow breathing, "fruity" odour of acetone on breath

Management of the hypothermic casualty depends entirely on the expedition scenario and the severity of the hypothermia, as well as many other problems (such as injuries resulting in immobility and/or shock)(see Chapter 25). No single symptom or sign is diagnostic of hypothermia other than an accurate measurement of core temperature. For symptoms of hypothermia see Table 25.2, page 286. In practice, mild/moderate and severe hypothermia are different problems, the latter being a medical emergency requiring intensive care, mainly because of the ease with which life-threatening cardiac rhythm abnormalities can be provoked. See Chapter 25 for full details.

TABLE 28.3 MANAGEMENT OF COMMON CAVING INJURIES (SEE ALSO CHAPTERS 13 AND 14)

Fracture	*Symptoms/signs*	*Treatment*
Feet/toes	Pain in foot (may follow "insignificant" impact). Pain from heel (calcaneus) fractures may prevent weight bearing	Usually splinted by well-fitting shoe or boot. Give painkillers
Ankle/lower leg	Deformity, crepitus (grating of bone ends), pain, swelling (latter may be greater with sprains). Minor fractures (e.g. lateral malleolus) may allow limited weight bearing	Immobilise with a splint. Straightening may be necessary first. Treat sprains as fractures until excluded by X-rays. Give painkillers
Thigh	Pain, deformity, haemorrhage (into fracture), painful muscle spasms	Immobilisation and traction (which controls haemorrhage and spasms) ideally with dedicated traction splint (e.g. Thomas splint). Avoid non-traction splints. Give painkillers
Hip	Pain, deformity (shortening and rotation of leg and foot to the outside) if displaced	Splint by binding to the other leg. Do not allow to walk. Give painkillers
Pelvis	Pain (especially with front-to-back or side-to-side pressure), major blood loss, damage to bladder (no or bloodstained urine) or other pelvic organs	No splinting required (pelvic muscles hold fragments together). Treat for major haemorrhage. Evacuate supine on stretcher; do not allow to sit or stand. Give antibiotics (if available)
Spine	Pain, tenderness along spine. Pain, tingling, weakness, numbness, loss of bladder control suggests nerve injury	If unconscious, assume cervical (neck) spine injury. For all cases, immobilise using rigid board or similar (e.g. ladder, rigid stretcher). Move casualty only by "log-rolling", keeping all sections of spine aligned. Consider waiting for specialist help and equipment
Chest (ribs)	Pain aggravated by breathing or movement. Breathlessness if pneumothorax (air leak in chest), haemothorax (blood in chest) or "flail chest" (section of ribs moving in the "wrong" direction with breathing). Extreme breathlessness and low blood pressure (tension pneumothorax). Open "sucking" chest wounds	Oxygen, antibiotics (if available). In extremis drain air from tension pneumothorax (both sides if unsure) – insert a large-bore cannula through the second intercostal space in the mid-clavicular line. Immobilise a flail segment with padding and adhesive tape (lie patient on flail segment in emergency). Seal "sucking" wounds immediately (e.g. with a square of polythene secured with tape)
Head	Unconsciousness, bleeding from ears and/or nose; 15% have broken neck. Lesser injuries cause drowsiness, confusion	Evacuate as emergency. If rescue of unconscious casualty is impossible, consider waiting a few hours in case consciousness returns. Maintain airway (recovery position). Search for other injuries; assume broken neck until proven otherwise in hospital

Trauma

Most fatal caving accidents result from falls causing multiple major injuries. Lesser injuries also occur and are not unique to caving. The lower limb and pelvis are most commonly affected, with upper limb, spinal and head trauma accounting for most of the remainder.

Figure 28.1 *Moulin Rouge Passage, Mulu, Sarawak (A. Eavis/RGS)*

SPECIFIC MEDICAL PROBLEMS OF CAVING

Histoplasmosis

Histoplasma capsulatum is a spore-forming fungus that is found in caves containing dry, dusty, bat or bird guano. Cavers may breathe in the airborne spores, resulting in a range of clinical manifestations depending on the individual's previous health and the quantity of spores inhaled. The disease is called histoplasmosis, but other names include cave fever and Darling's disease. It was identified in 1983 as a specific cave-related health hazard after a number of visitors to Church Cave in Wee Jasper, Australia and scientific investigators contracted the disease.

Several clinical varieties of this rare disease exist; members of caving parties are most likely to suffer from acute (epidemic) pulmonary histoplasmosis. After a latent period of 12–21 days, symptoms of tiredness, fever, dry cough and chest pain develop. Pain that migrates from joint to joint often occurs; occasionally a rash (erythema nodosum or erythema multiforme) appears. Chest X-rays show hilar lymphadenopathy and diffuse

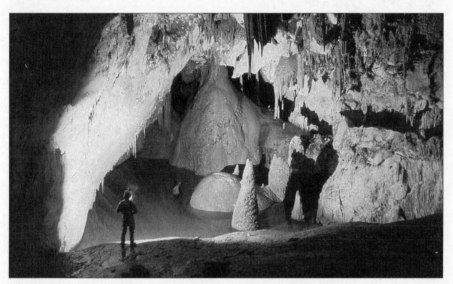

patchy consolidation. Skin tests may be negative; a rising antibody titre in an individual with a history of exposure is the best confirmation of the diagnosis. In most cases no specific therapy is required, but if symptoms are prolonged or lung function is significantly affected treatment with intravenous amphotericin B may be needed.

Leptospirosis (Weil's disease)

Leptospira interrogans causes a variety of disease states from a subclinical infection to jaundice and liver failure in the severe form known as Weil's disease. Rats and other rodents are the major reservoir of infection and excrete the organism continuously in urine. The organism can enter through skin abrasions or the mucous membranes of the eyes, nose and mouth, and infection can also occur through swallowing infected water. Cavers are obviously at risk from prolonged immersion in stream water and the abrasive nature of the cave environment. Cave divers are particularly at risk.

Leptospirosis is a rare disease, symptoms typically appearing 1–2 weeks after exposure. Most cases consist of non-specific fever with muscle pains (especially calf and lower back muscles) and nausea. In a few the disease progresses with abdominal pain, rashes, vomiting and conjunctivitis (septicaemic phase). Headache is usually intense and occasionally the patient becomes delirious. Jaundice indicates severe infection, and renal failure should be suspected. A tendency to bleed (e.g. nose bleeds) is also a sinister sign. The third (immune) phase occurs a week later and includes meningitis, nervous system problems and visual disturbances. Treatment is with appropriate antibiotics; benzylpenicillin (1.2g 6 hourly), doxycycline (200mg daily) and erythromycin (500mg 6 hourly) have all been used successfully. Maintenance of fluid and electrolyte balance is important, particularly when the patient is febrile. Most recover; kidney function may need to be supported temporarily (hence hospitalisation is mandatory). Prevention is best achieved by protective clothing; doxycycline 200mg weekly has also been used. Vaccination is impracticable for humans as numerous serotypes (strains) of the organism exist; however, this may be useful if repeated exposure to a known serotype is necessary.

Harness hang syndrome

Also known as compression–avascularisation–reperfusion (CARP) syndrome, this problem may be easily misdiagnosed as hypothermia or exhaustion while on rope. It occurs when a caver hangs immobile in a harness that occludes the blood supply to and from the legs. Tests using a variety of harnesses and body positions have shown that hypotension occurs in minutes and that reperfusion injury to the lower limb may result in the caver being unable to ascend further. The affected caver must be rescued from the rope; subsequent treatment is supportive.

Altered atmosphere ("bad air")

Sections of cave close to the surface tend to be well ventilated; deeper caves and sections sealed by water may not be sufficiently ventilated to prevent an alteration in atmospheric contents. "Air bells" in or between sumps are very often affected. The two components of most importance are oxygen and carbon dioxide.

Oxygen is essential for life and is produced by photosynthesising plants exposed to sunlight; no oxygen production therefore occurs in caves. Oxygen is used by the metabolic processes of the body and by combustion (e.g. carbide lamps). Exertion increases the body's use of oxygen. Features of hypoxia (lack of oxygen) *at normal atmospheric pressure* do not usually occur until the atmospheric concentration falls to below 12%. Symptoms of acute hypoxia include breathlessness, weakness, lack of coordination, euphoria and apathy, with the victim typically being unable to recognise his or her impairment. Unconsciousness may occur suddenly with no warning whatsoever. The traditional method used by cavers to detect "bad air" is the naked flame test, which is useful to prevent hypoxia as it has been shown that matches and butane lighters will not stay lit at oxygen concentrations below 14%.

The naked flame test does not reliably indicate high levels of carbon dioxide. This gas is produced by combustion, metabolism and also by the cave itself as water containing carbonic acid evaporates releasing carbon dioxide into the cave atmosphere. Being about 1½ times heavier than air it tends to sink into shafts and other low areas of the cave; particular caution should be observed by the first caver down a new pitch. The carbon dioxide concentration in normal air is 0.03% and levels of up to 0.5% are harmless. At carbon dioxide levels above 1% symptoms appear, which consist of headache, breathlessness (worse if there is associated hypoxia), sweating, vasodilatation, fatigue and, at sustained levels of more than 6%, unconsciousness. Provided there is no shortage of oxygen, carbon dioxide levels of up to 15–20% can be survived for periods of several hours.

Treatment for exposure to such an atmosphere consists of removal to a normal atmosphere. The principal danger is the likelihood of sustaining an injury (e.g. a fall) while incapacitated by an altered atmosphere.

Caving beyond sumps

Cave divers should be aware that any injury or equipment malfunction that prevents them from returning through a sump is extremely hazardous and potentially fatal. A very high degree of caution should therefore be used when caving beyond a sump that requires a significant dive. There are no hard-and-fast rules about rescues from beyond sumps; these depend on the limit of what may be achieved with any degree of safety. It is now generally agreed that it is better to try to assist injured cavers (with analgesia, splints and so on) to dive through the sump themselves than to try to stretcher them through with attached breathing apparatus, although the latter approach may be necessary with severely injured casualties. Any risk of loss of consciousness necessitates a full-face mask and such casualties should be taken under water only if there is no alternative.

29 CANOE, KAYAK AND RAFT EXPEDITIONS

Andy Watt

Water journeys can be expeditions, run by individuals, usually with some experience, who plan and carry out their own trip, or they can be commercial trips, where private companies take clients down white-water rivers (see page 338). Expeditions can be grouped into the following types.

Flat water

These expeditions are undertaken for pleasure or scientific purposes, on slow-flowing

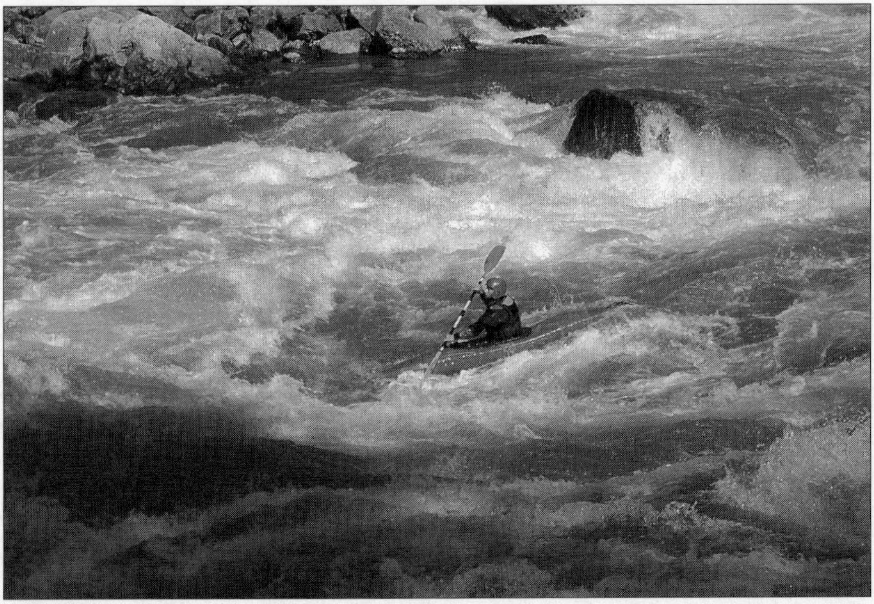

Figure 29.1 *Kayaker tackling white water (A. Watt)*

rivers or lakes, in any craft. The terrain they pass through, including jungle or arid areas (see Chapters 23 and 24), is often as important as the water they travel on.

River

These expeditions are undertaken by white-water kayakers to whom the terrain is often less important than the rapids they seek. With the growth in popularity of destinations like Nepal and Chile, increasing numbers of paddlers with little expedition or medical experience are travelling to remote, often mountainous, areas. The rivers are bigger, significantly faster and more powerful, they show marked seasonal variation and there is less information available on them compared with rivers at home.

Sea canoeing

Sea paddlers are often experienced in multi-day trips and in eliciting tidal and local weather information.

PREPARATION

As you will be paddling on long, multi-day trips, which are more physically and mentally demanding than day trips at home, you should be fit. Cardiovascular fitness – running and swimming – is better than weight training, but time in a boat (especially distance paddling) is best. Ensure that you practise your Eskimo roll in agitated water. In addition it is important that all expedition members should review resuscitation procedures and management of a near-drowned casualty.

Medical kit

Space is limited, especially in a kayak, so a lot of thought has to go into selecting items for your medical kit (see Chapter 3). A smaller spare medical kit should always be carried in another boat.

MEDICAL PROBLEMS SPECIFIC TO WATER-BASED EXPEDITIONS

Water quality

Iodine (see Chapter 11) is the preferred option for sterilising water among experienced paddlers, with each carrying their own personal supply. Rafts may have space for filters or extra fuel to boil water. The water in lakes or rivers in developing countries should always be considered unclean, but the concentration of bugs is usually low enough for your stomach acid to deal with small volumes of water (for example, from splashes). In countries with seasonal monsoons the rivers are most dirty immediately after the rains start, when the land gets "flushed".

TABLE 29.1 ESSENTIAL MEDICAL ITEMS FOR WATER-BASED EXPEDITIONS
Plastic dropper bottle for iodine solution (1 per paddler)
1 large bandage (+ cut to size required)
Paracetamol
Strong painkillers
Ziplock plastic bags and waterproof container/dry bags
Antibiotic drops for ears, cotton wool + Vaseline
Hand cream, lip salve
Calamine lotion for sunburn
Sea-sickness tablets (e.g. cinnarizine 15mg)
Tape, e.g. Elastoplast; better still duct tape
Antibiotics

Dehydration

Paradoxically, despite being surrounded by water, dehydration can be a problem, especially for raft groups in hot countries or sea kayakers in semi-tropical areas, who may not realise that water intake in the sun should be about 3–4 litres a day. The early signs of dehydration are vague symptoms such as headache, light-headedness, lethargy and just feeling unwell. These are difficult to recognise unless you are on the lookout for them.

Diarrhoea

If a paddler gets diarrhoea the group should tighten up its hygiene practices. Treatment for simple diarrhoea for the first few days is fluid replacement, not medicines. If the diarrhoea is accompanied by abdominal pain, blood or fever, or persists for more than 2–3 days, antibiotics, such as ciprofloxacin, may be considered (see Chapter 18). Paddlers with simple diarrhoea on harder rivers may consider antibiotics before 2–3 days have passed.

Accidents and bouyancy aids

The commonest threat to trips is accidents caused by foolishness or lack of foresight (campfire burns, twisted ankles due to inadequate footwear and so on) rather than natural incidents. The most important item of equipment on the water is a lifejacket/buoyancy aid, even for flat-water sections, where raft passengers especially can become careless. If for any reason you end up in the water, your chances of near-drowning are much higher if you aren't wearing a lifejacket/buoyancy aid.

Near-drowning

This term is more accurate than drowned (someone who is dead). Near-drowning ranges from a bad swim with a gasping but conscious victim to prolonged immersion with loss of consciousness. These stages can be with water inhalation or without (dry drowning, caused by the larynx or voice box closing in spasm and preventing both air and water getting to the lungs).

If the patient has suffered prolonged immersion, for example at sea, they should be lifted out horizontally (to stop the blood pressure dropping severely), and gently if they are hypothermic. (Rough handling can induce fatal rhythms in a hypothermic heart.)

Head injuries may be a cause of unconsciousness and are often accompanied by neck injuries. Removal of helmets should be done by two people, with one responsible for holding the head stable. If a neck injury is suspected, remember that establishing the airway means lifting the chin, not bending the neck. Clearly, if you are on your own on a slippery bank such advice is hard to follow. If there is only a low suspicion of neck injury, then absent breathing demands more urgent attention. The lungs cannot be emptied of water; besides, manoeuvres to do this precipitate vomiting.

TABLE 29.2 MANAGEMENT OF A "NEAR-DROWNED" BREATHING CASUALTY

- Place in the recovery position (note – likely to vomit)
- Keep warm, move as little as possible
- Start regular observations – respiratory + pulse rate, temperature, urine output (see Chapter 12)
- If water is dirty give antibiotics – amoxycillin or erythromycin, and metronidazole

Severe respiratory illness ("secondary drowning") is heralded by breathlessness and the patient looks very unwell. It occurs 12–24 hours after a near-drowning and is more likely if the near-drowning was severe, for example with unconsciousness, or if "crackles" can be heard when you put your ear to the patient's chest. These patients should be evacuated to a facility that has oxygen and artificial ventilation (usually only available in cities). In the wilderness, there is no difference in the management of near-drowning in salt or fresh water.

Hypothermia

Significant hypothermia can occur in water temperatures below 20°C, which covers most of the waters visited by expeditions. Water can be a big drain on the body's resources because it removes heat 25 times faster than the air trapped by our clothes. Hypothermia can be a hidden danger. Experienced paddlers will notice the subtle early signs of hypothermia in group members, especially those who have been rolling a lot or have had a swim. These include shivering, mild confusion and muscle incoordination.

Signs and symptoms of hypothermia

- Feeling cold
- Shivering – this can stop as temperature falls below 33°C
- Muscles are stiff, weak and less responsive – can lead to capsizes, failure to roll, inability to climb on to the bank
- Mental disorientation, inappropriate behaviour and slurred speech. Accidents then become inevitable
- Armpit feels "marble cold".

The group should stop and get the person warmed up. If it is the end of the day and you are close to your destination, with no ideal campsite, the temptation is to press on. But remember that the hypothermic person (and probably others in the group) will be markedly less competent at paddling.

Management of hypothermia

- Get the patient into dry clothes (sea kayaks especially should have these accessible) and put on a hat.
- Place the patient in a sleeping bag (alone).
- Insulate the patient from ground.
- Rewarm the patient.
- Give small, frequent amounts of warm fluids.
- Make the patient rest for a day after recovery.

Remember that the skin warms up before the inner (core) temperature, so early on the person feels inappropriately better. Allow plenty of time for rewarming. Seriously hypothermic patients should be handled carefully, as fatal heart rhythms can be precipitated. Unfortunately, in remote areas, not much more can be done to rewarm them beyond the measures outlined above.

Note: putting an extra person in the sleeping bag may not be as beneficial as was previously thought.

Resuscitation of a near-drowned paddler

The management of an unconscious, non-breathing casualty, pulled out of the water, is:

- **A** Airway
- **B** Breathing, start expired air resuscitation (EAR) if breathing is absent
- **C** Circulation – start external cardiac compression (ECC) if carotid pulse is absent.

If there is no immediate recovery, and hypothermia is not an issue, then there is a limited period within which recovery is possible. This period is affected by factors such as the efficiency of your resuscitation (one reason to practise before you go) and how long the heart has stopped. Even very efficient cardiopulmonary resuscitation (CPR) in optimum conditions can only keep a brain going for approximately 2 hours. If there has been no sign of life (pulse or breathing) after this period in a non-hypothermic casualty who has drowned without other medical conditions, then you may have done all that is possible for the casualty. If you are within 2 hours of a hospital, you may think of evacuation, but remember that your CPR will be much less efficient, if not impossible.

Whether successful or not, resuscitation can be followed by further problems – attention has to turn to management of a tired, cold, shocked group and the prevention of further accidents.

Hypothermia and immersion

If the victim is in very cold water, severe hypothermia can modify the advice about drowning. Hypothermia occurs after at least half an hour of immersion in very cold water.

Severe hypothermia can mimic death in that the body is cold, stiff, with white/blue skin, dilated pupils and barely detectable breathing or pulses, so your examination should be very thorough (for example, you should feel for a carotid pulse for 1 minute). If there is a chance that the victim is still alive, you should start EAR and rewarming (but not ECC – see below). If there is no recovery, the advice is that you cannot pronounce the patient dead (i.e. there is no pulse or breathing) until they have been rewarmed; theoretically, this means to 36°C, which may take 6 hours or more. In other words, they are not dead until they are warm and dead.

There are cases of hypothermia victims surviving prolonged immersion with no breathing (up to an hour) in very cold water, but these have been children who were subsequently taken to a high-tech medical facility

Figure 29.2 *Kayaking on open sea water (G. Bruce)*

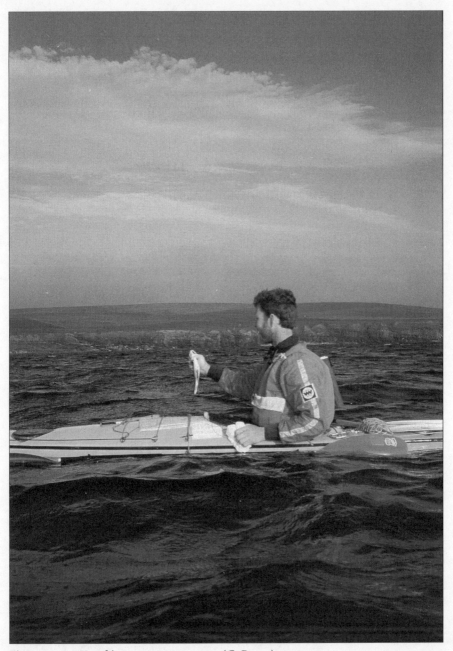

The heart is very unstable in severe hypothermia, and thus can be easily jolted into a fatal rhythm. This means that:

- ECC should probably not be started, as it may cause fatal rhythms in a heart that is beating. The heart has a slightly better chance of slowly improving by itself if treatment is limited to rewarming and EAR.
- The casualty should be moved only if it is strictly necessary, and then as carefully as possible.

Shoulder dislocation

Shoulder dislocations are probably the most serious injury that canoeists will experience. Intermediate kayakers, unfamiliar with the power of big water rivers, should be especially careful. Your future in white-water canoeing is limited if you have a dislocation, as subsequent dislocations happen a lot more easily. Dislocations occur when the arm is extended higher than the shoulder.

Good paddling technique prevents shoulder dislocation – keep arms below the level of your shoulders. Think of a box between the chin and spraydeck and "Keep your hands in the box".

In the wilderness, it is reasonable for you to try to put back ("reduce") a dislocated shoulder. The technique is simple, you are unlikely to cause more damage than has already been done, the healing process can start sooner, there is likely to be less damage to the shoulder in the long term, and the patient will be more comfortable during the evacuation. However, it is the patient's decision as to whether reduction is attempted. The diagnosis is usually obvious and patients realise the shoulder is "out": the elbow will lie away from their side and they cannot move their arm. From the front, the shoulder looks abnormally square compared with the other side and the head of the upper arm bone (humerus) can usually be felt in front of the "cup" of the joint (Figure 29.3).

Action must be swift. Relocation can most easily be done in the first few minutes, but becomes progressively more difficult during the next 2 hours as muscle spasm sets in.

Management of a dislocated shoulder

- Give your strongest painkiller and muscle relaxant (e.g. 5mg diazepam) to suck).
- Gently remove the buoyancy aid and paddle jacket.
- Carefully examine the arm and shoulder.
- Check and record – pulse, finger movement, numb "herald patch" and hand sensation.

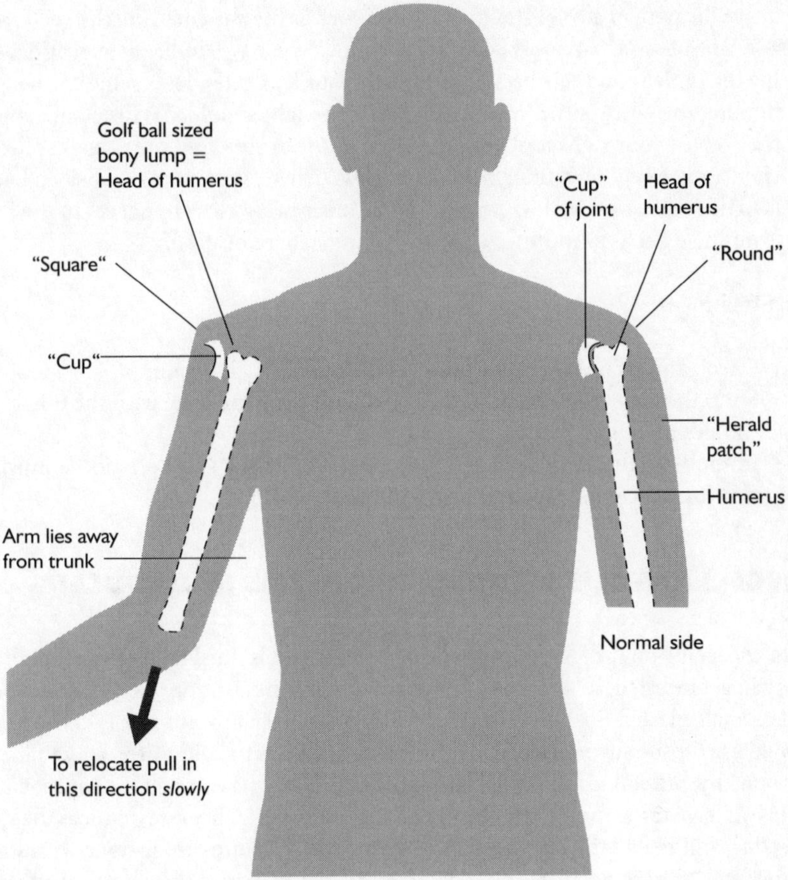

Figure 29.3 *Shoulder dislocation – diagnosis (A. Watt)*

The principle of good reduction is a *very slow continuous pull* to tease out the muscle spasm. When the humeral head comes to the edge of the cup of the joint it will suddenly "clunk" into place. If you pull too hard or too sharply, muscle spasm will worsen and grip the humeral head more firmly outside the cup.

There are several techniques, but the two easiest ones are shown in Figure 29.4:

1. Lie the victim face down on a flat boulder, rock ledge or similar with a table-like edge, so that their arm hangs down freely. Attach a helmet or bucket to their wrist. Add a weight (e.g. small stones) of around 2kg (3kg for a large patient) and very slowly increase this to double; if the patient has pain then decrease the weight.

Leave the patient alone; gravity does the work as the patient's muscles relax. After 5–15 minutes the patient should feel a "clunk" which will indicate relocation.

2. Lie the patient on their back and sit with your legs extended, facing the head, holding the wrist between your thighs. If the right shoulder is dislocated, place the arch of your right foot (not the toes) in the armpit and press against the chest wall. Keeping your arms straight (less tiring), very, very slowly lean back. (Do not press too hard with your foot as it is resting close to nerves in the armpit.) After 5–10 minutes a clunk will indicate relocation.

After treatment, whether or not relocated:

- Check and record the wrist pulse, and "herald patch" again;
- Strap the arm to the front of the chest with the hand level with the other shoulder (see Chapter 13, page 149);
- Immobilise the shoulder until the patient consults a good physiotherapist, so that long-term damage can be minimised.

MISCELLANEOUS MEDICAL PROBLEMS IN PADDLERS

Cuts

Cuts, especially on the legs, may not heal until the trip is finished. Even the smallest of cuts can get infected, so at the end of every day wash the cut, apply iodine or povidone and a small plaster. So-called waterproof dressings usually are not (although some people use Opsite successfully). My preferred option is the ubiquitous duct tape. It is not stretchy, but it does stick well and most canoeists carry some for boat repair.

If you have the training, the closure of cuts gives better healing, reduces the risk of infection and makes the cut waterproof after a day. Closure can be done with sutures or medical "superglue". On water-based trips you may find that Steri-strips do not stick well, even with the addition of sticky tincture of benzoin to the skin.

Hand blisters

These are fairly common on multiday trips, even among experienced paddlers who may not have paddled recently. If you feel a faint, early soreness it is worth trying some tape or Moleskin strapped over the friction point before a blister forms. Blisters usually de-roof with further paddling; then treat as you would a simple cut.

Burns

Wood fires are common on river trips and burn injuries are frequent. If the burn is severe enough to require a silver sulphadiazine dressing, then keeping it dry is important. The dressing probably does not need changing unless it gets drenched (see Chapter 13).

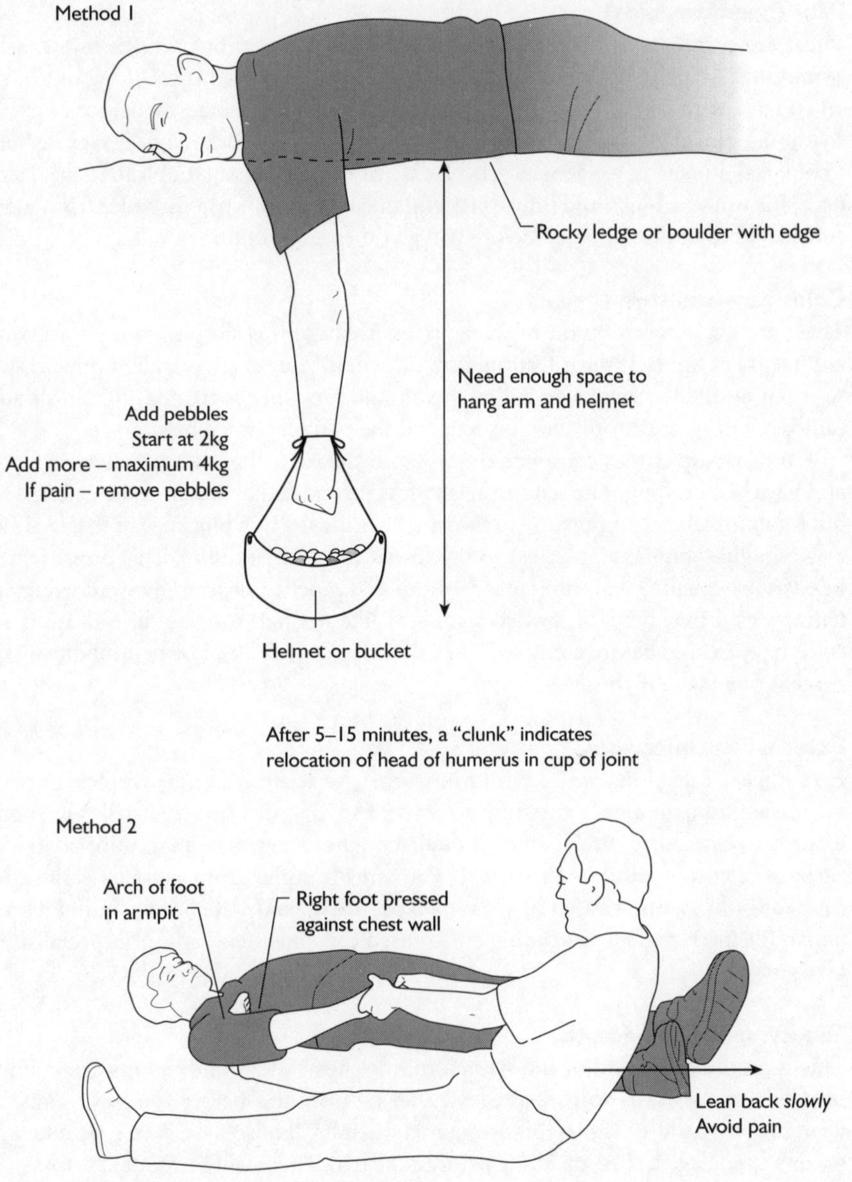
Method 1
Rocky ledge or boulder with edge
Need enough space to
hang arm and helmet
Add pebbles
Start at 2kg
Add more – maximum 4kg
If pain – remove pebbles
Helmet or bucket
After 5–15 minutes, a "clunk" indicates
relocation of head of humerus in cup of joint
Method 2
Arch of foot
in armpit
Right foot pressed
against chest wall
Lean back *slowly*
Avoid pain

Figure 29.4 *Relocation techniques for a dislocated shoulder*

Piles (haemorrhoids)

These are common in rafters, kayakers and mountaineers but no one knows why. Symptoms are pain, bright red bleeding on defecation or a lump sticking out of the anus. Treat with careful washing and application of a local anaesthetic, for example, Xyloproct ointment. If severe, lie patient flat, legs and buttocks slightly elevated and a cold pack in place. Paradoxically, both diarrhoea and constipation can make haemorrhoids worse; a high fluid intake is useful in either case. If you do suffer from them, consider getting them treated before you go on an expedition.

Colds ears and sore throats

These are fairly common on multiday trips. Treatment is simple, with paracetamol and plenty of fluids. If the infection moves down to your chest, purulent (green) sputum can result. Anything worse than this should probably be treated with antibiotics (amoxycillin or erythromycin), especially if the patient has a temperature.

Kayakers sometimes complain of "water in the ear", often when they have a cold and have been rolling. The sensation is in fact not caused by water in the external ear but by an imbalance of pressure in the inner ear caused by a blockage of the very narrow tube that joins the inner ear to the throat (eustachian tube). This pressure may be eased by exhaling against a closed mouth and pinched nose, or by swallowing. Inhaling steam may help, or try decongestants like Actifed. You should wait until any colds have cleared before going back to Eskimo rolls, and it can be painful during the descent of a plane flight.

External ear infections

External ear infections are common in warm, moist areas like the tropics. Encourage expedition members carefully to wash and dry the ear, then use Otosporin eardrops (two drops three times a day). On the water, you may want to try an earplug of cotton wool in Vaseline. If you already suffer from "surfer's ear" (exostoses, or bony lumps, caused by years of exposure to cold water), you should discuss a plan for its treatment (including customised earplugs) with an ENT specialist before you go.

Tenosynovitis (tendonitis)

This is an inflammation of the synovium, the sheath surrounding muscle tendons, usually at the wrist. If you are already suffering from this before you leave, consider changing to paddle feather or use cranked shafts. Those at risk are people who haven't spent much time paddling prior to the trip. There will be moderate-to-severe pain on slight wrist movement, sometimes with palpable "creaking". One point is very tender to touch, usually on the thumb side of the back of the wrist. Point tenderness can distinguish tenosynovitis from other wrist pains. This is an overuse injury and the only cure is complete rest, ideally in a splint. If you insist on paddling then try a wrist bandage (of neoprene, for example) and consider an anti-inflammatory drug like ibuprofen.

Back and muscle problems

Stiff bodies and knotted muscles, especially in your neck or between the shoulder blades, are common on multiday trips and when moving heavy craft. Doing warm-up stretches before and after paddling is a routine worth following, and so is getting someone firmly to massage the "knots". Sea paddlers can get leg strains through constantly sitting in the same position. Back trouble is common in paddlers, especially as the kayaking posture flexes the lower, lumbar spine against its natural curve. If you suffer from recurrent back trouble the hazards of becoming disabled in a remote area should stimulate you to remember proper lifting techniques, to review flexibility exercises with a physiotherapist before you go, to fit a proper backrest, and to consider lifting aids like straps or even portable trolleys.

Sea paddling

In the tropics be aware of the glare of the sun. Take sunglasses, spare hats and plenty of high-factor sun cream. Dry skin can be a problem, especially for hands that are constantly getting wet (through removal of natural oils), so carry something like Neutrogena hand-cream. In cold climates lips especially can suffer from chapping; a cap or hat for the head is important for hypothermia prevention. Sea sickness can happen in experienced as well as novice paddlers, especially when staring at a compass in poor visibility. Sea-sickness medicines (for example, cinnarizine tablets) are most likely to be effective if taken before the onset of nausea. Sore skin from friction on constantly wet skin (such as the armpits) can be prevented with Vaseline.

Burn-out and stress

If you do more than a couple of long trips your body may not recover fully before the next trip, and chronic mild exhaustion can result. Pushing ambitious schedules in developing countries just doesn't work; the pace of life is slower and you just burn out. On challenging sea trips, safe landings can be hours away, and all team members have to be able to face the consequent fatigue and fear.

COMMERCIAL WHITE-WATER RAFTING

White-water rafting is a thrilling activity. Multiday trips are true experiences, offering unique access to wilderness areas. People with no experience of rafting, or even of outdoor activities, can be guided safely down reasonably hard rapids. Certain places in the world have thus experienced a massive growth in white-water rafting, for example, the Zambezi in Zimbabwe, and Nepal. At these sites, experienced river

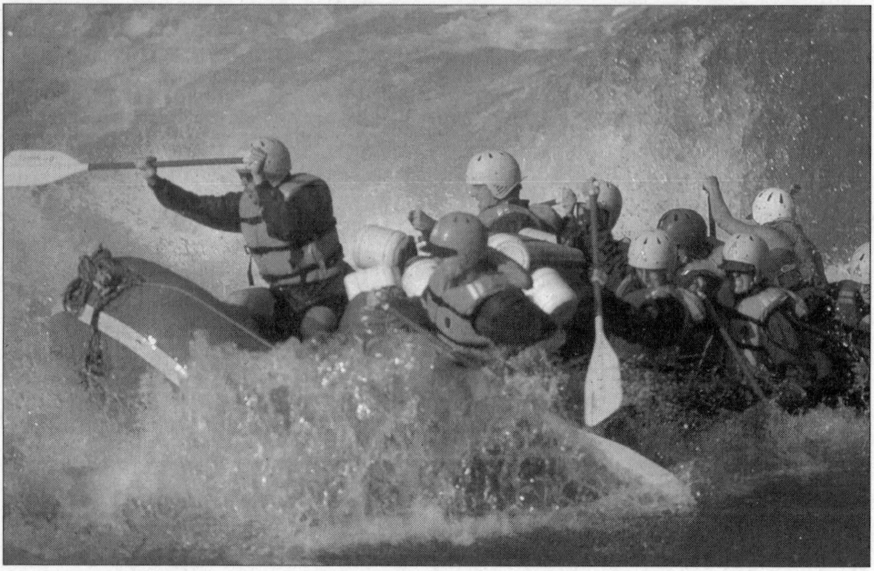

Fig. 29.5 *An inflatable raft (D. Allardice)*

runners can use their hard-earned skills in gainful employment as raft guides/safety kayakers.

Before going on a raft trip

You need to be reasonably fit, so running or swimming is ideal. An ability to swim is preferable, but at least you should not be scared of water. For developing country destinations, add hepatitis A to your list of vaccinations. Clothing items will be advised by your raft company, but should include a peaked sun cap and good river sandals with either buckles or Velcro with additional fastening. You should have your own small medical kit, including paracetamol, plasters and sun screen, and iodine for grazes, cuts and emergency water sterilisation.

Safety and raft companies

Although white-water rafting appears dangerous it is actually quite safe, with low accident rates, if basic safety rules are followed. However, this is an outdoor adventure activity and you are assuming the risk by signing on. Good companies run professional standard trips, but local competition can reduce prices to the detriment of safety. You should ask about the following:

- the experience of the guides, e.g. how often they've done the river, what guiding and first aid qualifications they have;

- the age and serviceability of the rafts ("self-bailers" are best);
- buoyancy aids and helmets provided;
- whether another craft (raft or kayak) will accompany your raft.

The provision of "safety kayakers" adds to the security of the trip. There should be a safety briefing before you start that covers paddling, holding on when not paddling, and what to do if you fall into white water.

On the river in hot developing countries do not forget suntan cream and remember to drink plenty of clean water to prevent dehydration. Your buoyancy aid is vital if you fall in the water, and it should therefore be worn when manoeuvring on any flowing water. Newcomers to foreign parts worry about exotic tropical diseases, but in fact the biggest threat to your health will come from factors that you control yourself:

- prevention of accidents (especially around the fireplace);
- hygiene, especially handwashing before meals.

The river guides will explain campsite and water sterilisation procedures. Enjoy it – white-water rafting is a great experience.

All water-based trips are an enjoyable and rewarding way to travel when abroad. However, do not neglect your preparation and make sure you are fit before you go.

AUTHOR BIOGRAPHIES AND ACKNOWLEDGEMENTS

Mukul Agarwal BA MRCP DTM&H Dip Sport & Exer Med

Born in the wilds of south London, Mukul then spent a number of years recovering in the shadows of the Indian Himalayas. His training in medicine and general practice has been interspersed with several spells as an expedition doctor, participating in research and youth development projects with able-bodied and disabled team members in a variety of terrains. As an instructor with Wilderness Medical Training and the RGS expedition medicine course, he has been actively involved in teaching lay people and health workers about medicine relevant to remote travel. He is completing specialist training in rehabilitation and musculoskeletal medicine while pursuing his interests in sports medicine and international health.

Sarah R. Anderson MA MB BChir MRCPI MRCGP DTM&H DFPHM

Sarah trained as a doctor in Cambridge and London. While at Cambridge, she led an expedition to Uganda, was President of the Cambridge Expedition Society and has been involved with expeditions ever since. She has a Diploma in Tropical Medicine and Hygiene and has worked in hospitals in Uganda, Zimbabwe and South Africa, and as a flying doctor with AMREF in Kenya. Sarah co-ordinates the Royal Geographical Society's Medical Cell, co-edits the book *Expedition Medicine*, is co-author of *Expedition Health and Safety – a risk assessment* (*JRSM* 2000; 93:557–562) and acted as medical officer to the RGS – Shoals of Capricorn Programme in 2001. Currently Sarah is training in public health medicine.

Clive Barrow

Clive has led or participated in sixteen expeditions in developing countries since 1983, including Chile, Guyana, Venezuela, Ecuador, Canada, Morocco, Kenya, Tanzania, Namibia, Zimbabwe, Pakistan, Papua New Guinea, Australia and New Zealand. He most recently led an expedition to Poland conducting community tasks and treks in the High Tatras for Endeavour Training. Clive was field director for Operation Raleigh 1985–89, operations director for World Challenge Expeditions 1989–96, and is currently running ITEC, an independent expedition consultancy which included a recruitment service for expedition staff and leaders. He is a YET trustee and a member of the John Hunt Exploration Group Executive Committee.

Hokey Bennett-Jones

Hokey trained as a nurse at Westminster Hospital, London, and attended an external course at the London School of Tropical Medicine; she did midwifery in Edinburgh and a family planning course at King's College Hospital, London. She has travelled in north and east Africa, Australia and the Caribbean, and was expedition nurse on Royal Geographical Society research projects in Mulu (Sarawak), Kora (Kenya) and Wahiba Sands (Sultanate of Oman). Hokey is now a full-time housewife and mother.

Charles Clarke MA MB BChir FRCP

Charlie is a consultant neurologist who has been climbing for 36 years and has visited the Himalayas on more than ten occasions. He was expedition doctor with Chris Bonington on the ascent of the south-west face of Everest in 1975; on Kongur in 1981; on the north-east ridge of Everest in 1982; and more recently in Tibet on the Sepu Kangri expedition in 1997. He is the founder of the UIAA Mountain Medicine Data Centre, now administered by the British Mountaineering Council.

Jon Dallimore MSc MRCGP DCH DRCOG

Jon is a general practitioner in Chepstow who has had a keen interest in expedition and travel medicine since 1988. He completed a Master's degree in travel medicine in 1998 and is medical adviser to six expedition companies. He also works part-time as a staff doctor in the accident and emergency department of Bristol Royal Infirmary. Jon has been doctor or leader on 21 overseas expeditions to environments such as the deserts of Namibia and the Sinai and the jungles of Sulawesi, Belize, Thailand and Ecuador. He has also acted as a doctor on many high-altitude climbs and treks to Nepal, the Andes, Kenya, Morocco and, in 1999, Arctic Greenland (which included four first ascents). Community project work includes an orphanage-building project in Kenya, irrigation work in Pakistan and nature conservation in Namibia. Jon's research interests include acute mountain sickness and the incidence of illness and injuries on expeditions. Jon is co-founder and medical director of Wilderness Medical Training.

Richard Dawood MD DTM&H

Richard has travelled to 80 countries and runs an independent travel clinic in Fleet Street, London. He is the editor of *Travellers' Health: how to stay healthy abroad* (OUP) and writes for newspapers and travel magazines in the UK and United States. His current interest is looking after journalists in high-risk environments.

Sundeep Dhillon MA BM BCh

On 25 May 1998 Sundeep reached the summit of Everest on his second attempt, and is the youngest person to have climbed the Seven Summits (the highest mountain on each continent). He trained in medicine at Oxford where he also ran the University Exploration Club. He is a major in the Royal Army Medical Corps and is a GP registrar serving with airborne forces. He has been involved with expeditions and military deployments worldwide.

Matthew S. Dryden MA MB BS MSc MD FRCPath

Matthew has travelled widely, often in a medical capacity. He has been an expedition doctor on several occasions, usually in jungle and desert environments including South America, the Sahara, Kenya, Botswana, Costa Rica, Sudan, Australia and Papua New Guinea. He is a member of the Royal Geographical Society Medical Cell. He has a particular interest in travel-related infection. His research interests include Lyme disease and novel antibiotics active against multiply resistant bacteria. Matthew is a consultant in microbiology and communicable disease at the Royal Hampshire County Hospital, Winchester.

Alistair Duff

Alistair is a partner in the Edinburgh law firm Henderson Boyd, Jackson, WS and specialises in sports law and reparation. He has published over 37 articles on sports law and is one of the Scottish Arbiters on the Sports Dispute Resolution Panel. He is company secretary of Medical Expeditions Ltd. He took part in the first Everest marathon in 1987 and has returned on four subsequent climbing trips to the Himalayas.

David Geddes

David Geddes is a dental surgeon who served with frontline troops and airborne forces field ambulances for many years. He has climbed and ski-mountaineered all round the world. David retired from the army in the 1980s and from general practice in the 1990s. Currently he runs an ISO 9000 Quality Assurance certification company for medical and dental practices, primary care groups and trusts, and an internet company delivering MSc-accredited distance learning to doctors, dentists, nurses and managers. He has set up dental projects and scholarships in Nepal and carries out remote dentistry there. The new Nepal National Dental Hospital and specifically the maxillofacial centre are his creations.

Larry Goodyer BPharm MPharm PhD MRPharmS

Larry is a lecturer in clinical pharmacy at the Department of Pharmacy, King's College, London. Apart from travel medicine, his research interests include clinical trials on over-the-counter medicines and multimedia computer presentation systems. In

1990 he helped set up and became a director of the Nomad Travel Pharmacy, which specialises in medical provision for people travelling overseas, from large sponsored expeditions to private individuals.

Paul Goodyer

Paul is the managing director of Nomad Traveller's Store and Medical Centre. He has travelled for the last 20 years and visited, among other areas, Africa, South America, the Middle East and south-east Asia. In his early travelling days he contracted infections such as dysentery through drinking contaminated water. He knows the secrets of staying healthy while travelling and passes this information on via his own travel store so that new travellers can avoid the pitfalls he has experienced.

Stephen Hearns MB ChB FRCSEd Dip IMC

Based in Glasgow, Stephen specialises in accident and emergency medicine and has an interest in pre-hospital care. He has been an active member of Arrochar mountain rescue team since 1998. He has acted as medical officer on a number of expeditions and now works on a regular basis for a commercial expedition company. Since 1999, through his company Frontlinemedics.com, Stephen has organised the ExpeMed expedition medicine course for doctors and nurses. Stephen also has an interest in event medicine and in 2001 organised the medical cover for the largest 2-day music festival in the UK. Stephen has written a number of publications relating to emergency medicine and mountain rescue medicine.

Robin Illingworth MA BM BCh FRCP FFAEM

Robin is a consultant in accident and emergency medicine at St James's University Hospital, Leeds. From 1974 to 1990 he was honorary medical adviser to the Brathay Exploration Group, which is based at Ambleside, Cumbria, and organises many expeditions. Robin has been on mountaineering and scientific expeditions to Iceland, Greenland, Alaska, Morocco, Nepal and Borneo, and has travelled in several other countries. He is the author of *Expedition Medicine, A Planning Guide* (3rd edition, 1984) and co-author and editor of books on accident and emergency medicine.

Chris Johnson MA MD FRCA

Chris was medical officer to the British Antarctic Survey at Halley Bay during 1979/80. On his return to the UK he worked at the Institute of Environmental and Offshore Medicine in Aberdeen where he completed his MD on the effects of cold on peripheral circulation. Chris has also been involved with epidemiological work on expedition medical problems. He is currently a consultant anaesthetist at Southmead Hospital, Bristol, but regularly goes cross-country skiing in Norway and the Canadian Rockies.

Michael Phelan BSc MB BS MRCPsych

Michael is a consultant psychiatrist at Charing Cross Hospital, London. He has previously worked at the Institute of Psychiatry, London, and at Prince Alfred Hospital, Sydney, Australia. His interest in expeditions started when he was invited to join an anthropological expedition to the highlands of Papua New Guinea. Since then he has been the doctor on a 3-month expedition in the Ecuadorian rainforest, where he ran out of suture material as a result of the over-enthusiastic use of machetes by team members. He also has extensive experience of long-distance sailing trips, where sea sickness and complete isolation often result in even greater strains and tensions than on land-based expeditions.

Andrew Pitkin MBBS MRCP

Andrew is an anaesthetist in Southampton. Until recently he was the Royal Navy's only civilian diving medical officer at the Institute of Naval Medicine in Gosport. He is an avid diver and has provided medical support as well as diving expertise to several scientific expeditions in Belize and Mexico which used technical diving to retrieve geological specimens with the purpose of investigating sea level change over the last 250,000 years.

Paul Richards MB ChB MRCGP DFFP MSc

Paul is a medical doctor with special interest in wilderness and expedition medicine who has practised in Africa and Nepal. He has travelled widely and been medical officer on several remote expeditions including expeditions involved in Mayan archaeology, discovering new rainforest species and mapping of Irian Jaya highlands. Latterly he has pursued research interests in high-altitude medicine and is a member of Medical Expeditions, a charity that is influential in promoting research and teaching of altitude physiology and medicine. Recently, he has completed the new MSc in travel medicine.

Charles Siderfin MB ChB BSc MSc MRCGP FACRRM

Charles is a general practitioner currently working in Orkney. He has previously worked in Antarctica, Africa and the Australian outback and undertaken a number of expeditions. His particular interests is are in expedition medicine and remote healthcare and he is currently developing posts for junior doctors training to become rural and remote general practitioners. He spent 3 years as a medical officer with the British Antarctic Survey, during which time he developed an integrated system of healthcare for expeditions. This included advanced training for non-medical personnel and 24-hour medical cover using low-technology communication systems.

Rod Stables TD MA DM BM BCh MRCP

Rod is a consultant cardiologist at the Cardiothoracic Centre, Liverpool. He has been involved in civilian expeditions and military operations over all types of terrain and in all climates from the Arctic Circle to the jungles of south-east Asia. He is an active mountaineer with experience in the UK, European Alps and Greater Ranges. He was the deputy of the UK Reserve Forces expeditions to Mt McKinley, Alaska, in 1991 and to Everest in the winter of 1992–3.

David A. Warrell MA DM DSc FRCP
David is professor of tropical medicine and infectious diseases and director of the Centre for Tropical Medicine, University of Oxford. He has lived and worked in Ethiopia, Nigeria, Sierra Leone, Kenya, Thailand, Burma, Sri Lanka, Papua New Guinea, Brazil and Ecuador. David is co-editor of the *Oxford Textbook of Medicine* and *Bruce Chwatt's Essential Malariology*, and author of articles on malaria, rabies, relapsing fever and venomous animals.

Andy Watt MB ChB MRCP BSc DTMH
Andy discovered white-water canoeing at Glasgow University and spent a year kayaking and raft guiding the rivers of the Indian and Nepalese Himalayas. He makes video programmes and teaches wilderness medicine with Wilderness Medical Training, and is the project director for the proposed artificial white-water course in Glasgow. His hospital speciality is care of elderly people, but he has a broad range of skills derived from time spent in surgery, obstetrics and a year in an Indian mission hospital.

Mark Whittingham
Mark has worked as an underwriter for the Zurich Insurance Company for 5 years and is presently employed as a senior account executive with Aon Risk Services where he has worked for 13 years. He is a chartered insurance practitioner and specialises in custom-made insurance programmes for expeditions and companies undertaking adventurous travel.

Acknowledgements
The editors would like to thank the following additional contributors:

Dr Rupert Bourne
Dr Charles Easmon
Dr Annabel Nickol
Roz Nurse
Dr Jane Wilson-Howorth

and the following first-edition authors:

Jon Buchan
Dr Tom Davies
Dr Victor De Lima
Dr Bobby Forbes
Dr Bev Holt
David Watt.

The antecedents of this book were the five successful earlier editions of *Expedition Medicine*, edited from 1986 to 1994 by Bent Juel-Jensen and published by the Royal Geographical Society. Much of Bent's wisdom survives in this edition. The editors would also like to acknowledge the assistance of the staff of the RGS–IBG's Expedition Advisory Centre, especially Tim Jones, Tom Martin, Annabelle Newbigging and Shane Winser.

ROYAL GEOGRAPHICAL SOCIETY

WITH THE INSTITUTE OF BRITISH GEOGRAPHERS

The Royal Geographical Society (with the Institute of British Geographers) is the learned society representing geography and geographers. It was founded in 1830 for the advancement of geographical science and has been among the most active of the learned societies ever since.

The Society supports research, education and training, together with the wider public understanding and enjoyment of geography. The Society has a membership of approximately 13,300, a world-renowned reputation and a programme of activities that extend far beyond its membership. Over 150 lectures and conferences are organised each year including a major 4-day residential conference and a highly popular programme of lectures for the geography enthusiast. There is a specialist unit, the Expedition Advisory Centre, devoted to training younger field scientists. The Society's information resources include its library, map room, manuscript archives and picture library. It also regularly publishes three scholarly journals, a research bulletin, a newsletter and a popular magazine. The Society is based in a listed building in its own grounds in Kensington opposite Hyde Park, and operates eight regional branches in the UK and one overseas. There is a permanent full-time staff of 50, together with part-time, temporary and volunteer staff.

Overseas field research and expedition support

The Society is one of the largest organisers in the UK of geographical field research overseas. It has run ten major multidisciplinary overseas expeditions during the last two decades. All of these have contributed geographical knowledge to conservation and development priorities at government level in the host ocuntry.

Expedition Advisory Centre

The Society's internationally acclaimed Expedition Advisory Centre (EAC), funded by Shell International Limited, provides training and advice to anyone embarking on an expedition. It is the leading such centre in the world. Each year it assists more than

500 teams, the majority of which are university based. The EAC publishes a range of training manuals on every aspect of expeditionary research and logistics, and runs regular workshops and seminars.
Website www.rgs.org/eac

Expedition Grants Programme

The RGS–IBG is also the country's main organisation for screening and funding small research expeditions through its Expedition Grants programme.
Website www.rgs.org/grants

Medical Cell

The Society's Medical Cell provides a forum for discussion, information and advice to those operating in remote and challenging environments. All expeditions are encouraged to contribute to an ongoing survey of expedition health and safety which began in 1995. It holds regular seminars and workshops on matters of expedition health and safety including wilderness medical training, off-site safety management, and risk assessment and crisis management. The Society helps expeditions recruit medical personnel for expeditions through its *Register of Personnel* and publicises opportunities for medical professionals to participate in expeditions and fieldwork overseas through its *Bulletin of Expedition Vacancies.*
Website www.rgs.org/medicalcell

For further information on the work of the Society please contact:
RGS–IBG Expedition Advisory Centre
1 Kensington Gore
London SW7 2AR
Tel. +44 20 7591 3030
Fax +44 20 7591 3031
Email eac@rgs.org
Website www.rgs.org/eac

APPENDICES

I PRE-EXPEDITION MEDICAL QUESTIONNAIRE

Name: **Date:**

Address:

Home telephone:
Work telephone:
Fax number:

Age: **Date of Birth:**

Passport details:

Nationality:
Passport number:
Place of issue:
Date of issue:
Date of expiry:

Next of kin:

Name:
Address:

Telephone/fax:
Relationship:

GP details:

Name:
Address:

Telephone/fax:

Current medical problems:

1.
2.
3.

Past medical problems:
1.
2.
3.

Past psychiatric history:

Current medication:

Allergies (drugs, food, environmental):

Immunisations (with dates):

Routine:	Diphtheria	....
	Polio	....
	Tetanus	....
Travel:	Hepatitis A	....
	Gamma-gobulin	....
	Hepatitis B	....
	Japanese encephalitis	....
	Meningoccocal meningitis	....
	Rabies	....
	Tick-borne encephalitis	....
	Tuberculosis (BCG)	....
	Typhoid	....
	Yellow fever	....

Blood group:

Itinerary:	**Country**	**Date**

Departure date: **Return date:**

Total length of trip:

2 CRISIS MANAGEMENT PLAN

Leader/Planner:
Expedition destination:
Expedition area:

Aim:

Objectives:
1.
2.
3.
4.
5.

PLANNING AREA	ACTION REQUIRED	Deadline	Completed	Revision date
1. Risk assessment	a. Agree objectives with team b. Risk assessment meeting c. Review objectives			
2. Legal and insurance	a. Legal status b. Contracts/Booking conditions d. Insurance coverage agreed c. Insurance arranged			
3. Team screening and selection	a. Application forms prepared b. Interviews/selection process c. Criteria for selection d. Insurance screening			
4. Briefing and training	a. Training/Briefing programme b. Key briefing documents and timetable c. Key training events and timetable			
5. Emergency procedures	a. Emergency contacts in place b. Action plans on emergencies c. Contacts briefed/trained d. Chain of responsibility/roles			

PLANNING AREA	ACTION REQUIRED	Deadline	Completed	Revision date
	e. Next of kin details f. Medical questionnaires completed g. Assistance agencies			
6. National and local contacts	a. Foreign Office b. Sponsors c. Local agents/reps			
7. Medical umbrella	a. Staff/participant skills b. Medical kit c. Local medical support d. National/international medical support e. Casualty evacuation procedures			
8. Communications	a. International b. National c. Local d. Network established			
9. UK back-up	a. UK liaison point b. Access (phone, email, etc.) c. Detailed knowledge of plans			
10. Share the experience	a. Plan for sharing data/learning b. Presentations/journals/reports c. How information will be shared (RGS/Uni/trade bodies, etc.)			

3 MEDICAL ASSESSMENT QUESTIONNAIRE (MAQ)

(A) PATIENT DETAILS

1. Name
2. Address
3. Date of birth
4. Age
5. Sex
6. Occupation
7. Time (at completion of form)
8. Date
9. Location of patient at present

(B) PATIENT'S MAIN COMPLAINT/COMPLAINTS

1.
2.
3.
4.

(C) A SHORT DESCRIPTIVE HISTORY OF THE ABOVE PROBLEMS IN THE ORDER THEY OCCURRED

(In the patient's own words, including how long ago the problem(s) started)

(D) PAIN

1. Is there any pain? (If no then pass to section E)	**No**	**Yes**
2. Site of the pain at onset or describe in words	*Use diagram 1a (front) or 1b (back)*	
3. Site of the pain now or describe in words	*Use diagram 2a (front) or 2b (back)*	
4. Time since pain began	.... hours	.... minutes
5. Severity of pain now (mild, severe, etc.)		
6. Since beginning has the pain	Got better/stayed the same/worsened?	
7. What is the pain like (dull, hot, sharp, etc)?		
8. Is the pain	Constant?	Variable?
9. Does the pain go anywhere?	No	Yes
10. Did it come on during activity?	No	Yes
11. How did the pain start?	Suddenly	Gradually
12. Does anything make it better? If yes, what?	No	Yes
13. Does anything make it worse? If yes, what?	No	Yes

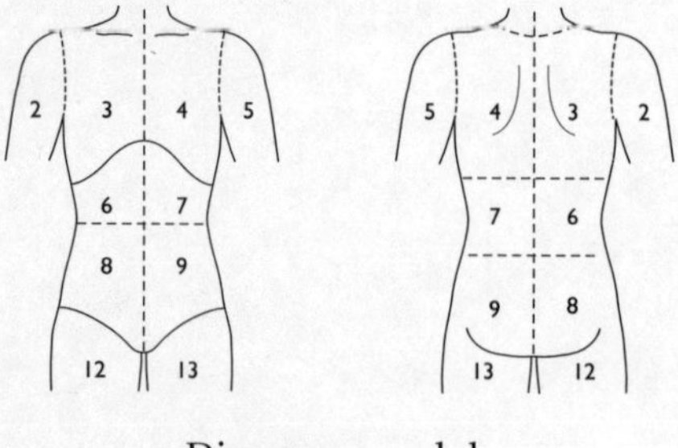

Diagram 1a and 1b
Site of pain at onset

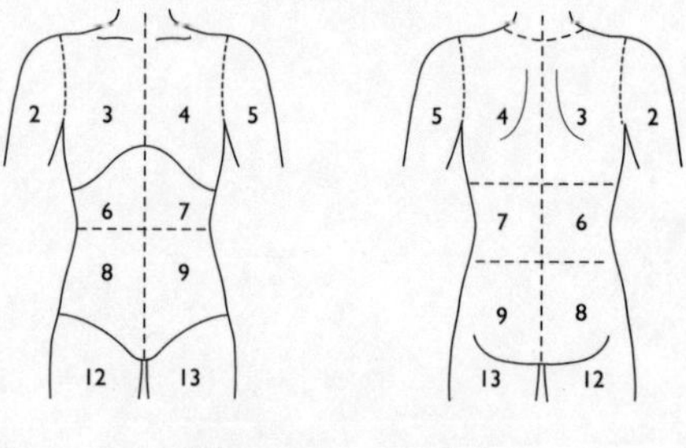

Diagram 2a and 2b
Site of pain now

(E) CHEST

1. Is there any shortness of breath (SOB)?	**No**	**Yes**
2. How severe is this SOB?	Very slight A little tight chested Short of breath at rest Gasping for air	
3. How long ago did this SOB start?	.... hours	.... minutes
4. Does anything make it better? If yes, what?	No	Yes
5. Does anything make it worse? If yes, what?	No	Yes
6. Is a cough present?	**No**	**Yes**
7. Is there any phlegm/spit?	**No**	**Yes**
8. Colour of phlegm/spit		
9. Is the heart pounding in the chest?	**No**	**Yes**

(F) SICKNESS AND BOWELS

1. Is there any feeling of sickness?	**No**	**Yes**
2. Time since this feeling began	.... hours	.... minutes
3. Has there been vomiting?	**No**	**Yes**
4. Time since vomiting began	.... hours	.... minutes
5. Colour of the vomit	Food Yellow/green/bile Red/blood/other	
6. Is the appetite changed?	**No**	**Yes**
7. Is the bowel habit changed?	**No**	**Yes, constipation** **Yes, diarrhoea**
8. Frequency of moving bowels	**Normally** **Now**	**.... times per day** **.... times per day**
9. Is this at all painful?	**No**	**Yes**
10. Colour of the bowel motion		

(G) URINE

1. Is there any pain on passing urine (PU)?	**No**	**Yes**
2. Where is this pain felt?		
3. Timing of pain when PU	During	After
4. Any blood seen when PU?	**No**	**Yes**
5. Frequency of PU	**Normally**	**.... /day**
		.... /night
	Changed to	**.... /day**
		.... /night

(H) OTHER COMPLAINTS

1. Headache present	**No**	**Yes**
2. Severity of headache	Mild, fully active	
	Moderate, non-restricting	
	Severe, restricting activity	
3. Blackout or collapse	**No**	**Yes**
4. Light-headed or faint	**No**	**Yes**
5. Sweating	**No**	**Yes**
6. Shaking or shivering	**No**	**Yes**
7. Feeling weak	**No**	**Yes**
8. Muscle ache	**No**	**Yes**
9. Vision blurred	**No**	**Yes**
10. Earache	**No**	**Yes**
11. Nose clear	**Yes**	**No, blocked**
		No, running
		No, bleeding
12. Sore throat	**No**	**Yes**
13. Skin rash present	**No**	**Yes, all body**
		Yes, trunk
		Yes, limbs
		Yes, head/neck
14. Is the rash itchy?	No	Yes

(I) WOMEN ONLY

1. Unusual vaginal bleeding	**No**	**Yes, spotting** **Yes, light** **Yes, heavy** **Yes, clots**
2. Is this linked to any pain?	**No**	**Yes**
3. Date of last period starting		
4. Was this a "normal" period?	**Yes**	**No**

(J) PAST MEDICAL HISTORY

1. Has this occurred before?	**No**	**Yes**
2. What was wrong then?	Date: Diagnosis:	
2. Has the patient been admitted to hospital before?	**No**	**Yes**
3. For what conditions?		
4. Any other significant episodes of illness or injury?	**No**	**Yes**
5. Dates and conditions		

(K) DRUG HISTORY

1. Is the patient taking any medications?	**No**	**Yes**
2. Drug name	Dosage	
3. Is the patient allergic to anything?	**No**	**Yes**
4. Allergies to what?		

CLINICAL EXAMINATION

(N) ALWAYS ANSWER THESE 13 QUESTIONS

1.	PATIENT LOOKS	Well	Unwell Ill Awful
2.	PATIENT APPEARS	Awake and alert	Awake but confused Drowsy Responds to pain only Unwakable
3.	TEMPERATURE		.... °Centigrade
4.	PULSE (AT REST)		beats/minute
5.	BREATHING RATE		breaths/minute
6.	BLOOD PRESSURE		..../.... mmHg
7.	SKIN COLOUR	Normal	Flushed Blue or cyanosed Pale or anaemic Yellow or jaundiced
8.	SKIN TEMPERATURE TO TOUCH	Warm or normal	Hot or fevered Cold and dry Cold and clammy
9.	A HEAVING CHEST ON BREATHING	No	Yes
10.	PERSPIRATION or SWEATING	No	Yes
11.	DEHYDRATION or DRY TONGUE	No	Yes
12.	PAIN or DISTRESS ON MOVING	No	Yes
13.	PAIN or STIFFNESS IN THE NECK	No	Yes

THESE BODY DIAGRAMS MAY BE USED FOR ILLUSTRATION IF REQUIRED

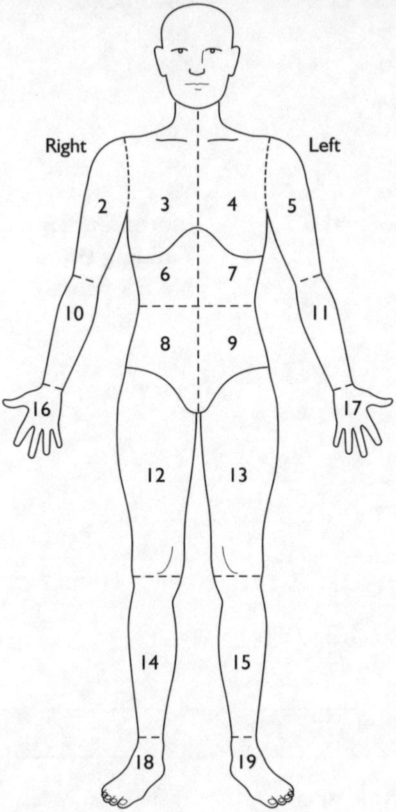

Diagram 3 *Front*

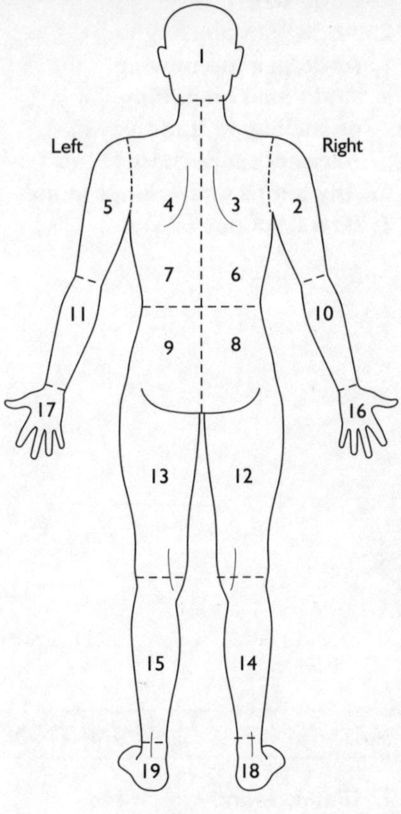

Diagram 4 *Back*

(O) CHEST (bare all chest, front and back)

1. Signs of injury to chest	**No**	**Yes**	
2. Tender chest wall	**No**	**Yes**	
3. Position of windpipe in neck	**Central**	**To right**	**To left**
4. Chest movement on breathing	**Relaxed**	**Heaving** **Painful** **Unequal**	
5. Air entry of chest (describe the position of any abnormality)	**Normal**	**Wheezy** **Crackly**	

(P) ABDOMEN (ABDO)

1. Abdo size	**Normal**	**Distended**
2. Abdo pain on coughing	**No**	**Yes**
3. Abdo pain on moving	**No**	**Yes**
4. Abdo pain on puffing out or sucking in tummy wall	**No**	**Yes**
5. Areas of tenderness found	**No**	**Yes**
6. Any lumps or swellings found	**No**	**Yes**
7. Bowel sounds (BS)	**Normal BS**	**Increased BS** **Tinkling BS** **No BS heard**

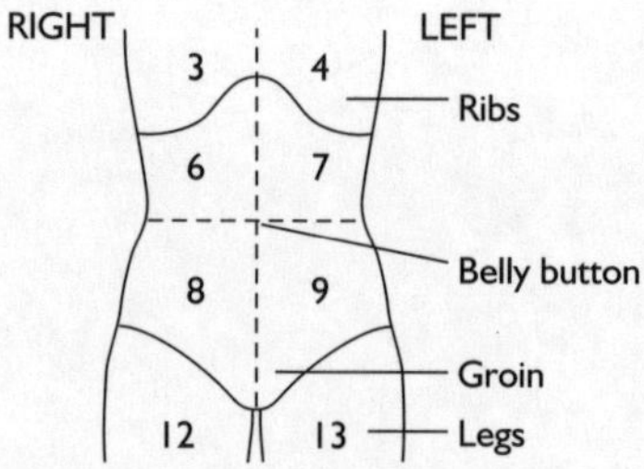

Diagram 5 *Abdomen*

(Q) GENERAL EXAMINATION

1. Glands found	**No**	**Yes, neck**	**R**	**L**
		Tender	**Yes**	**No**
		Yes, armpit	**R**	**L**
		Tender	**Yes**	**No**
		Yes, groin	**R**	**L**
		Tender	**Yes**	**No**
2. Ear discharge (If no pass to 4)	**No**	**Yes, from**	**R**	**L**

3. Colour of ear discharge	Clear Pus Blood

4. Throat colour	**Normal**	**Red**
5. Tonsil size	**Normal**	**Enlarged**
6. Skin rash found	**No**	**Yes**

7. Size of rash (in cm)
8. Colour
9. Surface (to touch)
10. Where rash found

(R) ANY OTHER COMMENTS OR FINDINGS

(S) POSSIBLE DIAGNOSIS

Examiner's signature

Name (printed) and qualifications

Source: Siderfin, C., Maclean, J. and Haston, W. (1995) The Medical Assessment Questionnaire for Radio. *Journal of Telemedicine and Telecare* 1: 57–60.

4 REFERENCES AND FURTHER READING

1 What is expedition medicine?

Auerbach, P. S. (1995) *Wilderness Medicine. Management of Wilderness and Environmental Emergencies.* 3rd edition. Mosby, St Louis

Robinson, W. A. and Oelz, O. (1990) *Wilderness and Environmental Medicine.* Wilderness Medical Society Periodical (001-317-6311745), PO Box 2463, Indianapolis, IN 46206

2 Vaccinations

Salisbury, D. M. and Begg, N. T. (1996) *Immunisation against Infectious Disease.* HMSO, London

Website:

www.who.int/ith/diseasemaps_index
World Health Organization maps showing areas with risk of infection from various diseases

3 Expedition medical kits

A'Court, C. H. D., Stables, R. H. and Travis, S. (1995) "Doctor on a mountaineering expedition". *British Medical Journal*, 310: 1248–1252. (This paper lists the medical supplies taken on the 1992 expedition to Everest in winter)

Bollen, S. (1999) *First Aid on Mountains.* British Mountaineering Council, Manchester

Illingworth, R. N. (1984) *Expedition Medicine, A Planning Guide.* 3rd edition. Blackwell Scientific Publications, Oxford

Pollard, A. J., Murdoch, D. R. (1997) *The High Altitude Medicine Handbook.* Radcliffe Medical Press, Oxford. (This is available as a micro edition weighing less than 60g for use on an expedition)

Steele, P. (1999) *Medical Handbook for Walkers and Climbers.* Constable, London.

Wilkerson, J. A. (2001) *Medicine for Mountaineering and Other Wilderness Activities.* 5th edition. The Mountaineers Books, Washington, Seattle

4 Expedition first aid training

American College of Surgeons (1997) *Advanced Trauma Life Support Course Manual.* 6th edition. American College of Surgeons, Chicago

Colquhoun, M. C. *et al.* (1995) *ABC of Resuscitation.* BMJ Publishing Group, London

Dunne, J. (ed.) (1997) *First Aid Manual. The Authorised Manual of the St John Ambulance, St Andrews Ambulance Association and The British Red Cross.* 7th edition. Dorling Kindersley, London

Goth, P. and Isacc, J. (1994) *Outward Bound First Aid Handbook.* Ward Lock, London
Paton, B. C., *et al.* (1998) *Wilderness First Aid. Emergency Care for Remote Locations.* Jones and Bartlett Publishers International, London
Renouf, J. and Hulse, S. (1989) *First Aid for Hillwalkers and Climbers.* Cicerone Press, Milnthorpe, Cumbria

5 Legal liability

Dinnick, S. (1996) "Antarctica revisited". *Summons: Journal for the Medical and Dental Defence Union of Scotland* 5
Whittingham, M. (2001) *Expedition Insurance.* Expedition Advisory Centre, London

7 Pre-existing medical conditions

ABC of Healthy Travel. (1997) BMJ Publishers, London
American College of Sports Physicians (1997) *Exercise management for Persons with Chronic Diseases and Disabilities.* Human Kinetics
American College of Sports Physicians (2000) *Guidelines on Exercise Testing and Prescription.* 6th edition. Lippincott, Williams & Wilkins, New York
Bruckner, P. and Khan, K. (2000) *Clinical Sports Medicine.* 2nd edition
Skinner, James S., (1993) *Exercise Testing and Exercise Prescription for Special Cases.* 2nd edition. Lea & Febiger
Townend, M. (2000) "Travelers with pre-existing conditions", *Family Medicine* Sept. pp. 32–35

8 Risk assessment and crisis management

Putnam, R. (1994) *Safe and Responsible Youth Expeditions.* Young Explorers' Trust, London
UK Health and Safety Executive (1996) *Five Steps to Risk Assessment Ind (G) 163L.* HMSO, London
UK Health and Safety Executive (1996) *Licensing Regulations. Pamphlet L77.* HMSO, London
Young Explorers' Trust (1994) *Code of Practice for Youth Expeditions.* London

10 Base camp hygiene and health

The Guide Association *Health and Hygiene.* Commonwealth Headquarters Shop, 17–19 Buckingham Palace Road, London SW1W 0PT, tel. +44 20 7834 6242
Wilson Howarth, J. (1999) *Bugs, Bites and Bowels.* Cadogan Books, London
Website:
The Centre for Alternative Technology www.cat.org.uk, tel. +44 1654 702400

11 Water purification

Epstein, O. (1997) *Clinical Examination.* Mosby-Year Book Inc., Boston, MA

Dunne, J. (ed.) (1997) *First Aid Manual. The Authorised Manual of the St John Ambulance, St Andrews Ambulance Association and The British Red Cross.* 7th edition. Dorling Kindersley, London

Siderfin, C. D. (1995) "Low-technology telemedicine in Antarctica". *Journal of Telemedicine and Telecare* 1: 54–60

Werner, D. (1979) *Where There Is No Doctor.* Macmillan Tropical Community Health Manuals, Macmillan Press, London. Available from TALC, PO Box 49, St Albans, Herts AL1 4AX

13 First aid and management of minor injuries

American College of Surgeons (1989) *Advanced Trauma Life Support Course Manual.* American College of Surgeons, Chicago

Benner, A. G. *et al.* (1987) *Emergency Medical Procedures for the Outdoors.* Menasha Ridge Press, Birmingham

Burge, P. (1989) *Limb Injuries.* JB Lippincott Co., Raven, New York

Dunne, J. (ed.) (1997) *First Aid Manual. The Authorised Manual of the St John Ambulance, St Andrews Ambulance Association and The British Red Cross.* 7th edition. Dorling Kindersley, London

Eaton, C. J. (1995) *Essentials of Immediate Medical Care.* Churchill Livingstone, Edinburgh

Ferguson, D. G. and Fodden, D. I. (1993) *Accident and Emergency Medicine.* Churchill Livingstone, Edinburgh

Goth, P. and Isacc, J. (1994) *Outward Bound First Aid Handbook.* Ward Lock, London

Huckstep, R. L. and Sherry, E. (1994) *Orthopaedics and Trauma.* Churchill Livingstone, Edinburgh

Kirby, N. G. (1985) *Field Surgery Pocket Book.* HMSO, London

Renouf, J. and Hulse, S. (1989) *First Aid for Hillwalkers and Climbers.* Cicerone Press, Milnthorpe, Cumbria

Skinner, D. *et al.* (1996) *ABC of Major Trauma.* BMJ Publishing Group, London

14 Management of the seriously injured casualty

American College of Surgeons (1997) *Advanced Trauma Life Support Student Course Manual.* 6th edition. American College of Surgeons, Chicago

Auerbach, P.S. (1995) *Wilderness Medicine.* 3rd edition. Mosby, St Louis

Hodgetts T. J. (1995) *Major Incident Medical Management and Support.* BMJ Publishing Group, London

Wyatt J. P. *et al.* (1999) *Oxford Handbook of Accident and Emergency Medicine.* Oxford University Press, New York

15 Remote medical emergencies

Auerbach, P. S. (1995) *Wilderness Medicine.* 3rd edition. Mosby, St Louis

Marx *et al. Rosen's Emergency Medicine.* 5th edition. Mosby, St Louis

Wyatt, J. P. *et al.* (1999) *Oxford Handbook of Accident and Emergency Medicine.* Oxford University Press, New York

16 Casualty evacuation

March, B. (1973) *Modern Rope Techniques.* Cicerone Press, Milnthorpe, Cumbria

17 Medical aspects of survival

Greenbank, A. (1976) *The Book of Survival.* Wolfe Publishing

Robertson, D. (1975) *Survive the Savage Sea.* Penguin Books, London

Wiseman, J. (1995) *The SAS Survival Handbook.* HarperCollins, London

18 Common infections

Dawood, R. (2002) *Travellers' Health: How to stay healthy abroad.* Oxford University Press, Oxford.

Wilson Howarth, J. (1999) *Bugs, Bites and Bowels.* Cadogan Books, London

19 Malaria and other tropical diseases

Bell, D. R. (1995) *Lecture Notes on Tropical Medicine.* 4th edition. Blackwell Science, Oxford

Bradley, D. J. and Warhurst, D. C. (1997) "Guidelines for the prevention of malaria in travellers from the UK." *CDR Review* (PHLS, Colindale, London) Vol. 7, Review No. 10 R1–152

British Medical Association (1995) *The BMA Guide to Rabies.* Radcliffe Medical Press, Abingdon

Cook, G. C. (1996) *Manson's Tropical Diseases.* 20th edition. W. B. Saunders, London

Gilles, H. M. and Warrell, D. A. (1993). *Bruce Chwatt's Essential Malariology.* 3rd edition. Edward Arnold, London

Weatherall, D. J., Ledingham, J. G. G. and Warrell, D. A. (1996) *Oxford Textbook of Medicine.* 3rd edition. Vol. I, Section 7, Infection. Oxford University Press, Oxford

20 Venomous and poisonous animals

Junghanss, T. and Bodio, M. (1996) *Notfall-Handbuch Gifttiere.* Georg Thième, Stuttgart (Rildigerstrasse 14, D-70469 Stuttgart). In German

Meier, J. and White, J. (1995) *Handbook of Clinical Toxicology of Animal Venoms and Poisons.* CRC Press, Boca Raton (2000 Corporate Bvd, NW Boca Raton, FL 33431)

Warrell, D. A. (1996). "Animal toxins", in Cook, G. C. (ed.) *Manson's Tropical Diseases.* 20th edition. W. B. Saunders, London: 468–515

Warrell, D. A. (1996) "Injuries, envenoming, poisoning and allergic reactions caused by animals", in Weatherall, D. J., Ledingham, J. G. G. and Warrell, D. A. (eds), *Oxford Textbook of Medicine.* 3rd edition. Oxford University Press, Oxford: 1124–1151

23 **Desert expeditions**

Ash, C. J. and Kashmeery, A. M. S. (1999) "Management of heatstroke", in Webb, A. R., Shapiro, M. J., Singer, M. and Suter, P. M. (eds), *Oxford Textbook of Critical Care.* Oxford University Press, Oxford: 808–811

Blatteis, C. M. (ed.) (1998) *Physiology and Pathophysiology of Temperature Regulation.* World Scientific Publishing, Singapore

Harding, M. (ed.)(2001) *Weather to Travel.* 3rd edition. Tomorrow's Guides. Worldwide guide to temperature, rainfall and humidity month-by-month

Hubbard, R. W., Gaffin, S. L. and Squire, D. L. (1995) "Heat-related illnesses", in Auerbach, P. S. (ed.) *Wilderness Medicine.* 3rd edition. Mosby, St Louis, 167–212

Maughan, R. J., Leiper, J. B. and Shirreffs S. M. (1999) "Factors influencing the restoration of fluid and electrolyte balance after exercise in the heat" in MacAuley, D. (ed.) *Benefits and Hazards of Exercise.* BMJ Books, London: 256–75

Noakes, T. D. (1998) "Fluid and electrolyte disturbances in heat illness". *International Journal of Sports Medicine*: S146–149

Scott, C. (2000) *Sahara Overland.* Trailblazer Publications
Contains detailed information including GPS waypoints for a range of expeditions. Also has a website (www.sahara-overland.com) with up-to-date reports from travellers

Stroud, M. (1998) "Marathon of the sands" in Stroud, M., *Survival of the Fittest.* Random House, London: 88–121

Websites:

www.nlm.nih.gov/medlineplus/heatillness.html
Information for the public on the prevention, recognition and treatment of heat illness

www.mindef.gov.sg/army/unit/gsi/_education/heat/heatprevent.pdf
Singapore Army guidelines for prevention of heat illness – incorporates UK and US military perspectives

www.graduateresearch.com/thermometry/
Useful discussion about the measurement of body temperature and the pros and cons of various devices and sites

24 **Tropical forest expeditions**

Auerbach, P. S. (ed.) (2001) *Wilderness Medicine.* Mosby, St Louis

Chapman, R. and Jermy, C. (1993) *Tropical Forest Expeditions.* Expedition Advisory Centre, London

Dawood, R. (2002) *Traveller's Health: How to stay healthy abroad.* Oxford University

Press, Oxford
Melville, K. E. M. (1984) *Stay Alive in the Desert.* Roger Lascalles, London
Schroeder, D. G. (1993) *Staying Healthy in Asia, Africa and Latin America.* Moon Publications, Chicago
Sheppard, T. (1988) *Desert Expeditions.* Expedition Advisory Centre, London

25 Polar expeditions

Adam, J. M. (1981) *Hypothermia: Ashore and Afloat.* Aberdeen University Press, Aberdeen
Auerbach, P. S. (1995) *Wilderness Medicine. Management of Wilderness and environmental emergencies.* 3rd edition. Mosby, St Louis
Dawson, B. (1994) "The removal of rock flour from glacial streams". *Island: Bulletin of the Iceland Unit,* Young Explorers' Trust 7: 7–8
Lloyd, E. L. (1996) "Accidental hypothermia". *Resuscitation* 32: 111–24
Lloyd, E. L. (1986) *Hypothermia and Cold Stress.* Croom Helm, London
Milne, A. H. and Siderfin, C. D. (1995) *Kurafid.* 4th edition. British Antarctic Survey, Madingley Road, Cambridge. Advanced first aid for well-equipped expeditions
Rivolier, J., Goldsmith, R., Lugg, D. J. and Taylor, A. J. W. (1988) *Man in the Antarctic.* Taylor & Francis, London. A summary of research work in polar areas

26 High-altitude and mountaineering expeditions

Bezruchka, S. (1994) *Altitude Illness, Prevention and Treatment.* The Mountaineers, Seattle and Cordee, Leicester
Hultgren, H. (1997) *High Altitude Medicine.* Hultgren Publications, fax +1 415 493 4225
Murdoch, D. R. and Pollard, A. J. (1997) *The High Altitude Medicine Handbook.* Radcliffe Medical Press, Abingdon, Oxon
UIAA Mountain Medicine Data Centre leaflets. Available from the British Mountaineering Council, 177–179 Burton Road, Manchester M20 2BB. Tel. +44 161 445 4747, fax +44 161 445 4500
Ward, M. P., Milledge, J. S. and West, J. B. (1994) *High Altitude Medicine and Physiology.* Chapman & Hall Medical, London
Wilkerson, J. A. (1985) *Medicine for Mountaineering.* The Mountaineers, Seattle. Frequently re-edited; available through Cordee, 3a De Montfort Street, Leicester LE1 7HD

27 Underwater expeditions

Bennet, P. B. and Elliot, D. H. (1982) *The Physiology and Medicine of Diving.* 4th edition. W. B. Saunders Co. Ltd, London
British Sub-Aqua Club (1993) *Sports Diving: The BSAC Diving Manual.* British Sub Aqua Club, Telford's Quay, Ellesmere Port, Cheshire L65 4FY, tel. +44 151 357 1951,

fax +44 151 357 1250

Flemming, N. C. and Max, M. D. (1996) *Scientific Diving: A general code of practice.* 2nd edition. UNESCO

Sisman, D. (1995) *The Professional Diver's Handbook.* Best Publishing, Arizona

Websites:

British Hyperbaric Association: www.hyperbaric.freeserve.co.uk/

Institute of Naval Medicine: www.royal-navy.mod.uk/static/pages/1152.html

28 Caving expeditions

"Advice for Cavers Concerning Hypothermia" (1993–4) *Plymouth Caving Group Newsletter and Journal* 119: 16–20

Ashford, D. A., Hajjeh, R. A., Kelley, M. F., Kaufman, L., Hutwagner, L. and McNeil, M. M. (1999) "Outbreak of histoplasmosis among cavers attending the National Speleological Society Annual Convention, Texas, 1994", *American Journal of Tropical Medicine and Hygiene* 60: 899–903

Ashford, D. A., Knutson, R. S. and Sacks, J. J. (1999) "Injury among cavers: results of a preliminary national survey". *Journal of Sports Medicine and Physical Fitness* 39(1): 71–73

Baguley, F. S. (1994–5) "Cryptosporidium in water", *Red Dragon Cambrian Caving Council Annual Journal* 21:

Bailey, D. (1994) "Hypothermia – when the shivering stops", *The Speleograph* 30: 112–113

Brocklebank, T. (1992) "Falls!!!", *British Caver* 115: 5–7

Buchan, J. (1976) "Medical report on British New Guinea Expedition", *Transactions of the British Cave Research Association* 3: 238–242

Cave Rescue Association. Annual Reports.

Fogg, T. (1989) "Mulu Caves 88 Expedition Report", *Cave Science* 16 (2): 57

Frankland, J. C. (1974) "Studies on the response of healthy English speleologists to exposure to histoplasmosis infection", *Transactions of the British Cave Research Association* 1(3): 153–158

Frankland, J. C. (1984) "Hypothermia in cavers", *Transactions of the British Cave Research Association* 11(3): 154–159

Lewis, W. (1989) "Histoplasmosis: a hazard to new tropical cavers", *National Speleological Society Bulletin* (Huntsville, Alabama) 51: 52–65

Lyons, T. (1984) "Medical equipment for caving expeditions". *Transactions of the British Cave Research Association.* 11: 171

Sacks, J. J., Ajello, L. and Crockett, L. K. (1986) "An outbreak and review of cave-associated histoplasmosis capsulatum", *Journal of Medical and Veterinary Mycology* 24: 313–325

Self, C. A., Iskrzynska, W. I., Waitkins, S. A., Whicher, J. W. and Whicher, J. T. (1989) "Leptospirosis amongst British cavers", *Cave Science* 14(3): 131–134

Valdez, H. and Salata, R. A. (1999) "Bat-associated histoplasmosis in returning

travelers: case presentation and description of a cluster", *Journal of Travel Medicine* 6(4): 258–260
Wilkerson, J. A. (ed.) (1986) *Hypothermia, Frostbite, and Other Cold Injuries.* The Mountaineers, Seattle, WA
Willis, D. W. (1993) *Caving Expeditions.* 2nd edition. BCRA/Expedition Advisory Centre
Websites:
British Cave Rescue Council information on UK cave rescues: www.managerie.co.uk/bcrc/IREPPDF/ANAL8998.pdf
Centers for Disease Control and Prevention–information on histoplasmosis: www.cdc.gov/ncidod/dbmd/diseaseinfo/histoplasmosis_g.htm
Centers for Disease Control and Prevention–information on leptospirosis: www.cdc.gov/ncidod/dbmd/diseaseinfo/leptospirosis_g.htm

5 USEFUL ADDRESSES

Air Ambulance International
San Francisco, CA, USA
Tel. +1 800 227 9996
+1 415 786 1592

Air Ambulance Network
Miami, FL, USA
Tel. +1 800 327 1966
+1 305 447 0458

Air Response
Box 109, Fort Plain, NY 13339, USA
Tel. +1 518 993 4153

Aventis Pasteur MSD Ltd
Tel. +44 1628 411412
Fax +44 1628 671722
Website www.aventis-pasteur-msd.com
Source of antivenom in the UK

BCB Limited
Morland Road, Cardiff CF24 2YL
Tel. +44 292 046 4464
Fax +44 292 048 1100
Website www.bcb.ltd.uk
Email bcb@bcb.ltd.uk
First aid kits and emergency medical supplies

Blood Care Foundation
PO Box 588, Horsham RH12 5WJ
Tel. +44 1403 262652
Fax +44 1403 262657
Website www.bloodcare.org.uk
Email bcfgb@compuserve.com
Emergency blood supplies

British Association for Immediate Care (BASICS)
BASICS Headquarters, Turret House, Turret Lane, Ipswich IP4 1DL
Tel. +44 870 165 4999
Fax +44 870 165 4949
Website www.basics.org.uk
Email admin@basics.org.uk

British Association of Ski Patrollers (BASP)
Contact: Fiona Gunn
Tel. +44 1855 811443

British Dental Association
64 Wimpole Street, London W1M 8AL
Tel +44 20 7935 0875
Website www.bda-dentistry.org.uk

British Medical Association
BMA House, Tavistock Square, London WC1H 9JP
Tel. +44 20 7387 4499
Fax +44 20 7383 6400
Website www.bma.org.uk
Email info.web@bma.org.uk

British Red Cross Society
9 Grosvenor Gardens, London SW1X 7EJ
Tel. +44 20 7235 5454
Website www.redcross.org.uk

Cega Air Ambulance Ltd
Goodwood Airfield, Chichester PO18 0PH
Tel. +44 1243 538888
Fax +44 1243 773169

Centre for Tropical Medicine, University of Oxford
Nuffield Department of Clinical Medicine, John Radcliffe Hospital, Oxford OX3 9DU
Founding Director (Emeritus): *Prof David Warrell*
Tel. +44 1865 220968
Fax +44 1865 220984
Email david.warrell@ndm.ox.ac.uk

Compagnie Générale de Secours
Paris, France
Tel. +33 1 47 47 66 66

Data (Southern) Enterprises Ltd
Unit 6, Fareham Enterprise Centre, Hackett Way, Newgate Lane, Fareham PO14 1TH
Tel. +44 1329 829268
Fax +44 1329 829276
Website http://www.999-supplies.co.uk

Department of Health (Medicines Division)
Market Towers, 1 Nine Elms Lane, London SW1 5NQ
Tel. (weekdays 09.00–17.00)
+44 20 7273 0000
Tel. (other times)
+44 20 7210 3000
Fax +44 20 7273 0353
For UK drug export certificates
Website www.open.gov.uk/mca
Email info@mca.gsi.gov.uk

Diving Diseases Research Centre
The Hyperbaric Medical Centre, Tamar Science Park, Research Way, Plymouth PL6 8BU
Emergency tel. +44 1752 209999
Fax +44 1752 209115
Website www.ddrc.org
Email enquiries@ddrc.org

East Africa Flying Doctors Society (AMREF)
11 Old Queen Street, London SW1H 9JA
Tel. +44 20 7233 0066
Fax +44 20 7233 0099

Europ Assistance
Sussex House, Perrymount Road, Haywards Heath RH16 1DN
Tel. +44 1444 411999
Fax +44 1444 415775

Expedition Advisory Centre
Royal Geographical Society (with the Institute of British Geographers)
1 Kensington Gore, London SW7 2AR

Tel.	+44 20 7591 3030
Fax	+44 20 7591 3031
Website	www.rgs.org/eac
Email	eac@rgs.org

The Fleet Street Travel Clinic
Dr Richard Dawood
29 Fleet Street, London EC4Y 1AA

Tel.	+44 20 7353 5678
Fax	+44 20 7353 5500
Website	www.fleetstreetclinic.com
Email	Info@fleetstreetclinic.com

Foreign and Commonwealth Office Travel Advice Unit
Old Admiralty Building, Whitehall, London SW1A 2PA

Tel.	+44 20 7008 0232/0233
Fax	+44 20 7008 0155
Website	www.fco.gov.uk

Frontline Medical Services Ltd

Tel./Fax	+44 1389 877811
Email	expemed@frontlinemedics.com
Website	www.frontlinemedics.com

Health Literature Line
The Library, Department of Health, Shipton House, London SE1 6LH

Tel.	+44 800 555777
Fax	+44 1623 724524
Website	www.equip.nhs.uk/support

Phone for individual copies of material produced by the Department of Health. If more copies are required, fax or write

Hospital for Tropical Diseases
Mortimer Market, Capper Street, Tottenham Court Road, London WC1E 6AU

Tel.	+44 20 7387 9300/4411
Healthline	+44 9061 337733
Fax	+44 20 7388 7645
Website	www.thehtd.org

HSE Books
PO Box 1999, Sudbury CO10 2WA
Tel. +44 1787 881165
Fax +44 1787 313995
Website www.hsebooks.co.uk

The Ieuan Jones First Aid Course for Mountaineers
Contact: Gerry Lynch
Tel. +44 1248 600589

InterHealth
157 Waterloo Road, London SE1 8US
Tel. +44 20 7902 9000
Website www.travelhealth.co.uk
Email Info@interhealth.org.uk
Long-term advice and treatment for aid workers and expatriates

International Assistance Services
32–42 High Street, Purley CR8 2PP
Tel. +44 20 8763 1550
Fax +44 20 8668 1262

International Health Exchange
134 Lower Marsh, London SE1 7AE
Tel. +44 20 7620 3333
Fax +44 20 7620 2277
Website www.ihe.org.uk
Email info@ihe.org.uk
Maintains a register of health professionals wanting to work in developing countries, and runs training courses on primary health care and refugee community health

International SOS
Box 11568, Philadelphia, PA 19116, USA
Tel. +1 800 523 8930
+1 215 244 1500

John Bell and Croyden
50–54 Wigmore Street, London W1V 2AU
Tel. +44 20 7935 5555
Fax +44 20 7935 9605
Website www.johnbellcroyden.co.uk
Pharmacy and medical supplier

Life Flight Hermann Hospital
Houston, TX, USA
Tel. +1 800 231 4357

Life Support Training Services
2 Underhill Cottages, The Hill, Millom LA18 5HA
Tel./Fax +44 1229 772708

Lifesystems Limited
4 Mercury House, Calleva Park, Aldermaston RG7 8PN
Tel. +44 118 981 1433
Fax +44 118 981 1406
Website www.lifesystems.co.uk
Email mail@lifesystems.co.uk
First aid and emergency dental kits

Liverpool School of Tropical Medicine
Pembroke Place, Liverpool L3 5QA
Tel. +44 151 708 9393
Fax +44 151 708 8733
Website www.liv.ac.uk/lstm/lstm.html

London School of Hygiene and Tropical Medicine
Keppel Street, London WC1E 7HT
Tel. +44 20 7636 8636
Fax +44 20 7436 5389
Website www.lshtm.ac.uk

London School of Tropical Medicine Malaria Reference Laboratory
Tel. +44 20 7636 3924
+44 9065 508 908 (24-hr)
Website. www.lshtm.ac.uk/centres/malaria

Medical Advisory Service for Travellers Abroad (MASTA) Travel Clinics
Tel. +44 1276 685040
Website www.masta.org
Email enquiries@masta.org

MedicAlert Foundation International
1 Bridge Wharf, 156 Caledonian Road, London N1 9UU
Tel. +44 20 7833 3034
Fax +44 20 7278 0647
Email info@medicalert.org.uk
Website www.medicalert.org.uk

National Jets
Fort Lauderdale, FL, USA
Tel. +1 305 359 9900
+1 800 327 3710

National Poisons Centre
Tel. +44 870 600 6266 (for clinically complex cases)
Website www.doh.gov.uk/npis.htm

National Poisons Information Service
Belfast – Royal Victoria Hospital, Grosvenor Road, Belfast BT9 7BL
Tel. +44 28 9033 5772
Birmingham – City Hospital, Dudley Road, Birmingham B18 7QH
Tel. +44 121 507 4123
Website www.npis.org/npis.htm
Cardiff – Llandough Hospital, Penarth, Cardiff CF64 2XX
Edinburgh – The Royal Infirmary, Edinburgh EH3 9YW
Tel. +44 131 536 2298
Website www.show.scot.nhs.uk/spib
London – Medical Toxicology Unit, Avonley Road, London SE14 5ER
Tel. +44 20 7771 5315
Newcastle – Wolfson Unit, Claremont Place, Newcastle upon Tyne NE2 4HH
Tel. +44 191 230 5460

Nationwide/Worldwide Emergency Ambulance Return (NEAR)
450 Prairie Avenue, Calumet City, IL 60409, USA
Tel. +1 800 654 6700

Nomad Traveller's Store and Medical Centre
3–4 Wellington Terrace, Turnpike Lane, London N8 0PX
Tel. +44 20 8889 7014
Fax +44 20 8889 9529
Website www.nomadtravel.co.uk
Email sales@nomadtravel.co.uk
Travel pharmacy. Medical kits made to order at a low cost

North American Air Ambulance
Blackwood, NJ, USA
Tel. +1 800 257 8180

Orion First Aid
Brownrigg Guide Road, Hesketh Bank, Nr Preston PR4 6XS
Tel./Fax +44 1772 812 277
Website www.oriontraining.co.uk

Public Health Laboratory Health Centres
London and the south-east:
Tel. +44 20 7725 2757
Fax +44 20 7725 2597
East:
Tel. +44 160 350 6900
Fax +44 160 350 1188
Midlands:
Tel. +44 174 326 1336
Fax +44 174 326 1192
Out of hours: +44 174 326 1000
North:
Tel. +44 191 261 2577
Fax +44 191 261 2578
Out of hours: +44 191 261 2577
North-west:
Tel. +44 151 529 4900
Fax +44 151 529 4918
South-west:
Tel. +44 145 230 5334
Fax +44 145 230 7213
Trent:
Tel. +44 115 981 5544
Fax +44 115 981 5500
Wales:
Tel. +44 292 074 6410/4515
Fax +44 292 074 6403
Out of hours: +44 292 074 7747
Website www.phls.co.uk

Royal College of Nursing
20 Cavendish Square, London W1G 0RN
Tel. +44 845 772 6100
Website www.rcn.org.uk

Royal Society for the Prevention of Accidents
Edgbaston Park, 353 Bristol Road, Edgbaston, Birmingham B5 7ST
Tel. +44 121 248 2000
Fax +44 121 248 2001
Email help@rospa.co.uk
Website www.rospa.co.uk

SP Services (UK)
Unit D4, Hortonpark Estate, Hortonwood 7, Telford TF1 7GX
Tel. +44 1952 288999
Fax +44 1952 606112
Website www.999supplies.com
Emergency medical and rescue supplies

Specialist First Aid Training
Nyth yr Hebog, Llandyrnog, Denbigh LL16 4HB
Tel./Fax +44 1824 790195
Website www.mtn.co.uk/sherriff

St Andrew's Ambulance Association
St Andrew's House, 48 Milton Street, Glasgow G4 0HR (national headquarters)
Tel. +44 141 332 4031
Fax +44 141 332 6582
Website www.firstaid.org.uk
Email firstaid@staaa.demon.co.uk

St John Ambulance
27 St John's Lane, London EC1M 4BU (national headquarters)
Tel. +44 8700 10 49 50
Fax +44 8700 10 40 65
Website www.sja.org.uk

St John Supplies
PO Box 707B, Friend Street, London EC1V 7NE
Tel. +44 20 7278 7888
Fax +44 20 7837 1642
Website www.stjohnsupplies.co.uk

Swiss Air Ambulance
Zurich, Switzerland
Tel. +41 22 383 11 11

TALC (Teaching-aids At Low Cost)
PO Box 49, St Albans AL1 5TX
Tel. +44 1727 853869
Fax +44 1727 846852
Website www.talcuk.org

Trailfinders Travel Clinics
Tel. +44 20 7938 3999 (London)
Tel. +44 141 429 0913 (Glasgow)

UIAA Mountain Medicine Data Centre
Patients seen through the NHS at: The National Hospital for Neurology and Neurosurgery, Queen Square, London WC1N 3BG
Website www.thebmc.co.uk/world/mm/mmo.htm
Email (serious altitude emergency) raa07@dial.pipex.com

Wilderness Expertise Ltd
The Octagon, Wellington College, Crowthorne RG45 7PU
Tel. +44 1344 774430
Fax +44 1344 774480
Email rec@wild-expertise.demon.co.uk
Website www.wild-expertise.demon.co.uk

Wilderness Medical Training (WMT)
The Coach House, Thorny Bank, Skelsmergh, Kendal LA8 9AW
Tel./Fax +44 1539 823183
Website www.wildernessmedicaltraining.co.uk
Email enquiries@wildernessmedicaltraining.co.uk

World Health Organization
World Health Organization, Avenue Appia 20, 1211 Geneva 27, Switzerland
Tel. +41 22 791 21 11
Fax +41 22 791 31 11
Website www.who.int
Publishers of the *WHO Weekly Epidemiological Record, Global Epidemiological Surveillance and Health Situation Assessment, International Travel and Health*

USEFUL WEB ADDRESSES

Asian Collaborative Training Network for Malaria
www.actmalaria.org
Asian malaria website

British Travel Health Association
www.btha.org

Centers for Disease Control (CDC) USA
www.cdc.gov

Department of Health
Advice for Travellers
www.doh.gov.uk/traveladvice

E-Med
www.e-med.co.uk

Fit for travel
www.fitfortravel.scot.nhs.uk

International Society for Infectious Diseases
www.promedmail.org
For disease alerts

International Travel Health Association
www.istm.org

McGill University Center for Tropical Disease
http://sprojects.mmi.mcgill.ca/tropmed

Public Health Laboratory Service
www.phls.org.uk
Excellent malaria guidelines

Travel Health Online
www.tripprep.com

Travel Screening Services
www.travelscreening.co.uk

The Travellers' Health website
www.travellershealth.info
Has news and links to over 200 travel health-related sites

Tropical Medicine Bureau Ireland
www.tmb.ie

6 GLOSSARY

Abdomen	Body cavity which contains the liver, spleen, kidneys and bladder
Abrasion	Superficial wound caused by damage to the outermost layers of skin or cornea
Abscess	A localised collection of pus (infection)
Airway	The passage through which air moves from the nose and mouth via the throat to the lungs
Airway, lower	Trachea, bronchi, alveoli
Airway, upper	Mouth, nose, throat
Altitude sickness (AMS or acute mountain sickness)	A condition caused by the lack of oxygen at high altitude
Alveoli	Small sacs of air in the lungs where gas is exchanged with the blood
Anaphylaxis	Severe allergic reaction involving widespread oedema and shock
Aspiration	The breathing in of foreign liquid or solid into the lungs
Basic life support (BLS)	The process of supporting a person's respiratory and circulatory function using artificial ventilation, chest compressions and bleeding control
Cardiac arrest	The loss of an effective pumping action of the heart
Cardiogenic shock	Shock caused by an inadequate pumping action of the heart
Cardiopulmonary resuscitation (CPR)	A technique using artificial respiration and chest compressions to circulate oxygenated blood in the absence of an effectively pumping heart
Capillaries	The narrowest blood vessels in the body where gases and nutrients are exchanged between circulating blood and tissue cells
Carotid pulse	The pulse felt on either side of the neck at the site of the carotid artery
Central nervous system (CNS)	The brain and spinal cord
Cervical spine	The portion of spine in the neck between the skull base and the top of the thorax
Conjunctiva	The membrane that covers the front of the eye and the inside of the eyelids
Conjunctivitis	Inflammation (swelling and redness) of the conjunctiva due to irritation, infection or injury

Consciousness, level of	Describes the level of brain function in terms of responsivenesss to specific stimuli (the AVPU scale): A = Awake and Alert V = responds to Voice P = responds to Pain U = Unresponsive to any stimulus
Cornea	The clear part of the eye which covers the iris and the pupil
Dental abscess	Infection at the base of a tooth
Diagnosis	The specific identification of an injury or illness by name
Diaphragm	A dome-shaped muscle that separates the chest from the abdominal cavity
Discharge	Excess fluid escaping from the site of infection or inflammation
Dislocation	Disruption of a normal joint's position
Drowning, near-	At least temporary survival of water inhalation. Often associated with the protective effects of hypothermia in cold water
Evacuation	The removal of a patient from the scene of injury or illness to a place of expert medical care
Extension	A movement that is the opposite of flexion
Exudate	Discharge
Femoral artery	A large artery found in the thigh alongside the femur
Femur	Long bone of the thigh
Fits	The movement of an unconscious patient as a result of unco-ordinated electrical activity in the brain
Flexion	The bending of a joint to bring the bones forming it closer together
Fracture	Broken bone or cartilage
Frostbite	Frozen tissue
Frostnip	Loss of blood flow to the skin during the early stages of tissue freezing as a result of blood vessels narrowing (vasoconstriction)
Heart attack	An episode of ischaemia or lack of oxygen to the heart muscle caused by a blood clot or spasm of the coronary arteries
Heat stroke	Severe elevation of body temperature (over 40°C)

High-altitude cerebral oedema (HACE)	The accumulation of excess fluid within the brain owing to a lack of oxygen at high altitude
Hyperextension	The extension of a joint beyond its normal range of movement
Hyperventilation syndrome	Symptoms usually associated with acute stress caused by reduced carbon dioxide in the blood as a result of overbreathing
Hypothermia	The lowering of body temperature below the normal body core temperature (below 35°C). Can be mild (35°C) or severe (<35°C)
Infection	Invasion of body tissues by harmful organisms such as bacteria, viruses or fungi
Intracranial	Inside the skull
Intravenous fluids	Fluids given directly into the blood through a needle inserted into a vein
Ischaemia	A lack of blood flow to a part of the body
Ligament	A tough band of tissue that joins two bones across a joint
Lumbar spine	The lower portion of the spine between the thorax (chest) and the pelvis
Monitor	To reassess a patient regularly and repeatedly for the purpose of revising treatment plans as the situation changes
Neutral position	The position halfway between flexion and extension
Oedema	The accumulation of excess fluid within body tissue
Open fracture	A broken bone with an associated break in the skin
Oxygenation	To saturate the blood with oxygen. This takes place in the lungs
Patella	Knee cap
Penicillin	An antibiotic drug
Perfusion	The flow of blood through blood vessels in body tissues
Peripheral nerves	The nerves running from the central nervous system (brain and spinal cord) to the body tissues (periphery)
Pneumonia	Infection of the lungs
Pneumothorax	A collection of free air in the chest cavity, usually from a puncture to the chest wall or lung
Pulmonary oedema	The accumulation of excess fluid within the air spaces of the lung

Reduction	Restoration of a dislocated joint or a displaced fracture to normal anatomical position
Resuscitation	The process of trying to revive a person who appears to be dead
Scene survey	After an accident, this is the assessment in which you look for dangers to the rescuer and patient, and assess the mechanism of injury
Sexually transmitted disease (STD)	Infection passed from person to person by sexual activity
Shock	A condition associated with inadequate blood supply leading to circulatory collapse; the patient is pale and sweaty, has a weak rapid pulse, irregular breathing and a reduced flow of urine
Sinuses	Hollow spaces in the bones of the skull
Spasm	Involuntary contraction of muscle
Spinal cord	The portion of the central nervous system running from the base of the brain to the lower spine, encased within the bones of the spinal column
Spine	The column of vertebral bones extending from the base of the skull to the pelvis
Stethoscope	An instrument used to listen to body sounds and transmit them to the ears of the examiner via rubber tubes
Survey	A systematic examination
Swelling	An excess of fluid in body tissues from bleeding or oedema
Symptoms	The problems complained of by the patient, e.g. pain, shortness of breath
Systemic	Involving the whole body
Thorax	The region of the body between the top of the abdomen and the base of the neck
Tourniquet	A constricting band used to restrict and prevent the flow of blood to an extremity
Traction	Tension applied along the long axis of bone
Trauma	Injury
Ventilation	The movement of air in and out of the lungs
Vertebrae	The bones of the spine
Vital signs	The measurement of body functions including pulse, blood pressure, respiration, consciousness, skin colour and temperature

INDEX

NOTES

NOTES

NOTES

NOTES

NOTES

NOTES